PSYCHOLOGICAL ASPECTS OF WOMEN'S HEALTH CARE

THE INTERFACE BETWEEN PSYCHIATRY AND OBSTETRICS AND GYNECOLOGY

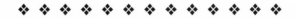

PSYCHOLOGICAL ASPECTS OF WOMEN'S HEALTH CARE

THE INTERFACE BETWEEN PSYCHIATRY AND OBSTETRICS AND GYNECOLOGY

Edited by

Donna E. Stewart, M.D., D.Psych., F.R.C.P.C.
Associate Professor of Psychiatry and Obstetrics and Gynecology
Co-Director, Program in Women's Mental Health
University of Toronto
Acting Chief of Psychiatry
Chief of the Psychiatric Consultation-Liaison Service
St. Michael's Hospital
Toronto, Ontario, Canada

Nada L. Stotland, M.D.
Associate Professor of Clinical Psychiatry and Obstetrics
  and Gynecology
The University of Chicago
Chicago, Illinois

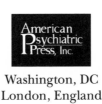

American Psychiatric Press, Inc.

Washington, DC
London, England

Note: The authors have worked to ensure that all information in this book concerning drug dosages, schedules, and routes of administration is accurate as of the time of publication and consistent with standards set by the U.S. Food and Drug Administration and the general medical community. As medical research and practice advance, however, therapeutic standards may change. For this reason and because human and mechanical errors sometimes occur, we recommend that readers follow the advice of a physician who is directly involved in their care or the care of a member of their family.

Books published by the American Psychiatric Press, Inc., represent the views and opinions of the individual authors and do not necessarily represent the policies and opinions of the Press or the American Psychiatric Association.

Copyright © 1993 American Psychiatric Press, Inc.
ALL RIGHTS RESERVED
Manufactured in the United States of America on acid-free paper
96 95 94 93   4 3 2 1
First Edition

American Psychiatric Press, Inc.
1400 K Street, N.W., Washington, DC   20005

Library of Congress Cataloging-in-Publication Data
Psychological aspects of women's health care: the interface between
psychiatry and obstetrics and gynecology /
   edited by Donna E. Stewart, Nada L. Stotland.
      p.   cm.
   Includes bibliographical references and index.
   ISBN 0-88048-421-7
   1. Gynecology—Psychosomatic aspects. 2. Obstetrics—
Psychosomatic aspects. I. Stewart, Donna E., 1943–   .
II. Stotland, Nada Logan.
   [DNLM: 1. Genital Diseases, Female—psychology. 2. Pregnancy
  Complications—psychology. 3. Reproduction. 4. Women—psychology.
  WP 140 I603]
  RG103.5.I54 1993
  618.1′001′9—dc20
  DNLM/DLC
  for Library of Congress   92-48771
                                       CIP

British Library Cataloguing in Publication Data
A CIP record is available from the British Library.

CONTENTS

SECTION I: PREGNANCY

SECTION II: GYNECOLOGY

SECTION III: GENERAL ISSUES

CONTRIBUTORS

Barbara L. Andersen, Ph.D.
Professor, Department of Psychology and Department of Obstetrics and Gynecology, The Ohio State University, Columbus, Ohio

Sheila B. Blume, M.D., C.A.C.
Medical Director, Alcoholism, Chemical Dependency, and Compulsive Gambling Programs, South Oaks Hospital, Amityville; and Clinical Professor of Psychiatry, State University of New York at Stony Brook, Stony Brook, New York

Melanie L. Carr, M.D., F.R.C.P.C.
Assistant Professor of Psychiatry, University of Toronto; and Women's Clinic, Department of Psychiatry, The Toronto Hospital, Toronto, Ontario, Canada

Mary Ann Chiasson, Dr.P.H.
Assistant Commissioner, Disease Intervention Research, New York City Department of Health, New York, New York

Jennifer Downey, M.D.
Assistant Professor of Clinical Psychiatry, Department of Psychiatry, and Consultant, Department of Obstetrics and Gynecology, Columbia University College of Physicians and Surgeons; and Research Psychiatrist, New York State Psychiatric Institute, New York, New York

Susan Doyle-Mirzadeh, M.A.
Graduate Student, Department of Psychology, The Ohio State University, Columbus, Ohio

Mindy Thompson Fullilove, M.D.
Associate Professor of Clinical Psychiatry and Public Health, Columbia University; and Research Psychiatrist, New York State Psychiatric Institute, New York, New York

Elisabeth K. Herz, M.D.
Associate Professor of Obstetrics and Gynecology and Director,
Psychosomatic Obstetrics and Gynecology, George Washington
University Medical Center, Washington, DC

Paula J. A. Hillard, M.D.
Associate Professor of Obstetrics and Gynecology and Director of
Ambulatory Care, University of Cincinnati College of Medicine,
Cincinnati, Ohio

Margaret F. Jensvold, M.D.
Director, Institute for Research on Women's Health, Washington,
DC; and private practice, Washington, DC, and Bethesda, Maryland

Carola Marte, M.D.
Director of HIV Services, Beth Israel Methadone Program, Beth
Israel Medical Center, New York, New York

Cheryl F. McCartney, M.D.
Associate Professor of Psychiatry, Adjunct Associate Professor of
Obstetrics and Gynecology, and Associate Dean for Student Affairs,
University of North Carolina School of Medicine, Chapel Hill,
North Carolina

Laura J. Miller, M.D.
Assistant Professor, Department of Psychiatry, University of Illinois,
Chicago, Illinois

William H. Miller, Jr., M.D.
Medical Director, Kootenai Psychiatric Center, Coeur d'Alene, Idaho

Carol C. Nadelson, M.D.
Professor and Vice-Chair, Department of Psychiatry, Tufts–New
England Medical Center, Boston, Massachusetts

Malkah T. Notman, M.D.
Clinical Professor of Psychiatry, Harvard Medical School; and Acting
Chair, Department of Psychiatry, The Cambridge Hospital,
Boston, Massachusetts

Robert O. Pasnau, M.D.
Professor, Department of Psychiatry, University of California, Los Angeles, School of Medicine, Los Angeles, California

Gail Erlick Robinson, M.D., F.R.C.P.C.
Associate Professor in Psychiatry and Obstetrics and Gynecology and Co-Director, Program in Women's Mental Health, University of Toronto; and Director, Program in Women's Mental Health, The Toronto Hospital, Department of Psychiatry, Toronto, Ontario, Canada

Deborah S. Rose, M.D.
Clinical Assistant Professor of Psychiatry, Department of Psychiatry and Behavioral Sciences, Stanford University School of Medicine, Stanford, California

Miriam B. Rosenthal, M.D.
Associate Professor of Psychiatry and Reproductive Biology, Case Western Reserve University School of Medicine; and Chief of Behavioral Medicine, Department of Obstetrics and Gynecology, University MacDonald Women's Hospital, Cleveland, Ohio

Marcia Russell, Ph.D.
Senior Research Scientist, New York State Research Institute on Alcoholism; and Clinical Associate Professor, Department of Social and Preventive Medicine, State University of New York at Buffalo, Buffalo, New York

K. B. Segraves, Ph.D.
Assistant Professor of Psychiatry, Case Western Reserve University; and Director, Behavioral Medicine Unit, MetroHealth Medical System, Cleveland, Ohio

R. T. Segraves, M.D., Ph.D.
Professor of Psychiatry, Case Western Reserve University; and Associate Director, Department of Psychiatry, MetroHealth Medical System, Cleveland, Ohio

Barbara B. Sherwin, Ph.D.
Associate Professor, Departments of Psychology and Obstetrics and
Gynecology, McGill University; and Co-Director, McGill Menopause
Clinic, Jewish General Hospital, Montreal, Quebec, Canada

John F. Steege, M.D.
Clinical Professor, Department of Obstetrics and Gynecology,
University of North Carolina at Chapel Hill, Chapel Hill,
North Carolina

Donna E. Stewart, M.D., D.Psych., F.R.C.P.C.
Associate Professor of Psychiatry and Obstetrics and Gynecology and
Co-Director, Program in Women's Mental Health, University of
Toronto; Acting Chief of Psychiatry and Chief of the Psychiatric
Consultation-Liaison Service, St. Michael's Hospital, Toronto,
Ontario, Canada

Nada L. Stotland, M.D.
Associate Professor of Clinical Psychiatry and Obstetrics and
Gynecology, The University of Chicago, Chicago, Illinois

Anna L. Stout, Ph.D.
Associate Clinical Professor, Division of Medical Psychology,
Department of Psychiatry, Department of Obstetrics and
Gynecology, Duke University Medical Center, Durham,
North Carolina

Pauline Thomas, M.D.
Director of AIDS Surveillance, New York City Department of Health,
New York, New York

Katherine L. Wisner, M.D., M.S.
Assistant Professor of Child Psychiatry and Medical Director,
Pregnancy and Infant/Parent Center, University of Pittsburgh,
Pittsburgh, Pennsylvania

Dooley Worth, Ph.D.
Director of Ethnographic Research, WHEEL Project (NIDA),
NOVA Research Company, Bethesda, Maryland

FOREWORD

The relationship between mental and reproductive functions has fascinated scientific thinkers for centuries. In almost every culture and religion, one can find customs and beliefs that affect the lives and health of men and women in the present century. The belief of many 19th-century gynecologists that oophorectomy could cure some forms of mental disorders in women influenced psychophysiological research in the early 20th century. Psychiatrists have functioned in liaison and consultation roles with obstetricians and gynecologists for over 50 years, but very few texts have been written in this area in the United States since Kroger and Freed's volume, *Psychosomatic Gynecology: Including Problems of Obstetrical Care,* in the 1950s. More scholarly and sophisticated publications have been appearing in recent years, but there has been no recent attempt to bring them all together in one comprehensive book.

This volume is a welcome example of what has been long overdue. It is devoted to the psychiatric aspects of female reproductive issues and the psychiatric interface with the field of obstetrics and gynecology. Drs. Stewart and Stotland have solicited chapters from the major leaders in the fields of both psychiatry and obstetrics and gynecology and have compiled a remarkable set of chapters covering almost every major area of contemporary concern. It sets a very high standard for those who will follow.

The first section of the book is devoted to obstetrics and reproduction. It includes a review of the psychological aspects of normal and complicated pregnancy, fetal anomalies, perinatal loss, postpartum psychiatric disorders, adolescent pregnancy, and psychiatric disorders during pregnancy, with special attention to psychopharmacology. The second section of the book is devoted to the psychological aspects of gynecology. With the possible exception of psychiatry, no field of medicine is so inevitably involved in the sensitive psychopolitical and ethical-religious issues of our day—induced abortion, sexual dysfunction, sexual assault, rape, harassment, menstrual cycle disorders, infertility, menopause, pelvic pain, hysterectomy, and sterilization—as well as the life-and-death issues of emergency surgery, acquired immuno-deficiency syndrome (AIDS), and cancer.

The third section of the book deals with general issues in the field of women's health care: reproductive choices and development, sexual disorders, the male perspective, substance abuse, eating disorders, breast cancer, sexual assault, domestic violence, incest, medical ethics, and minority women. The penultimate chapter is devoted to the interface itself: psychiatric consultation and liaison to obstetrics and gynecology. This chapter, as is true for those preceding it, is well written and referenced. The style is free and readable. The approach is eclectic, as befits contemporary psychiatrists. Both the editors and contributors have done their parts in producing an excellent, useful, and valuable book.

Robert O. Pasnau, M.D.

REFERENCE

Kroger WS, Freed SC: Psychosomatic Gynecology: Including Problems of Obstetrical Care. Philadelphia, PA, WB Saunders, 1951

Chapter 1

THE INTERFACE BETWEEN PSYCHIATRY AND OBSTETRICS AND GYNECOLOGY: AN INTRODUCTION

Donna E. Stewart, M.D., D.Psych., F.R.C.P.C.
Nada L. Stotland, M.D.

❖ ❖ ❖ ❖ ❖ ❖ ❖ ❖ ❖ ❖ ❖ ❖ ❖ ❖

T̲he interface between psychiatry and obstetrics and gynecology may be conceptualized as a narrow subspecialty of the psychiatric study of somatic events and diseases (Alexander 1950). From another perspective, however, psychosomatic obstetrics and gynecology includes a realm both broad and deep. It begins with men's and women's feelings and behaviors related to female reproductive physiology (Benedek and Rubenstein 1942). It ranges from the events surrounding conception—or its frustration—to reactions to the terminal gynecologic malignancies that are so tragically common in our population. It encompasses the joyous embodiment of romantic love and the enactment of the most brutal victimization. Although only a small percentage of psychiatric and other mental health professionals explicitly devote their clinical or academic practices to this area, virtually all encounter these issues in their work with patients and their families, with medical students, and with residents.

While every organ system and its pathology are associated with psychological meanings, dynamics, conflicts, and symptoms, the relationship between psychiatry and obstetrics and gynecology is especially rich. "Hysteria" designates a psychiatric illness derived from the putative wanderings of the uterus from its proper site in the pelvis. This

1

term was coined over 2,000 years ago and is still in use (Pomeroy 1975). Long after dissection had demonstrated the realities of the anatomy of uterine connections, Sigmund Freud linked hysteria to forbidden sexual wishes and sexual frustration (Freud 1931).

One hundred years ago, the *Journal of the American Medical Association* published "Can the Gynecologist Aid the Alienist in Institutions for the Insane?" (1891). Portions were reprinted in a 1991 issue. The author or editor, unnamed, cites the work of several others alleging links between the functions, dysfunctions, and removal of the ovaries and uterus and psychiatric illness and cure. A quoted assertion (p. 3230) that "oophorectomy may be relied upon generally to cure insanity limited to the menstrual period" presages very recent attempts to treat late luteal phase dysphoric disorder. Other recent controversies were also foreshadowed. Bemoaning the "indisposition of alienists to accord the gynecologist a place in cooperation with them" (p. 3230) the article explains,

> There was said to have been too keen a desire to try oophorectomy as a panacea for all kinds of insanity in women. There was also an effort made to introduce female physicians upon this tide of so-called necessity, and thus were blended disadvantageously questions of public policy, or expediency, with what should have been scientific inquiry. . . . (p. 3230)

Clinical work and experimental studies performed in the years after Freud's major contributions have in turn disproved some of his assumptions. At the same time, new facets of patients' sexual histories prove to be as important in the etiology of psychiatric illness as those asserted in the past, albeit in a different way. Many patients with personality disorders and other diagnoses have histories of sexual and physical abuse. Sexually transmitted diseases and new reproductive technologies challenge the psychological coping mechanisms of patients and their psychiatrists today.

Acquired immunodeficiency syndrome (AIDS) introduces the possibility of a lingering and inevitable death into many sexual encounters (and into gynecologic care). The discrepancy between cognitive knowledge of the technically simple methods by which disease transmission can be reduced and the implementation of that knowledge into interpersonal behavior is an unsolved dilemma that has affected women and their children differentially. Women and children are the fastest-growing population infected with human immunodeficiency virus (HIV). Public health workers must be informed by knowledge of the psychology, sociology, and anthropology of female reproductive behavior in order to design and implement strategies to reduce the transmission of HIV (see Chapter 16). Breast and pelvic malignancies raise many of the same issues. The exchange of knowledge between psychiatrists and obstetrician-gynecologists might improve the diagnosis and effective treatment of breast and gynecologic malignancies by elucidating the factors that deter women from self-examination and regular medical screening and by using the knowledge of those factors to enhance compliance. The same knowledge can enable the psychiatrist to help patients understand and cope with the dread of pelvic examination and help gynecologists to adapt examination technique so as to minimize the emotional distress it elicits in women in general.

In other arenas, improvements in outcomes and discoveries at the cutting edge of theory and practice may have paradoxical effects. Among the middle and upper classes, maternal and perinatal mortality rates have been drastically decreased, anesthetic techniques improved, and parents-to-be informed of and participant in obstetric decisions. Obstetricians feel that every couple now demands a perfect childbirth and child. The fact that, in the United States, 80% of obstetricians have been sued for malpractice at least once is one social embodiment of that demand (Charles and Kennedy 1985).

The demands, in many cases, begin not only before birth, but before conception. Astounding, previously unimaginable developments in reproductive technology seem to offer the possibility of biological parenthood to every infertile woman or couple (Christie and Pawson 1987). These developments pose a host of problems whose resolutions will demand knowledge of biology, psychology, sociology, anthropology, ethics, and law, but the clinical dilemmas face psychiatrists in the field right now (Dickstein 1990). At what point in the diagnostic and treatment process for infertility does continued expense, life disruption, and bodily intrusion constitute an obsession? How can the psychiatrist help the patient and the treatment team to make prospective policy and ongoing decisions? What ethical and psychiatric issues are raised by the voluntary and paid donations of gametes and gestational services by one woman to another (Lantos 1990)? What roles, if any, ought psychiatrists to play in screening, support, and treatment? Unprecedented family constellations could offer us the opportunity to discern how family dynamics and psychological development are shaped by genetics and environment.

The dialogue between obstetrics and gynecology and psychiatry, and among obstetrician-gynecologists, patients, and psychiatrists, is interwoven with social change (Stotland 1988). Tensions are reflected in language: *doctor* and *patient,* with their rich associations of mutual obligations founded in age-old relationships, become *provider* and *consumer. Primum non nocere* ("First, do no harm") transmutes into *caveat emptor* ("Let the buyer beware"). Obstetrician-gynecologists are often women's primary care physicians and the experts on their most intimate bodily parts and behaviors. As such, they have become the object of the strongest negative and positive attitudes and of transferences of patients toward nonpsychiatric clinicians. As documented here, they are transferentially endowed with magical technical and emotional powers. Most obstetricians' offices are bedecked with photographs of infants they have delivered, testimony to a mutual emotional investment beyond the expert skills of the accoucheur.

On the other hand, women have reacted with vituperation to the actual and perceived arrogance, insensitivity, psychological ignorance, and authoritarianism of obstetrician-gynecologists. Lay persons and medical gadflies have published books with titles including *Male Practice* (Mendelsohn 1982), *Seizing Our Bodies* (Dreifus 1978), and *Immaculate Deception* (Arms 1975), alleging and sometimes documenting the negative physical and emotional effects of gynecologic interventions unsupported by scientific evidence. The ubiquitous book *Our Bodies, Ourselves* embodies in title and content the message that the self-esteem and physical health of women can be improved by knowledge about their own anatomy, physiology, pathology, and treatment, and that this knowledge need not remain the arcane preserve of physicians, but can also be explained and understood by the reading public (Boston Women's Health Collective 1984).

Meanwhile, social scientists and other professionals have documented physicians' demeaning attitudes toward women in articles such as "A Funny Thing Happened on the Way to the Orifice: Women in Gynecology Textbooks" (Scully and Bart 1973) and "The Training of a Gynecologist: How the 'Old Boys' Talk About Women's Bodies" (Hellerstein 1984). Artists like Judy Chicago have forced questions about women's bodily shame by producing works of art explicitly depicting the perineum, while in some women's consciousness-raising groups women have examined their own and each other's bodies in a more prosaic and immediate attempt to demystify, inform, and accept themselves. Self-help groups teaching and performing menstrual extraction and suction abortions as well as routine examinations have moved into the previous professional preserve. Other self-help or consumer groups have focused on the provision of information, support, and preparation for reproductive experiences (Bing 1973; La Leche League 1987; Seiden 1978).

The American College of Obstetricians and Gynecologists was so concerned about the negative image of obstetrician-gynecologists that it produced a packet of brochures and questionnaires that individual clinicians could adapt to their own practices (1986). Obstetrician-gynecologists, practicing in conscious good faith, have been hard put to fathom the skepticism, rage, and litigiousness of patients. Few, if any, specialties require such mastery of a combination of ever-increasing scientific knowledge, technical skills, long hours, legal liability, and exposure to clinical situations of such immediate emotional intensity (Friedman 1986).

Training programs in obstetrics and gynecology have tended to include little instruction in psychodynamics, psychopathology, and interpersonal skills, either by didactics or example. Often the patient population in teaching hospitals consists of disadvantaged women whose social circumstances distance them from the upper-middle-class doctors who are in training, prevent them from seeking timely care, disincline them to complain, and interfere with the pleasures of a successful outcome (as when a resident delivers a baby to an overwhelmed young teenager who will take it home to a dangerous housing project). Trainees are brought face to face with the medical outcomes of social problems (domestic violence, rape, incest, sexual abuse), which they do not have the time, knowledge, support, or resources to address (Adler 1972). All these factors conspire to increase their focus on the cognitive knowledge and technical agility that their mentors reward. Thus they emerge as private practitioners or as teachers in turn.

The changing circumstances of medical practice further erode opportunities for doctors and patients to get to know and trust one another. Health maintenance and preferred provider organizations, coupled with choices made at the employer, rather than at the consumer, level, inhibit or obliterate patients' choices of physicians with whom they feel comfortable. People make frequent geographic moves. Doctors have little motivation to understand their own responses to patients and medical situations, to examine patients' responses to them, and to develop skills that put patients at ease. Physicians practice in groups and subspecialties, both of which decrease continuity of care. In fact, it might be said that the sicker and/or more distressed a woman is, the less likely it is that she will obtain care from a physician who is familiar with her personality, defenses, usual responses to illness, family, and religious and social supports and other coping mechanisms. The psychiatrist's role in providing this sort of information and enhancing these skills is ever more important under these circumstances (Dunbar 1954; Karasu et al. 1979; Lipowski 1986; Stotland and Garrick 1990).

Contraception and induced abortion are areas in which personal feelings about sexuality, reproduction, and sex roles, as well as religious and cultural rules and values, color and politicize medical practice. Abortion has been practiced throughout recorded history and was permitted until a few centuries ago, even by the Roman Catholic Church (Newman 1991). New physicians, sworn by the Hippocratic and other oaths to protect "life," are arrayed opposite each other as they define life and the priorities of one form of life over another. Government, often swayed by single-issue lobbying blocs, sails one way and another, leaving a wake of social disruption and medical adaptation or protest. Legalization and the improvement of medical techniques have reduced the gynecologic complications of induced abortion to a small fraction of those of childbirth. It would seem that the same is true for major psychiatric sequelae. The decision to terminate a pregnancy is a weighty one, however, necessarily made under the pressure of time and best made with support and without coercion in either direction. An abortion represents a failure and a loss. The feelings surrounding it may stem as much from the circumstances that shape the decision as from the procedure itself. Governmental restrictions on abortion have powerful implications for the practice of all of medicine and for the practice of gynecology and psychiatry in particular. They limit the options for poor and psychiatrically ill patients and for the professional autonomy of psychiatrists and gynecologists to discuss those options with their patients (*Webster v. Reproductive Health Services*, 1989).

This volume is a clinical and theoretical sourcebook for the practitioner facing the many universal and specific issues of obstetrics and gynecology that arise in psychiatric practice. Such an issue may be a presenting symptom, as when a patient is referred for care after suffering a rape or being diagnosed with infertility or malignancy. In many other cases, the role of the obstetric-gynecologic event or condition in the psychiatric illness is not volunteered or even recognized. Sexual abuse is a frequent feature of the history of patients with several major psychiatric disorders but may require particularly informed and expert diagnostic skills, or several years of building trust in a psychotherapeutic relationship, to reveal itself. The fact that a psychotic, manic, or depressed inpatient is postpartum may be apparent only when one learns her children's ages from the family or reproductive history. Feelings about a hysterectomy or the loss or termination of a pregnancy may play a role in the dynamics of a current conflict. Women also have questions and concerns about the psychiatric aspects of menstruation and menopause. The editors and authors hope that this work will serve to remind readers of the many rich connections between psychiatry and obstetrics and gynecology and to inform their research, teaching, and clinical work.

The choice of topics to be addressed in this book was determined by three guiding principles: 1) What issues specific to women are seen by psychiatrists and other mental health workers? 2) What psychologic issues should be considered in providing women's health care? 3) What are the special problems encountered in a consultation or liaison service to an obstetric-gynecologic program? Notman and

Nadelson's (1978) pioneering work in this area is an excellent starting point, but the last decade has seen rapid technological and theoretical developments in the area of women's health that require a fresh look at some of the old issues and an attempt to explore some of the new dilemmas. Nowhere is this more apparent than in the rapidly developing field of new reproductive technologies. While trying to present an unbiased overview of the area, we have tried to emphasize those topics in which new developments have occurred as well as those in which new diseases, such as AIDS, have emerged. We have been guided in our choice of subjects by our clinical work, in which we daily see women patients referred by obstetrician-gynecologists as well as women referred by psychiatrists for problems specific to their sex. Our research in psychosomatic obstetrics and gynecology and our teaching of medical students and residents has helped to focus our attention on those issues that are most common and problematic.

This book is divided into three sections: "Pregnancy," "Gynecology," and "General Issues." The "Pregnancy" section consists of seven chapters that cover a range of topics, from normal gestation to physical and psychiatric complications during and following pregnancy. Robinson and Wisner's chapter on fetal anomalies (Chapter 3) examines the new prenatal diagnostic techniques as well as the management of the psychological issues that emerge when abnormalities are detected. Stewart and Robinson discuss the use of psychotropic drugs and electroconvulsive therapy in pregnancy and lactation, review current knowledge about the risks entailed, and provide clinical guidelines for the use of psychotropic drugs during these periods in Chapter 5. Rosenthal's chapter on adolescent pregnancy (Chapter 6) explores the factors responsible for this epidemic and offers guidelines to health care providers who assist these young women. Herz's chapter on perinatal loss (Chapter 8) describes the tragedy of infant death and offers practical advice to those who seek to help bereaved couples.

The "Gynecology" section consists of eight chapters dealing with both common gynecologic problems and some of the more controversial issues, such as induced abortion and the new reproductive technologies. Jensvold explores the role of the menstrual cycle in exacerbating, as well as initiating, psychologic symptoms in a biologic and social context in Chapter 9. Sherwin gives a comprehensive account of the psychological aspects of menopause in Chapter 12 and reviews studies on the controversial effects of hormone replacement therapy. In Chapter 13, Steege and Stout discuss the management dilemmas of chronic pelvic pain and offer practical treatment suggestions to aid the gynecologist and mental health professional. In Chapter 15, McCartney presents a thoughtful overview of the psychologic issues of women with gynecologic cancer that is helpful to psychiatrists in addressing the pain of the patient and the feelings of the oncology team. The new psychologic dilemmas for women raised by HIV infection are considered by Chiasson et al. in Chapter 16.

The section "General Issues" addresses 10 topics considered to be of current importance. Although some readers may not agree with our choice of topics or the views presented by the authors, we have tried to present a broad and balanced picture of issues within the confines of the space allowed. A psychodynamic perspective on reproductive choices and development is offered by Notman and Nadelson in Chapter 17. The role of sexuality is explored by Segraves and Segraves in Chapter 18, and Miller gives a unique perspective on women's issues from the male point of view in Chapter 19. The often overlooked role of substance abuse and eating disorders in the practice of obstetrics and gynecology is addressed by Stewart and Robinson in Chapter 21. Andersen and Doyle-Mirzadeh's chapter on breast disorders (Chapter 22) is an important contribution, particularly in view of epidemiologic data showing the rising prevalence of breast cancer in the Western world. The role of violence as experienced within the home and community or in sexual assault is discussed by Rose in Chapter 23. The numerous and complex ethical and legal issues in women's health care in a rapidly changing health care scene are addressed by Nadelson in Chapter 24. Stotland discusses the provision of psychiatric consultation-liaison services to obstetric-gynecologic programs in Chapter 25. Finally, the important experience of minority-group women in the health care system is ably expounded by Fullilove in Chapter 26.

We hope this book is a useful and important reference for health care professionals who provide services for women and that it will result in increased sensitivity and improved care.

REFERENCES

Adler G: Helplessness in the helpers. Br J Med Psychol 45:315–326, 1972

Alexander F: Psychosomatic Medicine. New York, WW Norton, 1950

Arms S: Immaculate Deception: A New Look at Women and Childbirth in America. Boston, MA, Houghton Mifflin, 1975

Benedek T, Rubenstein B: The Sexual Cycle in Women (Psychosomatic Medicine Monographs, Vol 3). Washington, DC, National Research Council, 1942

Bing E: Six Practical Lessons for an Easier Childbirth. New York, Bantam, 1973

Boston Women's Health Collective: The New Our Bodies, Ourselves. New York, Simon & Schuster, 1984

Can the gynecologist aid the alienist in institutions for the insane? JAMA 16:870–873, 1891. Reprinted in JAMA 100 Years Ago. JAMA 265(24):3230, 1991

Charles SC, Kennedy E: Defendant. New York, Free Press, 1985

Christie GL, Pawson ME: The psychological and social management of the infertile couple, in The Infertile Couple. Edited by Pepperell RS, Hudson B, Wood C. New York, Churchill Livingstone, 1987, pp 35–50

Dickstein LJ: Effects of the new reproductive technologies on individuals and relationships, in Psychiatric Aspects of Reproductive Technology. Edited by Stotland NL. Washington, DC, American Psychiatric Press, 1990, pp 123–139

Dreifus C (ed): Seizing Our Bodies: The Politics of Women's Health. New York, Vintage Books, 1978

Dunbar HF: Emotions and Bodily Changes: A Survey of Literature on Psychosomatic Interrelationships. New York, Columbia University Press, 1954

Freud S: Female sexuality (1931), in The Standard Edition of the Complete Psychological Works of Sigmund Freud, Vol 21. Translated and edited by Strachey J. London, Hogarth Press, 1961, pp 223–243

Friedman EA: The obstetrician's dilemma: how much fetal monitoring and cesarean section is enough? N Engl J Med 315:641–643, 1986

Hellerstein D: The training of a gynecologist: how the "old boys" talk about women's bodies. Ms. 13(5):136–137, 1984

Karasu TB, Plutchnik R, Conte H, et al: What do physicians want from a psychiatric consultation service? Compr Psychiatry 18:73–81, 1979

La Leche League International: The Womanly Art of Breastfeeding. Franklin Park, IL, La Leche League International, 1987

Lantos JD: Second-generation ethical issues in the new reproductive technologies: divided loyalties, indications, and the research agenda, in Psychiatric Aspects of Reproductive Technology. Edited by Stotland NL. Washington, DC, American Psychiatric Press, 1990, pp 87–96

Lipowski ZJ: Consultation-liaison psychiatry: the first half century. Gen Hosp Psychiatry 8:305–315, 1986

Mendelsohn R: Male Practice: How Doctors Manipulate Women. Chicago, IL, Contemporary Books, 1982

Newman LF: Historical and cross-cultural perspectives on abortion, in Psychiatric Aspects of Abortion. Edited by Stotland NL. Washington, DC, American Psychiatric Press, 1991, pp 39–49

Notman M, Nadelson C (eds): The Woman Patient: Sexual and Reproductive Aspects of Women's Health Care. New York, Plenum Press, 1978

Pomeroy SB: Goddesses, Whores, Wives and Slaves: Women in Classical Antiquity. New York, Schocken Books, 1975

Scully D, Bart P: A funny thing happened on the way to the orifice: women in gynecology textbooks, in Changing Women in a Changing Society. Edited by Huber J. Chicago, IL, University of Chicago Press, 1973, pp 283–288

Seiden A: The sense of mastery in the childbirth experience, in The Woman Patient: Sexual and Reproductive Aspects of Women's Health Care, Vol 3. Edited by Notman M, Nadelson C. New York, Plenum, 1978, pp 87–105

Stotland NL: Social Change and Women's Reproductive Health Care. New York, Praeger, 1988

Stotland NL, Garrick TR: Manual of Psychiatric Consultation. Washington, DC, American Psychiatric Press, 1990

Webster v Reproductive Health Services, 109 S.Ct. 3040 (1989)

Section I

Pregnancy

Chapter 2

NORMAL AND MEDICALLY COMPLICATED PREGNANCIES

Melanie L. Carr, M.D., F.R.C.P.C.

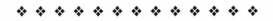

PSYCHOLOGY OF NORMAL PREGNANCY

The ability to conceive and bear a child has been considered to be important to women in all cultures and in all times. Pregnancy alters the course of a woman's life irreversibly; once having been pregnant, there is no return to a prepregnant psychology (Bibring et al. 1961). Even in women who choose induced abortion to terminate their pregnancies, the knowledge of fertility confirms a woman's gender identity and awareness of the essential "femaleness" of her biology.

Numerous authors have spoken of the "developmental crisis" or "critical phase" (Benedek 1970) that pregnancy affords to the woman. Old conflicts, particularly in relationship to her own mother, may be revived and reworked as a woman prepares to become a mother herself. Depending on how these conflicts are resolved, pregnancy can offer a chance to find new solutions and can propel her forward toward increasing psychological growth and maturity. Although the historical psychoanalytic literature focuses on the difficulties encountered in the experience of pregnancy, especially a first pregnancy, it is worth noting that for most women this is generally a time of excitement and anticipation. Most women handle this developmental task very well, although the test is made more arduous by circumstances such as an unwanted or unanticipated pregnancy, financial worries, a tumultuous or unsupportive spousal relationship, and realistic concerns about the developing fetus.

Although many authors have commented on the increasingly internalized focus established by the pregnant woman, the state of blissful calmness postulated by Freud is not borne out in clinical experience. Freud believed that until the oedipal phase, the psychosexual development of little girls paralleled that of little boys, both having a "masculine character" (Freud 1905, p. 219). In his formulation, when the little girl realizes she is "castrated," she turns to her mother in anger and disappointment for not having given her the gift of a penis and further devalues her for not having one herself (Notman 1990). The girl then looks to the father to repair this "mistake." According to this theory, the wish for a child—the father's child—is a substitution for the wish for a penis (Freud 1925, p. 256). In this hypothesis, pregnancy becomes the ultimate fulfillment for a woman and accounts for Freud's assumption that pregnant women are neither in need of nor accessible to psychoanalysis.

Freud's view permeated analytic thought on pregnancy until subtle changes were introduced by writers such as Deutsch and Bibring. Although Deutsch (1945) also espoused the belief that a baby was a substitute for the missing penis, she began to explore the "active ingredient" of motherhood and the sense of mastery involved in giving birth. To some extent, this took the woman beyond the essentially passive role ascribed to her by Freud. Deutsch, however, also believed that, having fulfilled her wish for a substitute penis, the woman would put aside her aggressive, "masculine" drives. Her step beyond classical analytic thought was, therefore, tentative at best.

Bibring (1961) set about to study women longitudinally throughout the course of pregnancy to determine whether theory was supported by clinical experience. She found that pregnancy evoked regressive responses and reactivated feelings about the original mother-daughter relationship. Rather than seeing this as a passive, uninterpretable state, however, Bibring and others following her felt that pregnancy provided an opportunity for significant maturation. Bibring also extended the framework of the psychological work of pregnancy beyond the individual to include a redefining of the marital relationship and a developing relationship with the future child.

Although foreshadowed by other authors, Benedek (1970) was the first person to conceptualize and develop the idea of pregnancy as a "critical phase" carrying a developmental function. She saw pregnancy as a basic biological drive in a woman and not merely as serving a substitutive function (p. 139):

> Thus motherhood is not secondary, not a substitute for the missing penis, nor is it forced by men upon women "in the service of the species," but the manifestation of the all-pervading instinct for survival in the child that is the primary organizer of the woman's sexual drive, and by this also her personality.

These ideas have been further developed by recent authors who have seen the wish for motherhood to be based not only on an inherent biological drive, but also on an identification with what is essentially female.

Kestenberg (1976) felt that pregnancy and the concomitant development of maternal feelings were central to female sexuality and fulfillment. Rather than seeing the woman as a castrated male, she postulated an "inner genital phase" based on libido arising from an awareness of the vagina. She saw this awareness as forming the wellspring of maternal feelings.

Whereas traditional analytic thinking focused on the oedipal nature of pregnancy, current thought has shifted the focus to the preoedipal period. Emphasis on the importance of positive feminine identification and the early relationship with the mother has led to an exploration of the importance of the maternal relationship with the child. Motherly feelings are not formed in a vacuum, but rather require an interaction with an infant to develop. Authors such as Stern (1974) and Thomas et al. (1963) have written of the infant's ability to elicit caretaking behavior from those around him or her. In the reciprocal relationship that develops as the mother responds to her infant's needs, the mother-child bond is strengthened and the woman finds increasing self-confidence and reassurance in her role.

Cultural expectations and the process of socialization undergone by the young girl cannot be ignored in considering the wish for motherhood and the adjustment to the pregnant state. Both Thompson (1973) and Kohut (1978) have elaborated on the interaction between biology and culture in these regards. Kohut described a woman's wish for a child as "a manifestation of her nuclear self, central ambitions and ideals that can occur when biological and cultural factors are supported" (Robinson and Stewart 1989, p. 862).

Although the ability to conceive and the state of being pregnant are seen to be important parts of the concept of femininity, recent authors have stressed the centrality of choice in reproductive decisions (Friedan 1981). A woman does not have to have children to achieve a complete sense of her feminine identity. That having been said, the developmental task associated with the milestone of pregnancy can provide the opportunity for a reworking of a woman's self-concept.

HORMONAL ASPECTS OF NORMAL PREGNANCY

In addition to the major psychological adaptation that accompanies childbearing, the pregnant woman also experiences profound physiologic alteration in every organ system, tissue, and cell in her body (Friedman 1978). These changes are predominantly the result of the unique hormonal environment of pregnancy.

The hormonal and physiologic changes of normal pregnancy are accompanied by multiple psychological concomitants. When pregnancy is diagnosed, most women experience a range of emotions, from elation to fear and ambivalence, as the enormity of the life change is glimpsed. In the first trimester, fatigue, nausea, and vomiting are common and may dampen the initial excitement that the knowledge of the pregnancy brings (Nadelson 1978). Women may also experience increased emotional lability in early pregnancy. Whether this is hormonally based or the result of the psychological adaptation required to adjust to the pregnant state is not clear.

As the pregnancy becomes more visible, the woman has to deal with both her own altered body image and the reactions of those around her, both to her pregnancy specifically and to pregnant women in general. Most women have had the experience of having their pregnant abdomen patted by people who would not consider such a gesture while she was in the nonpregnant state. In some respects, then, the pregnancy seems to be in the public domain, with many others having investment in its outcome, including spouse, parents, in-laws, other relatives, and friends. The stirring-up of feelings in others that is elicited by pregnancy is heightened for the woman therapist, who must deal with a plethora of reactions from patients. These feelings include envy, hostility, fear of abandonment, and denial.

The second trimester is usually accompanied by greater physical well-being and emotional quiescence. The experience of quickening is reassuring and begins the process of acknowledging the fetus as a separate being. Most studies of the psychological effect of experiencing fetal movement point to a concomitant increase in maternal-fetal attachment (Leifer 1977; Lerum and LoBiondo-Wood 1989; Reading et al 1984; Rubin 1975). The pregnant woman becomes more inward-focused, and heightened passivity and dependency are noted (Nadelson 1978).

As labor and delivery approach with the third trimester, most women report an increase in apprehension and anxiety. Fears that the baby will be abnormal become more pronounced. Concerns about loss of control during the delivery culminate in fears of being ripped apart or even of death. The individuation of the fetus from the mother continues during the third trimester and is aided by the increasing physical discomfort experienced by the mother. Restlessness, insomnia, and fatigue correlate with the desire for the pregnancy to be over. At the same time, concerns about her ability as a parent, reluctance to extend the spousal relationship to a triad, and sadness over the loss of the very intimate pregnant state may contribute to the ambivalence and emotional upheaval often experienced by the woman as her pregnancy draws to an end.

PRENATAL PREPARATION

Given the enormity of the psychological and physiological processes involved in labor and delivery, it is easy to see why prenatal preparation has gained increasing popularity in the last 50 years. The pioneer of the preparatory methods was Grantly Dick-Read (1944), who introduced the term *natural childbirth* and initially postulated that labor was not in itself an inherently painful process. By the time of the publication of his book, *Childbirth Without Fear,* however, he had modified his thoughts about the etiology of the pain of labor. He later outlined a process he called "the fear-tension-pain syndrome," which postulated that there are two distinct kinds of pain, that caused by the ischemia produced by prolonged uterine muscle tension and that caused by fear and subsequent sympathetic arousal. Dick-Read believed that labor pain could be ameliorated through education, relaxation training, breathing, and muscle exercises (Beck et al. 1979).

The second major theory regarding childbirth preparation was developed in Russia (Velvovsky et al. 1960). The Russian school claimed to base their theory on Pavlovian principles and also used education and "pain prevention techniques" in their program. These techniques included deep breathing, massaging of the abdomen or back combined with deep breathing, and pressure applied to points along the back and iliac crest. More recently, the Soviets have embellished this approach to include gymnastic training, hydrotherapy, and exposure to ultraviolet light (Beck et al. 1979).

Ferdinand Lamaze popularized childbirth education in the Western world. Lamaze modified Russian breathing techniques by including rapid breathing during the second stage of labor and panting just prior to delivery. He also recommended "controlled neuromuscular relaxation" (Lamaze 1958).

In the last decade, some of the early radicalism of the natural childbirth method and the guilt associated with the failure of women to have a "painless childbirth" have been tempered. The more realistic aims of helping a woman to cope with her pain and to participate actively in the childbirth experience are now proposed in the various "prepared" childbirth methods. As Beck and Hall (1978) have indicated, most of these methods include three distinct components: 1) accurate information regarding the processes of labor and delivery, 2) training in relaxation to reduce anxiety and cope with pain, and 3) breathing techniques. Different schools advocate additions to these basic tenets; the most frequent of these is participation of the father.

Unfortunately, many of the claims made by advocates of prenatal preparation, including claims for a shorter duration of labor, decreased perception of pain, decreased incidence of postpartum depression, reduced use of analgesics, and decreased neonatal morbidity and mortality, are not supported by well-designed studies (Beck and Hall 1978). In summary, it seems that the evidence for the efficacy of psychoprophylaxis is not very strong. As Wolkind (1981) points out, however, many authors speak of the "better subjective experiences of the prepared woman" (p. 203). Since one of the fears of women entering labor is loss of control, it makes sense that the provision of control offered by the psychoprophylactic methods would be helpful in increasing self-esteem and confidence. The encouragement of participation by the father can also foster the relationship between the couple. Future directions for research involve integrating the body of knowledge already available on pain, anxiety, and stress reduction and a variety of cognitive-behavioral and biofeedback approaches (Beck and Siegel 1980).

MEDICAL COMPLICATIONS OF PREGNANCY

Whereas a normal pregnancy results in considerable emotional and physiologic stress, a "high-risk" pregnancy may generate altered and intensified psychological and physical responses. Complications may develop at any stage of the pregnancy as a result of preexisting maternal disorders, obstetric difficulties, or fetal compromise. A cursory overview of these complications follows in order to set the stage for discussion of the psychological aspects of high-risk pregnancy. Although a more detailed description lies beyond the scope of this chapter, appropriate references are included. It behooves the psychiatrist working at the interface of psychiatry and obstetrics and gynecology to have a working knowledge of the medical complications that can develop in pregnancy in order to have a full appreciation of the patient's course and to provide effective liaison services.

The maternal factors associated with increased risk during pregnancy include hypertension, diabetes, cardiovascular disease, renal disease, and malignancies. Hypertension is a complicating factor in approximately 7% of all pregnancies, preeclampsia accounting for the majority of cases. The remaining 30% of cases involve chronic essential hypertension, which can have a wide range of consequences in pregnancy, from a normal outcome to increased fetal and maternal morbidity and perinatal mortality (Anderson and Sibai 1986). Before the availability of insulin, the risk of fetal and maternal death was approximately 50% in women with diabetes (Goldberg et al. 1985). Through the discovery of insulin, increasing knowledge of the pathophysiology of diabetes in pregnancy, and improved perinatal and neonatal care, this mortality rate has plummeted to 2%–5% for the offspring of diabetic mothers (Samuels and Landon 1986).

Cardiac disease complicates 1% of pregnancies and is the most frequent nonobstetric cause of maternal mortality during pregnancy and immediately postpartum (Meller and Goldman 1985). The effect of cardiac disease on the pregnancy will differ, depending on the severity of the underlying disorder.

The outlook for women with chronic renal disease who desire pregnancy has improved considerably: more than 85% of women with mild to moderately impaired renal function have a successful pregnancy outcome. When renal insufficiency is severe or complicated by significant hypertension, however, the prognosis is much more dismal.

A diagnosis of cancer coincident with pregnancy is relatively uncommon but is a subject of much emotion and concern. Breast cancer, the most common cancer in women, is sometimes found in pregnant women. Estimates of the incidence of pregnancy in women with breast cancer range from 0.2% to 2.9% (Malamud and Holland 1985). With prompt diagnosis and treatment, survival rates for pregnant and nonpregnant woman are thought to be equal (King et al. 1985).

In all discussions of high-risk pregnancy, it is important to appreciate first that most pregnancies proceed normally and with little need for any intervention aside from adequate, routine prenatal care. It has been estimated that in an average mixed obstetric practice, approximately 30% of patients may be considered high risk. Despite rating systems and subsequent increased surveillance, 25% of poor perinatal outcomes are unanticipated. The obstetric factors that increase pregnancy risks and can be detected prenatally include cervical incompetence, habitual abortion, preeclampsia, multiple gestation, placenta previa, and abruptio placentae.

The incidence of cervical incompetence is approximately 1 in 1,000 pregnancies (Thomason et al. 1982). Once the diagnosis is established, usually following a pregnancy loss, the primary treatment for subsequent pregnancies is cervical cerclage (Cherry 1985).

Miscarriage is a common problem in pregnancy, but most women will go on to deliver a healthy, normal baby in a subsequent pregnancy. A small subset of women, however, will repeatedly lose their pregnancies, a condition known as habitual abortion. Possible contributing factors include chromosomal abnormalities, dysfunction of the maternal endocrine system, infection, structural anomalies of the reproductive tract, and underlying maternal disease (Simpson 1986).

Preeclampsia is characterized by hypertension, edema, and proteinuria and develops with increasing frequency after the 20th week of gestation. Eclampsia is preeclampsia with convulsions. The only specific treatment is delivery, but temporization with bed rest and careful monitoring may be justified if the patient is remote from term (Wynn 1983).

It is well known that the presence of more than one fetus increases the complications associated with pregnancy. Early diagnosis of multiple gestation with ultrasound and increased surveillance during the pregnancy may help to achieve a more positive outcome (Berkowitz 1986).

Placenta previa, which occurs in 1 of every 200 pregnancies, is the implantation of the placenta in the lower segment of the uterus so that it extends to the margin of the internal os of the cervix or partially or completely obstructs it (Brenner et al. 1978). It presents in the third trimester as painless vaginal bleeding, and diagnosis is established by ultrasound evaluation. Management of placenta previa depends on gestational age, amount of bleeding, and fetal well-being and presentation.

The other major cause of third-trimester bleeding is abruptio placentae, in which the placenta begins to separate from the interior uterine wall too early in gestation. Signs and symptoms depend on the degree of placental separation and its duration. With significant bleeding, there may be signs of fetal distress or, if severe, fetal demise. Fetal monitoring is essential if the diagnosis of abruptio placentae is suspected (Wynn 1983).

In some cases, complications develop during the intrapartum period in a pregnancy that had progressed smoothly until term. Dystocia, literally meaning "abnormal labor" and sometimes referred to as "failure to progress," is caused by one of three main factors or a combination of them: 1) uterine dysfunction, 2) abnormalities of pelvic size or structure, and 3) abnormal presentation, size, or development of the fetus. Dystocia is the most common reason for primary cesarean deliveries, and although many of these are clearly indicated, it appears that conservative management and vaginal delivery can safely be undertaken in some cases.

The use of cesarean section is one of the most controversial areas in obstetrics. In 1970, the rate of abdominal delivery in the United States was approximately 5%. In the ensuing decade, that rate more than tripled, although there is great variation depending on the population and the attitude of the obstetrician toward variables such as vaginal birth after cesarean delivery. The increase in cesarean deliveries is the result of many factors, including increased safety of the procedure, a greater ability to detect fetal distress, and improved chances of survival with neonatal intensive care. Certainly, the current litigious climate has also contributed to the reluctance to allow trials of labor in any ambiguous circumstance (Hibbard 1986).

Fetal complications that qualify a pregnancy as high-risk include intrauterine growth retardation and intrapartum fetal distress. Intrauterine growth retardation complicates 3%–7% of all pregnancies. Many factors are associated with retarded growth, including intrauterine infection, multiple gestation, poor nutrition, chromosomal abnormalities, congenital malformation, maternal hypertension, and maternal smoking and drug and alcohol abuse. Once growth retardation is diagnosed, serial determinations of growth should be undertaken, treatment initiated that is aimed at contributing factors, or delivery considered if fetal compromise is evident (Gabbe 1986).

During the last 30 years, significant steps have been taken to identify fetal compromise during labor. Lowered morbidity and mortality have resulted, primarily through the determination of which fetus is at risk for hypoxia. The great benefit of intrapartum surveillance is that it allows for confirmation of fetal well-being, thus preventing unnecessary obstetric intervention. Unfortunately, some false-positive results still occur, and cesarean delivery is sometimes undertaken unnecessarily. The advantages of increased technology must be weighed against the disadvantages, including the psychological aspects of a monitored labor. It seems, however, that when adequate information is given to patients regarding the need for such intervention, most adjust to the added stress (Petrie 1986).

PSYCHOLOGICAL CONCOMITANTS

In all pregnancies, a level of uncertainty exists with which the woman must cope. This level of uncertainty is heightened to various degrees with the diagnosis of a high-risk pregnancy. High-risk pregnancy can be defined as "any pregnancy in which there is a factor—maternal or fetal—that will adversely affect the outcome of pregnancy" (Queenan 1985, p. xix). The patient's reaction to the diagnosis is affected by the stage at which the pregnancy is identified as high-risk, the etiology of the risk, and the personality structure and defenses of the pregnant woman (Wolreich 1986). Kemp and Page (1987) also reported that the degree of stress associated with the diagnosis depended on the nature of the risk, the nature of the treatment, and the woman's perception of the danger to the pregnancy.

Because the notion of motherhood carries so many social expectations and feelings, a woman's self-esteem may be affected by the knowledge that she is carrying an "imperfect" pregnancy (M. B. Jones 1986). She might even feel like a failure as a woman. With her own sense of identity shaken, negotiating the developmental tasks of pregnancy may become more difficult (Penticuff 1982). Since it is postulated that prenatal attachment to the fetus is important to the subsequent maternal-infant relationship (Cranley 1981), the disruptive effect of the high-risk pregnancy may extend well beyond the gestational period. There is little empirical research looking at the effect of the label of *high-risk* on a woman's view of herself or her pregnancy. Merkatz (1976), however, found that hospitalized high-risk women reported at least as much concern for their fetus as for themselves, and Kemp and Page (1987) reported that women experiencing a high-risk pregnancy had lower levels of self-esteem but equal degrees of attachment as did their "normal" counterparts. Kemp and Page also speculated that denial might be operative as a way of protecting the woman from the perception of actual threat to the pregnancy, allowing her to continue with the usual process of attachment. Further understanding of the psychological impact of this diagnosis is important, particularly in light of research suggesting that heightened anxiety and life stress might adversely affect pregnancy outcome (Berkowitz 1983; Chalmers 1982; Gorsuch and Key 1974; A. C. Jones 1978; Lederman 1978).

The nature of the risk to the pregnancy is also important in determining the effect of the diagnosis. A woman with a chronic medical illness such as diabetes, renal disease, or cardiovascular disease may experience a wide array of divergent emotions about her pregnancy. On the one hand, pregnancy may offer a "second chance" to start life anew and defeat the illness (Wolreich 1986, p. 56). In such instances, the pregnancy may be particularly highly valued. Clearly, the degree to which the woman has come to terms with her own disorder will affect how she responds to her pregnancy. Such women have often had long-term associations with doctors, hospitals, and medical procedures and may have conflicting feelings about such involvement. The increased surveillance that will be part of their pregnancies may result in reawakened feelings of distrust, anxiety, and anger as they confront their own suboptimal medical status and the risk that might be posed to their fetus (Wolreich 1986).

In making the decision to become pregnant, a woman with a chronic medical disease needs to consider her potentially shortened life span, whether the pregnancy will jeopardize her own health, and whether, in the case of genetically acquired diseases, there is a risk of passing on a heritable disorder to the fetus. In conditions requiring treatment during pregnancy, the effect of medication on the fetus is also a source of concern. Heightened anxiety, guilt, or denial may be present as the woman struggles to come to terms with these added variables.

One of the developmental tasks of the pregnant woman is to reassess the nature of her relationship with her own mother. Negotiating a new kind of interaction may be especially arduous for a woman who has had a longstanding medical disorder. Frequently, the mother-daughter relationship has been subject to overinvolvement and overprotection, which might make separation and the formation of a new alliance difficult.

A distinct group of high-risk patients are those with a previously poor obstetric history, including those with a history of infertility, miscarriage, genetic termination, or stillbirth. If there are unresolved issues and grief about previous pregnancies, the new pregnancy will be colored by those experiences, leading to increased anxiety, fears, or guilt. Kumar and Robson (1984) reported an increased incidence of postpartum depression in this group, although their findings have not been replicated.

Some pregnancies start out normally and then acquire the label of high-risk. Examples include diagnoses of preeclampsia, intrauterine growth retardation, abruptio placentae, and gestational diabetes. Ironically, those women most likely to have overdetermined feelings about their pregnancies, such as women with diabetes, patients of advanced maternal age, or those with prior obstetric complications, are also most likely to develop complications as the pregnancy progresses. In a well-designed study of the psychological impact of the diagnosis of gestational diabetes, Spirito et al. (1989) found that most pregnant women coped very well with that unanticipated diagnosis. This may be due to the fact that their group was interviewed several weeks after the diagnosis was established, allowing for a period of adjustment. In any event, presumably women who begin their pregnancy in good health and without increased risk are able to undertake the developmental tasks of pregnancy unfettered with extra emotional baggage and are in an improved position to cope with an unexpected turn of events.

Once the label of high-risk has been applied to the pregnancy, obstetric care is altered, both in terms of frequency of visits and application of technology. The woman may feel torn between wanting to have available every medical resource to monitor the baby and not wanting to know of the development of further complications. Many medications used in high-risk pregnancies, such as tocolytic agents, have their own psychoactive effects that mimic or augment the psychological effects of the increased stress and anxiety already present (Wolreich 1986). Prolonged rest or inability to perform her usual tasks may further add to the woman's distress.

For various reasons, women with high-risk pregnancies might require hospitalization. In these cases, the normal regression of pregnancy may be intensified by the enforced abandonment of usual activities and the provision of all aspects of daily care in a hospital milieu (Rogers 1989). White and Ritchie (1984) studied the effect of antepartum hospitalization on psychological functioning and found that the separation from the usual supports of spouse and family, concern about health, and a shaken self-image contributed to their finding of considerable stress and anxiety in these women. In a pilot study, Kramer et al. (1986) found a high number of "adverse reactions" in hospitalized women with high-risk pregnancies. These negative reactions, including distress and noncompliance, increased when the hospitalization was prolonged. The authors concluded that only women with "better than average social resources and very good psychic functioning and short length of stay were able to comply with their medical regimen without incident" (p. 37). This study was limited, however, by a very small sample size and the confounding variable of other social stressors for many of the subjects. In any event, ambivalent feelings about the pregnancy are not unusual in this circumstance and may be demonstrated through noncompliant behavior. Additionally, each new difficulty in management may add to existing fears and disillusionment, resulting in the feeling that it is not worth trying. Such resignation can be easily misinterpreted as noncompliance or hostility.

From the preceding discussion, it is easy to see how medical personnel can play a crucial role in the patient's response to an unwanted and stressful situation. Most helpful to patients and families is accurate and current information, delivered in understandable language. Good cooperation between what might become a number of physicians, including obstetricians, internists, and perinatologists, is essential so that the patient receives consistent messages and is able to trust her health care team (Rogers 1989). Opportunities for discussion of the myriad feelings related to her high-risk status can be immensely reassuring and helpful to the pregnant woman. Frank discussion and an understanding of the commonality of ambivalent and even hostile feelings may diminish the woman's sense of guilt and isolation (Kemp and Page 1987). Allowing the woman and her family to grieve in the event of an unfortunate outcome is a recognition of the fact that bonding occurs prenatally, even if the pregnancy has been in jeopardy.

Medical personnel can also, however, unwittingly add to the stress for the patient. For example, the complexities underlying noncompliant behavior may not be appreciated and the woman subsequently blamed for her lack of caring. As Kramer et al. (1986) comment, women of lower socioeconomic status are more at risk for complicated pregnancies and more likely to engage in problematic behaviors. Medical staff often have difficulty working with this group and are therefore likely to become frustrated and angry with the very patients who are most in need of their support. Although most obstetricians are aware that there are two patients, unacknowledged feelings may lead to an overidentification with either the fetus or the mother. With the benefit of improved neonatal care and the great decrease in maternal mortality, the focus in some instances has shifted from the pregnant woman as the patient to the fetus, and objective care can be compromised as a result.

In many high-risk pregnancies, increased surveillance leads to an intensification of the doctor-patient relationship. This, too, can have multiple effects. The usual dependency of late pregnancy may be heightened, resulting in the physician feeling annoyed or burdened by what seem like unreasonable demands. Alternatively, there may be an overinvestment in the pregnancy by the physician, leading to false reassurances and a lack of tolerance for anything other than optimism in the patient. This can increase the woman's sense of isolation and guilt at her own ambivalence. If unable to deal with their own feelings of powerlessness and distress in response to a worsening prenatal course, medical caregivers may inadvertently blame the patient, exacerbating an already stressful situation.

It should be said that, given the additional level of coping required of a pregnant woman who receives the diagnosis of high-risk pregnancy, most manage fairly well. Wolreich (1986) hypothesizes that there are several factors particular to pregnancy that aid in this adjustment. The heightened dependency feelings mentioned above may make the frequency of visits and intensive testing more tolerable than usual. In addition, the regression and passivity of pregnancy may allow for an increased compliance with all parental figures, including medical personnel. Women may endure considerable discomfort and hardship "for the sake of the child." This can both allow the pregnant woman to see herself as a good mother, partially undoing the feeling of inadequacy brought by the label of high-risk, and can act as a means of punishment for the ambivalence toward the pregnancy that might be felt in these situations. Finally, the time-limited nature of pregnancy can allow the woman to put up with difficult circumstances, knowing that an end to medical intervention is in sight.

Although most women seem to cope well with their high-risk status, Powers et al. (1986) found a greatly increased rate of psychiatric disorders in their sample population. Two-thirds of their high-risk patients had DSM-III diagnoses (American Psychiatric Association 1980); many patients had multiple diagnoses. The findings from this study must be generalized cautiously, however, as their sample contained an overrepresentation of women from a lower socioeconomic group and of those with chronic medical illnesses. Both of these groups are known to be predisposed to psychiatric disorders. Furthermore, their study did not utilize a control group of normal pregnant women. Clearly, further research is needed in this important area.

Although much has been written about the woman's response to carrying a high-risk pregnancy, her spouse and family also have reactions that need to be considered. The father may share the mother's anxiety about the fetus and may also be concerned about the effect of the pregnancy on the mother's health status. He may feel unable to voice his worries for fear of adding to the mother's burdens. On the other hand, he may feel resentful toward the mother and her ill health for jeopardizing his child (Rogers 1989). Fathers may also feel guilty and responsible for being instrumental in creating the pregnancy in the first place. If the woman is hospitalized during the pregnancy or has to stop working, financial pressures may be added to the emotional pressures already experienced. The father may need to take on increased responsibilities around the house, in some cases with existing children adding to his strain. To a greater or lesser extent, all members of the family can exhibit psychological reactions to the jeopardized pregnancy that are similar to those of the woman, including denial, ambivalence, guilt, and grief.

PSYCHIATRIC INTERVENTION

The role of the psychiatrist may begin even before conception. In women with chronic, sometimes severe, diseases, prepregnancy counseling can be very helpful. An open discussion in which the obstetrician outlines the risks to both the fetus and the woman is essential. The couple may need to feel that they have permission not to have a child or may need help exploring their feelings about options such as adoption. Encouraging each individual in the couple to voice his or her anxieties, expectations, and concerns about the other can help both arrive at a mutual, supportive decision. Nadelson (1978) has offered several suggestions to which the obstetrician can attend while eliciting the patient's history that may signal perinatal psychiatric difficulties. Many of these are particularly applicable in a high-risk pregnancy, including previous obstetric mishap, infertility, familial or congenital diseases, conflicts around separation from parents, and poor relationships with physicians. A psychiatric assessment in such instances may prove very useful to both the woman and the obstetric team and may play a preventive role.

Working with obstetric personnel can be challenging for the consultation-liaison psychiatrist. The medical team may have their own reactions to the jeopardized pregnancy that can interfere with providing optimal medical care and emotional support to the pregnant woman. Helping the staff understand their responses can assist in modifying unhelpful, overinvolved, or even hostile behavior. Allowing a forum for staff to ventilate their own stresses, fears, and disappointments can help reduce denial and distancing from patients who need their support.

Once a patient is referred, the first task of the psychiatrist is to undertake a complete history, looking particularly for underlying psychiatric disorders and emotional adjustment to both the pregnancy and the diagnosis of high-risk status. The time-limited course of pregnancy can be especially suited to short-term psychotherapeutic intervention aimed at improving adjustment to high-risk management and resolving conflicting feelings about the developing fetus (Wolreich 1986). Medication may be required during psychiatric treatment in this setting and requires a risk-benefit analysis (see Chapter 5).

In order to be most effective, the psychiatrist working in this multifaceted area must have an understanding of the psychology of normal pregnancy, a familiarity with the medical and obstetric complications of high-risk pregnancy and principles of its management, and an appreciation of the psychological reactions associated with high-risk status for the pregnant woman and her family. This complex role can be a rewarding one, for as Wolreich (1986) states, "the potential benefits include not only improved obstetric patient care, but also risk reduction in the mother-child relationship that follows" (p. 66).

REFERENCES

American Psychiatric Association: Diagnostic and Statistical Manual of Mental Disorders, 3rd Edition. Washington, DC, American Psychiatric Association, 1980

Anderson GD, Sibai BM: Hypertension in pregnancy, in Obstetrics: Normal and Problem Pregnancies. Edited by Gabbe SG, Niebyl JR, Simpson JL. New York, Churchill Livingstone, 1986, pp 819–863

Beck NC, Geden EA, Brouder GT: Preparation for labor: a historical perspective. Psychosom Med 41:243–258, 1979

Beck NC, Hall D: Natural childbirth: a review and analysis. Obstet Gynecol 52:371–379, 1978

Beck NC, Siegel LJ: Preparation for childbirth and contemporary research on pain, anxiety and stress reduction: a review and critique. Psychosom Med 42:429–447, 1980

Benedek T: The psychobiology of pregnancy, in Parenthood: Its Psychology and Psychopathology. Edited by Anthony EJ, Benedek T. Boston, MA, Little, Brown, 1970, pp 137–151

Berkowitz RH: Multiple gestations, in Obstetrics: Normal and Problem Pregnancies. Edited by Gabbe SG, Niebyl JR, Simpson JL. New York, Churchill Livingstone, 1986, pp 739–767

Berkowitz GS, Kasl SV: The role of psychological factors in spontaneous preterm delivery. J Psychosom Res 27:283–290, 1983

Bibring G, Dwyer T, Huntington D, et al: A study of the psychological processes in pregnancy and the earliest mother-child relationship. Psychoanal Study Child 16:9–72, 1961

Brenner W, Edelman D, Hendricks C: Characteristics of patients with placenta previa and results of expectant management. Am J Obstet Gynecol 132:180–191, 1978

Chalmers B: Psychological aspects of pregnancy: some thoughts for the eighties. Soc Sci Med 16:323–331, 1982

Cherry SH: The incompetent cervix, in Medical, Surgical, and Gynecologic Complications in Pregnancy. Edited by Cherry SH, Berkowitz RL, Kase NG. Baltimore, MD, Williams & Wilkins, 1985, pp 408–419

Cranley MC: Development of a tool for the measurement of maternal attachment during pregnancy. Nurs Res 39:281–284, 1981

Deutsch H: The Psychology of Women, Vol 2. New York, Grune & Stratton, 1945

Dick-Read G: Childbirth Without Fear. New York, Harper & Brothers, 1944

Freud S: Three essays on the theory of sexuality (1905), in The Standard Edition of the Complete Psychological Works of Sigmund Freud, Vol 7. Translated and edited by Strachey J. London, Hogarth Press, 1962, pp 261–285

Freud S: Some psychical consequences of the anatomical distinction between the sexes (1925), in The Standard Edition of the Complete Psychological Works of Sigmund Freud, Vol 19. Translated and edited by Strachey J. London, Hogarth Press, 1962, pp 248–258

Friedan B: The Second Stage. New York, Summit Books, 1981

Friedman E: The physiological aspects of pregnancy, in The Woman Patient, Vol 1. Edited by Notman M, Nadelson C. New York, Plenum, 1978, pp 55–71

Gabbe SG: Intrauterine growth retardation, in Obstetrics: Normal and Problem Pregnancies. Edited by Gabbe SG, Niebyl JR, Simpson JL. New York, Churchill Livingstone, 1986, pp 769–785

Goldberg JD, Jornsay DL, Hausknecht RV: Diabetes in pregnancy, in Medical, Surgical, and Gynecologic Complications in Pregnancy. Edited by Cherry SH, Berkowitz RL, Kase NG. Baltimore, MD, Williams & Wilkins, 1985, pp 408–419

Gorsuch R, Key M: Abnormalities of pregnancy as a function of anxiety and life stress. Psychosom Med 36:352–362, 1974

Hibbard LT: Cesarean section and other surgical procedures, in Obstetrics: Normal and Problem Pregnancies. Edited by Gabbe SG, Niebyl JR, Simpson JL. New York, Churchill Livingstone, 1986, pp 517–546

Jones AC: Life changes and psychological distress as predictors of pregnancy outcome. Psychosom Med 40:402–412, 1978

Jones MB: The high-risk pregnancy, in Nursing Assessment and Strategies for the Family at Risk, 2nd Edition. Edited by Johnson SH. Philadelphia, PA, JB Lippincott, 1986, pp 111–128

Kemp VH, Page C: Maternal self-esteem and prenatal attachment in high-risk pregnancy. Matern Child Nurs J 16:195–206, 1987

Kestenberg J: Regression and reintegration in pregnancy. J Am Psychoanal Assoc 24:213–250, 1976

King RM, Welch JS, Martin JK, et al: Carcinoma of the breast associated with pregnancy. Surg Gynecol Obstet 160:228–232, 1985

Kohut H: The Search for the Self. New York, International Universities Press, 1978

Kramer PP, Coustan D, Krzeminski J, et al: Hospitalization on the high-risk maternity unit: a pilot study. Gen Hosp Psychiatry 8:33–39, 1986

Kumar R, Robson K: A prospective study of emotional disorders in childbearing women. Br J Psychiatry 144:35–47, 1984

Lamaze F: Painless Childbirth. Translated by Celestin LR. London, Burke, 1958

Lederman R, Lederman E, Work B, et al: The relationship of maternal anxiety, plasma catecholamines, and plasma cortisol to progress in labor. Am J Obstet Gynecol 132:495–500, 1978

Leifer M: Psychological changes accompanying pregnancy and motherhood. Genet Soc Gen Psychol Monogr 95:55–96, 1977

Lerum CW, LoBiondo-Wood G: The relationship of maternal age, quickening and physical symptoms of pregnancy to the development of maternal-fetal attachment. Birth 16:13–17, 1989

Malamud SC, Holland JF: Neoplasia and pregnancy, in Medical, Surgical and Gynecologic Complications of Pregnancy. Edited by Cherry SH, Berkowitz RL, Kase NG. Baltimore, MD, Williams & Wilkins, 1985, pp 502–521

Meller J, Goldman M: Cardiovascular disease in pregnancy, in Medical, Surgical and Gynecologic Complications of Pregnancy. Edited by Cherry SH, Berkowitz RL, Kase NG. Baltimore, MD, Williams & Wilkins, 1985, pp 110–123

Merkatz RB: Behavior of hospitalized high-risk maternity patients. Unpublished Master's thesis. Cleveland, OH, Case Western Reserve University, 1976

Nadelson CC: "Normal" and "special" aspects of pregnancy: a psychological approach, in The Woman Patient, Vol 1. Edited by Notman M, Nadelson C. New York, Plenum, 1978, pp 73–86

Notman MT: Reproduction and pregnancy: a psychodynamic developmental perspective, in Psychiatric Aspects of Reproductive Technology. Edited by Stotland NL. Washington, DC, American Psychiatric Press, 1990, pp 13–24

Penticuff J: Psychological implications in high-risk pregnancy. Nurs Clin North Am 17:69–78, 1982

Petrie RH: Intrapartum fetal evaluation, in Obstetrics: Normal and Problem Pregnancies. Edited by Gabbe SG, Niebyl JR, Simpson JL. New York, Churchill Livingstone, 1986, pp 379–412

Powers PS, Johnson T, Knuppel R, et al: Psychiatric disorders in high-risk pregnancy. Compr Psychiatry 27:159–164, 1986

Queenan J: Management of High Risk Pregnancy, 2nd Edition. Oradell, NJ, Medical Economics, 1985

Reading A, Cox D, Sledmere C, et al: Psychological changes over the course of pregnancy: a study of attitudes toward the fetus/neonate. Health Psychol 3:211–221, 1984

Robinson GE, Stewart DE: Motivation for motherhood and the experience of pregnancy. Can J Psychiatry 34:861–865, 1989

Rogers MP: Psychological aspects of pregnancy in patients with rheumatic disease, in Rheumatic Disease Clinics of North America, Vol 15 (2). Philadelphia, PA, WB Saunders, 1989, pp 361–374

Rubin R: Maternal tasks in pregnancy. Matern Child Nurs J 4:143–153, 1975

Samuels P, Landon MB: Medical complications, in Obstetrics: Normal and Problem Pregnancies. Edited by Gabbe SG, Niebyl JR, Simpson JL. New York, Churchill Livingstone, 1986, pp 865–977

Simpson JL: Fetal wastage, in Obstetrics: Normal and Problem Pregnancies. Edited by Gabbe SG, Niebyl JR, Simpson JL. New York, Churchill Livingstone, 1986, pp 651–673

Spirito A, Williams C, Ruggiero L, et al: Psychological impact of the diagnosis of gestational diabetes. Obstet Gynecol 73:562–566, 1989

Stern D: Mother and infant at play: the dynamic interaction involving facial, vocal and gaze behavior, in The Effect of the Infant on Its Caregiver. Edited by Lewis M, Rosenblum L. New York, Wiley, 1974, pp 187–215

Thomas A, Chess S, Birch H, et al: Behavioral Individuality in Early Childhood. New York, University Press, 1963

Thomason JL, Sampson MB, Beckmann CR, et al: The incompetent cervix: a 1982 update. J Reprod Med 27:187–192, 1982

Thompson C: Cultural pressures in the psychology of women, in Psychoanalysis and Women. Edited by Miller JB. New York, Brunner/Mazel, 1973, pp 49–64

Velvovsky I, Platonov K, Ploticher V, et al: Painless Childbirth Through Psychoprophylaxis. Translated by Myshne DA. Moscow, USSR, Foreign Languages Publishing House, 1960

White M, Ritchie J: Psychological stressors in antepartum hospitalization: reports from pregnant women. Matern Child Nurs J 13:47–56, 1984

Wolkind S: Psychological intervention in pregnancy, in Pregnancy: A Psychological and Social Study. Edited by Wolkind S, Eajicek E. New York, Grune & Stratton, 1981, pp 195–218

Wolreich MM: Psychiatric aspects of high-risk pregnancy. Psychiatr Clin North Am 10:53–68, 1986

Wynn RM: Obstetrics and Gynecology: The Clinical Core. Philadelphia, PA, Lea & Febiger, 1983

Chapter 3

FETAL ANOMALIES

Gail Erlick Robinson, M.D., F.R.C.P.C.
Katherine L. Wisner, M.D., M.S.

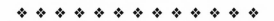

Fetal anomalies may be genetic-ally programmed at conception by the transmission of defective genes or chromosomes, or they may arise during pregnancy as a result of maternal illness or exposure to harmful substances. Prenatal genetic counseling and diagnostic techniques have made possible the in utero detection of a large number of these fetal defects. These technological advances also bring psychological stresses in the form of decisions about whether to have testing, anxiety related to the tests and the wait for results, and the possibility of having to choose whether to terminate a pregnancy.

This chapter discusses these reactions, as well as the emotional consequences and management of elective genetic terminations or of giving birth to a child with a defect. The psychiatrist may have a role in direct counseling of patients who are in the process of adjusting to the emotional trauma of losing a wanted pregnancy or who are adapting to having a child with abnormalities. The psychiatrist may also be involved in supervising or assisting other members of the treatment team.

We acknowledge the valuable assistance of Dr. Elaine Hutton in reviewing the information on genetics.

PREPREGNANCY

Risk of Hereditary Disorders

Geneticists and genetic counselors advise patients who are at risk for a hereditary disorder about the consequences of the disorder, the probability of developing the disease or transmitting the gene, and the ways in which this may be prevented. Ideally, this information is given before pregnancy so that the couple can make informed decisions about childbearing.

Counselors also provide general information on the risk of chromosome abnormalities for women of late maternal age. The risk of chromosomal abnormalities being detected at 16 weeks of gestation in a woman who is age 35 years is 1/250 for Down's syndrome and 1/130 for all chromosome abnormalities. These risks increase until, at age 46 years, they are 1/15 and 1/10, respectively (Hook et al. 1983). If a woman has previously given birth to an abnormal child, the geneticist uses clinical assessment of the affected infant, confirmation from medical records, and the construction of a family genetic tree in order to make an accurate diagnosis and estimate the risk for future pregnancies.

Single-gene, or Mendelian, disorders have three inheritance patterns: autosomal dominant, autosomal recessive, and X-linked recessive or dominant genes. When one parent has an autosomal dominant disorder (such as tuberous sclerosis or Huntington's disease), there is a 50% probability that the offspring will be affected. Autosomal recessive disorders include the hemoglobinopathies and a number of progressive metabolic disorders, such as Tay-Sachs disease. When both parents are carriers of an autosomal recessive condition, there is a 25% risk of transmission to their children, and each child has a 50% risk of being a carrier. When the mother carries an X-linked recessive disorder (such as hemophilia or Duchenne's dystrophy), there is a 50% risk that each son will be affected, as well as a 50% probability that each daughter will be a carrier.

Most common birth defects, such as cleft lip and palate and neural tube defects, involve multifactorial inheritance. The recurrence risk of these disorders is rarely over 5% when only one parent is affected

(Harper 1983). Chromosome disorders may involve numerical abnormalities caused by nondisjunction (e.g., Down's syndrome due to trisomy 21) or structural abnormalities such as chromosome translocations (e.g., Down's syndrome due to a translocation between chromosomes 14 and 21). The risk of nondisjunction after one occurrence is approximately 1%. With translocations, chromosomal material may be neither lost nor gained, but merely out of place; in these cases, the translocation is said to be "balanced," and the individual will be a carrier (i.e., not symptomatic). Asymptomatic carriers of balanced translocations, however, have a 5%–20% risk of transmitting the unbalanced chromosome complement (i.e., too little or too much genetic material) to the child, who will therefore exhibit symptoms (Jackson 1980).

Psychological Reactions to Discovery of Risk Factors

The parents' perceived risk for any genetic disorder differs from the statistical risk (Swerts 1987). Five major factors influence this perceived risk: 1) the potential degree of harm or lethality, 2) the degree to which the risk can be controlled through safety or rescue measures, 3) the number of people affected, 4) the degree of familiarity with the consequences and effects of the disorder, and 5) the degree to which the parents' exposure to the risk is voluntary.

Couples who have an increased risk for giving birth to a child with a genetic disorder are faced with the complications of a "natural" biologic process that is usually taken for granted. They may suffer from a strong sense of being defective. This presents a narcissistic threat to their self-esteem, to the extent that self-esteem is based on the expectation of creating a normal, healthy child (Blumberg 1975). There may also be a sense of guilt associated with being a carrier of a genetic disease. It is common for these couples to feel anger toward women who are enjoying normal pregnancies and to feel guilt because of difficulties with reproduction (G. E. Robinson and Stewart 1989). They may undergo a grieving process for the loss of their idealized family. Their sexual enjoyment may be affected by both the couple's distress and the realization that the procreative act can result in tragedy. Marital distress caused by this crisis complicates decisions regarding future pregnancies.

Genetic counseling and the possibility of detecting fetal defects prenatally play an important role in making decisions about further pregnancies (Bouie et al. 1991). Over half of counseled families with infants with Down's syndrome and up to 80% of those with a child with neural tube defects reported that they were positively influenced in their decision to have more children by the information received during counseling sessions. Preconception counseling may reduce the couple's guilt, their sense of defectiveness, and their grief.

PREGNANCY

Indications for Prenatal Genetic Testing

The goals of prenatal diagnosis are detection of fetal genetic disorders and improvement of outcome, provision of information to prepare parents, and identification of severely affected pregnancies that parents can elect to terminate. Indications for prenatal testing include advanced maternal age (women over age 35), a known balanced translocation in one of the parents, a previous child with a chromosome disorder or with a neural tube defect, a mother who is a carrier for an X-linked disease (to determine fetal sex and to provide molecular diagnosis, where applicable), and parents who are both carriers of recessively inherited metabolic disorders (Golbus et al. 1974). Some examples of the types of disorders that are common indications for prenatal diagnostic testing are shown in Table 3–1. This list is not exhaustive, as hundreds of conditions can now be diagnosed through prenatal testing.

The type of prenatal diagnostic test, the timing of testing, and the approximate waiting time for results are depicted in Table 3–2. Couples may not be willing to undergo prenatal diagnostic testing because of lack of information about the test, a perception of being at low risk for a fetal abnormality, concern about fetal injury or loss following the test, religious beliefs, or an unwillingness to consider elective termination as an option (Davies and Doran 1982; Dixson et al. 1981).

Table 3–1. Indications for prenatal diagnostic testing

Type of disorder	Example	Diagnostic ultrasound	MSAFP	CVS/Amniocentesis		
				DNA analysis	Chromosome analysis	Enzyme analysis
Single-gene disorders, known or suspected	Cystic fibrosis			X		
Multifactorial disorders, known or suspected	Neural tube disorders	X	X			
Chromosomal disorders in the consultand or a family member	Fragile X syndrome			X	X	
Abnormal trait or carrier state	Tay-Sachs disease			X		X
Prenatal diagnosis for late maternal age or other causes	Down's syndrome	X	X		X	
Teratogen exposure	Fetal alcohol syndrome	X				

Note. CVS = chorionic villus sampling; MSAFP = maternal serum alpha-fetoprotein.

Table 3–2.   Prenatal diagnostic testing

Type of test	Time of testing (weeks of gestation)	Waiting time for results (weeks)
Early amniocentesis	10–14	2–3
CVS	9–12	1–2
Diagnostic ultrasound (routine screening)	18–19	Immediate
Midtrimester amniocentesis	16–18	2–4
MSAFP	15–21	1

Note.   CVS = chorionic villus sampling. MSAFP = maternal serum alpha-fetoprotein.

Prenatal Diagnostic Tests

Maternal serum alpha-fetoprotein.   Alpha-fetoprotein (AFP) is normal human fetal protein that is found in high concentrations in the fetal serum throughout gestation. Rising levels of AFP can be detected in the sera of pregnant women as early as 7 weeks of gestation, and levels increase steadily until at least 30 weeks of gestation (Burton 1988). Elevated levels of maternal serum AFP (MSAFP) can be used to detect 80%–85% of open neural tube defects and other malformations, including omphalocele or gastroschisis, intestinal atresias, congenital nephrosis, and Turner's syndrome. MSAFP levels are approximately 25% lower when the fetus has Down's syndrome (Knight et al. 1988).

MSAFP screening can be done with reasonable reliability between 15 and 21 weeks of gestation. About 4.0% of women will have an elevated MSAFP level on initial testing, and 30% of these women will have a normal result on repeat testing. Patients who have an elevated MSAFP level and are found, through an ultrasound examination, to have a single, viable fetus at the anticipated gestational age may be advised to undergo amniocentesis. Using a combination of low MSAFP levels and maternal age to devise a Down's syndrome screening protocol, Palomaki (1986) found that 3.6% of women were classified as being at high risk for Down's syndrome. After ultrasound, this risk dropped to 2.1%, primarily due to a correction of gestational age. Women still considered at risk after ultrasound should undergo amniocentesis.

MSAFP testing may create unnecessary maternal anxiety, since some women will be falsely identified as having high-risk pregnancies (Evans et al. 1988). Patients undergoing genetic testing due to MSAFP levels have been found to have higher state anxiety than women undergoing testing because of advanced maternal age. This anxiety returns to normal levels only after assurance of a definitively negative amniocentesis result (J. O. Robinson et al. 1984). Women who undergo screening have significantly lower anxiety levels in the third trimester of pregnancy than women who have not been screened (Marteau et al. 1988).

Ultrasound. Two main types of ultrasound are in common use: *continuous ultrasound* is used to detect moving structures such as the fetal heart, whereas *pulse ultrasound* is used to outline structures within the uterus. In obstetrics, ultrasound is used for the screening and diagnosis of fetal age, multiple pregnancy, intrauterine growth retardation, and fetal malformations, including craniospinal defects such as anencephaly, cardiac defects, and musculoskeletal, gastrointestinal, and renal abnormalities. Diagnostic ultrasound has no known risks to the fetus or mother and produces little anxiety in low-risk women (Campbell et al. 1982). It may promote maternal-fetal bonding (Campbell et al. 1982) and may lead to a decrease in behaviors such as smoking and drinking (Reading et al. 1982), especially in women who receive a high level of feedback during the ultrasound examination (Reading et al. 1988).

Midtrimester genetic amniocentesis. Midtrimester genetic amniocentesis is carried out at approximately 16 weeks of gestation. After the exact positions of the placenta, fetus, and umbilical cord are determined by ultrasound, a needle is inserted through the abdomen into the amniotic sac. Amniotic fluid is withdrawn for AFP and karyotype testing.

In several studies, the rates of total fetal loss in the group receiving midtrimester amniocentesis (3.5%) and in nonrandomized control subjects (3.2%) were not significantly different. It is estimated that the risk of fetal loss due to midtrimester amniocentesis does not exceed 0.5% in experienced hands (Lowe et al. 1978). Serious fetal injury and bacterial infection within the uterus are extremely infrequent. The results are usually available 2–4 weeks later, at approximately 20 weeks of gestation.

Early genetic amniocentesis.   Early genetic amniocentesis can be performed between 10 and 14 weeks of gestation, although accuracy is greater at 12–14 weeks (Rooney et al. 1989). Preliminary reports suggest that early genetic amniocentesis is safer than chorionic villus sampling (Godmilow et al. 1988). Rates of spontaneous abortion have been reported to be 0.7% (Lui et al. 1991) to 4.7% (Shulman et al. 1991), with an average rate of 2.7%.

Chorionic villus sampling.   Chorionic villus sampling (CVS) is another method of obtaining fetal cells for genetic analysis. By using ultrasound as a guide, a catheter inserted through the cervix or a needle passed through the abdominal wall is used to aspirate chorionic tissue from the developing placenta. The material obtained is then sent for karyotype determination and other studies, where indicated. In a multicenter, randomized, clinical trial of CVS and midtrimester genetic amniocentesis, the difference between the rates of pregnancy loss with the two procedures was determined to be no greater than 2.8% for women ages 35 years and older (Canadian Collaborative CVS-Amniocentesis Clinical Trial Group 1989). The most likely risk is probably 1%–1.5%. There is also a possible association with fetal limb defects when CVS is performed at less than 10 weeks of gestation (Firth et al. 1991).

Psychological Consequences of CVS and Midtrimester Genetic Amniocentesis

Couples who undergo prenatal diagnostic testing may experience significant psychological stress. Prior to testing, women often worry that the procedure will be painful, cause injury to the fetus, or result in miscarriage. They may also be concerned about the results of the test

(Evers-Kiebooms et al. 1988; Finley et al. 1977). Women with decreased social support have increased anxiety (J. Robinson et al. 1975). Beeson and Golbus (1979) found increased anxiety in women who already had children with chromosomal disorders, but other investigators have not (Evers-Kiebooms et al. 1988; Tabor and Jonsson 1987). Fava et al. (1983) noted that women undergoing prenatal testing were more hostile than were control subjects. There was no increase in anxiety in women who had been adequately counseled, although counseling done immediately prior to the test was not beneficial (Nielson 1981).

Anxiety levels are also elevated in women prior to undergoing CVS (G. E. Robinson et al. 1988; Spencer and Cox 1987). A drop in anxiety immediately after testing has been noted for patients who underwent either midtrimester amniocentesis (Tabor and Jonsson 1987) or CVS (G. E. Robinson et al. 1988). Tabor and Jonsson (1987) found this to be especially true for younger women and women who perceive themselves to be at low risk for an abnormality. Older women remained anxious until the results were obtained. Beeson and Golbus (1979) found an immediate drop in anxiety with a subsequent rise during the wait for a possible miscarriage and test results. Women undergoing CVS experienced anxiety reduction much earlier than the group receiving midtrimester genetic amniocentesis (G. E. Robinson et al. 1988). Even after obtaining the results, about 25% of women receiving midtrimester genetic amniocentesis remained concerned about the outcome of the pregnancy (Dixson et al. 1981). McCormack et al. (1990) found that most patients had a better experience with CVS than with previous midtrimester genetic amniocentesis. Women who undergo CVS develop an increase in maternal-fetal bonding earlier than those having midtrimester genetic amniocentesis (Caccia et al. 1991).

Pregnancy Loss After Testing

Women who have a miscarriage after a genetic procedure experience grief, guilt, and anger. Women who have CVS may perceive the procedure to be more risky and may feel additional guilt over having chosen it (G. E. Robinson et al. 1991). Also, because of the early timing of

CVS, a miscarriage that would have occurred spontaneously may be falsely attributed to the procedure and create needless guilt.

Reactions to Detection of Fetal Anomaly

The detection of a fetal anomaly is a disturbing event. A pregnancy that has been desired and perhaps long sought may suddenly lose its value. The first reaction is one of shock and denial, either expressed openly or masked by an apparent calm acceptance of the diagnosis (Jackson 1980). It is often difficult for the couple to absorb information during this period of shock. The second stage is characterized by anxiety as they try to come to terms with future plans and alternatives for care. Many individuals have problems grasping the meaning of probability figures and using them for decision making (d'Ydewalle and Evers-Kiebooms 1987). Either parent may exhibit hostile and angry behavior that may be directed at the other partner, the physician, or the counselor. The parents may then enter a phase of depression as they deal with this difficult problem. The stages vary in length and severity and may fluctuate before the parents reach a stage of acceptance and equilibrium.

Reactions to Genetic Termination

Reproductive loss for any reason is always a distressing event. In an elective termination due to genetic disorders (i.e., genetic termination), the couple has to face not only the loss of a wanted pregnancy but the fact of making a conscious decision to end it. Ideally, discussion about the actions to be taken if an abnormal result is discovered occurs during pretest counseling. If the disorder is incompatible with life, the decision may be reasonably straightforward. For many others, a clear identification of a problem with known consequences such as Down's syndrome will allow them to make the choice despite ambivalence and pain. Problems in decision making increase with the identification of mosaicism or sex chromosomal disorders, in which the outcome is not clearly a severe abnormality. Acute grief reactions are experienced by 77%–92% of women and 82% of men following a genetic termination (Blumberg et al. 1975; Lloyd and Lawrence 1985).

Couples often feel guilty about their decision to terminate a pregnancy. Couples who are at risk of having a child with an X-linked disorder and who terminate a pregnancy based on knowledge of male sex only must deal with the added guilt of knowing that there is a 50% probability that the fetus would not have had the disorder (Blumberg et al. 1975). Couples may experience marital problems caused by projection of their anger onto each other or by isolation due to depression. The woman may have stronger feelings about the loss or may be more open about expressing her feelings. In an attempt to handle his own sadness as well as deal with his partner's grief, the man may suppress his own feelings.

The woman who has an induced abortion following genetic amniocentesis has probably experienced fetal movement, has usually been visibly pregnant, and has to undergo delivery in order to terminate the pregnancy. It has been hypothesized that elective terminations following CVS may be less traumatic, but G. E. Robinson et al. (1991) found that women who had an elective termination following either method had equally elevated levels of depression.

Couples who terminate a pregnancy for genetic reasons experience a grief reaction and mourn for their unborn child (Magyari et al. 1987). Protocols for the management of neonatal death have been proposed (Langer and Ringler 1989; Magyari et al. 1987; Phipps 1981). According to the protocol of Magyari et al. (1987), the finding of an abnormality is discussed immediately with the parents in the context of a nondirective planning meeting. The couple is given a factual description of the termination procedure. Mothers who choose termination are admitted to a private room on a nonmaternity ward where the spouses can remain during the procedure. The psychological management of pregnancy loss is discussed in more detail in Chapter 8 of this volume.

Selective Termination

Selective termination may be considered in multiple gestations in which one or more fetuses are severely abnormal or when continuation of the multiple pregnancy presents a risk to the mother or the pregnancy (Zaner et al. 1990). This problem is more common in infertility patients who achieve pregnancy after ovulation induction. Zaner et al. (1990) have argued that restricting selective termination to pregnancies of three or more fetuses provides the greatest chance of causing the least harm. They also advise early counseling for couples involved in ovulation induction to prepare them for the possibility of selective termination.

Fetal Sex Determination

Fetal sex determination can be done via ultrasound or chromosomal examination. In cases of X-linked recessive disorders, if the fetus is male and molecular analysis cannot detect whether it is affected, the couple may elect to terminate the pregnancy, knowing that there is only a 50% chance that it would be affected. Termination of fetuses of a particular sex merely for sociocultural reasons presents an ethical problem. Some physicians suggest that the sex of the fetus should be kept from the parents unless it is related to a genetic disorder. Others believe that caregivers do not have the right to withhold this information. Termination for the purpose of sex selection rarely occurs after midtrimester genetic amniocentesis (Johnson and Elkins 1988).

Psychological Reactions to Perinatal Death

Genetically caused stillbirth or neonatal death elicits not only grief reactions but guilty feelings on the part of the parents for having produced a defective child. Waiting for the autopsy results to confirm or allay their fears of having passed on a chromosomal defect to their baby is painful. Carrying a chromosomal defect that may harm future children is emotionally distressing.

Children also react to the death of a sibling. The parents can assist by providing accurate information about the death, explaining that it was not the surviving child's fault, including the child in mourning ceremonies, and sharing parental grief (Leon 1990). Children's repetition of questions parallels the same phenomenon seen in parents' questioning of doctors. For a sibling who is free of a genetic illness, the child can be reassured that the fatality is not contagious and cannot happen to him or her.

POSTPARTUM

Psychological Reactions to the Malformed Baby

The birth of a malformed baby constitutes an intense narcissistic injury for parents. Already coping with the psychophysiological depletion that follows labor and delivery, the couple must also grieve over the loss of the expected infant and accept the malformed child (Solnit and Stark 1961). They must attempt self-regulation in the face of chronic depression and rage when confronted with the disappointment inherent in producing a damaged child (Fajardo 1987). The couple may feel unable to accept the child because the narcissistic injury is intolerable, or alternatively, they may experience severe guilt leading to overinvolved parental dedication (Solnit and Stark 1961). This stress intensifies any preexisting difficulties in the relationship.

Mourning over a malformed infant does not take place in the usual manner because of continuation of the child's life and the increased demands for physical care that preoccupy most parents. Drotar et al. (1975) found that, despite reassurances, concern that the baby would die interfered with parental attachment to the child. This premature mourning for a child who subsequently recovers requires the parent to reverse psychological energy and reintegrate the child into the family. Difficulty accomplishing this task can result in disturbed parent-child relationships and behavioral dysfunction in children (Green and Solnit 1964; Naylor 1982). The continuation of mourning into a persistent, depressed, self-reproachful state is more likely if the mother's mourning reaction is not understood and if the care and planning for the child are carried out without her active participation.

Parents of a malformed infant experience guilt and shame and frequently seek causal connections between the defect and their prior thoughts, fantasies, wishes, or actions (Kessler et al. 1984). This guilt may or may not be realistic. Defenses against guilt include repression (behaviors such as substance abuse), intellectualization and rationalization, and isolation of affect. A common way for couples to handle the guilt is to decide against further reproduction.

Shame is frequently associated with responses to the anticipated or actual disapproval of others. Common defenses against shame include denial, reaction formation, compensation, or displacement, such as focusing on the deficiencies of the medical caregivers.

The parents must begin a lifelong reconciliation to the ongoing disappointments and special care required by the limitations of a child with a genetic defect. The child may be at risk of abuse, particularly if there is a history of child abuse in either parent or extreme social isolation from family and friends (Fost 1981).

Parents of children born with malformations may not remember the rational content of the first conversation with their doctor (Solnit and Stark 1961). They need repeated contact with their physician in order to accomplish the task of mourning. Parents also need assistance with decision structuring as they take responsibility for evaluative judgments and accept-reject decisions (Vlek 1987).

Psychotherapy

In the initial stages of work with families in which a child is malformed, Solnit and Stark (1961) recommended support and clarification of the reality of the child's condition as the parents are able to discuss their questions and fears. Avoidance of interpretation of unconscious conflicts during mourning was recommended. Group support for parents of children with fatal genetic illnesses can decrease parental isolation, allow discussion of the parents' need for both closeness and distance from the infant, and calm their fears about events immediately preceding their child's death (Mack and Berman 1988). In such a group, the parents may be able to admire the lovable qualities about each other's children and to share in each other's grief when the children die.

Zuskar (1987) advocated a short-term family crisis intervention model for the management of the psychological reactions to a baby born with genetic defects. This model includes multiple short meetings; initial work with the couple alone, followed by placement into couples groups; an empathic and accepting therapeutic style to facilitate adaptation; provision of a supportive environment for emotional work; direct confrontation of beliefs about the fetus's impairment as causality; and attention to the marital relationship.

Attention to biological information and reproductive technology, the parents' psychological capacities to receive information and use coping skills, and the parents' social milieu will allow the therapeutic team to develop a comprehensive treatment plan and achieve the most successful outcome.

REFERENCES

Beeson D, Golbus MS: Anxiety engendered by amniocentesis, in Risk, Communication and Decision Making in Genetic Counselling (March of Dimes Birth Defects: Original Articles Series, Vol 15[SC]). Edited by Epstein CJ, Curry CJ, Packman S, et al. New York, Alan R Liss, 1979, pp 191–197

Blumberg BD, Golbus MS, Hanson KH: The psychological sequelae of abortion performed for a genetic indication. Am J Obstet Gynecol 12:799–808, 1975

Bouie J, Muller F, Simon-Bouy B, et al: Consequences of prenatal diagnosis of cystic fibrosis on the reproductive attitudes of parents of affected children. Prenat Diagn 11:209–214, 1991

Burton BK: Elevated maternal serum alpha-fetoprotein (MSAFP): interpretation and follow up. Clin Obstet Gynecol 31:293–305, 1988

Caccia N, Johnson JM, Robinson GE, et al: Impact of prenatal testing on maternal-fetal bonding: chorionic villus sampling versus amniocentesis. Am J Obstet Gynecol 165(4 part 1):1122–1125, 1991

Campbell S, Reading AE, Cox DN, et al: Ultrasound scanning in pregnancy: the short-term psychological effects of early real-time scans. Journal of Psychosomatic Obstetrics and Gynaecology 1:57–61, 1982

Canadian Collaborative CVS-Amniocentesis Clinical Trial Group: Multicentre randomized clinical trial of chorion villus sampling and amniocentesis. Lancet 1:1–6, 1989

Davies BL, Doran TA: Factors in a woman's decision to undergo genetic amniocentesis for advanced maternal age. Nurs Res 31:56–59, 1982

Dixson B, Richards T, Reinsch S, et al: Midtrimester amniocentesis: subjective maternal responses. J Reprod Med 26:10–16, 1981

Drotar D, Baskiewicz A, Irvin N, et al: The adaptation of parents to the birth of an infant with a congenital malformation: a hypothetical model. Pediatrics 56:710–717, 1975

d'Ydewalle G, Evers-Kiebooms G: Experiments on genetic risk perception and decision making: explorative studies. Birth Defects 23:209–225, 1987

Evans MI, Bottoms SF, Carlucci T, et al: Determinants of altered anxiety after abnormal maternal serum alpha-fetoprotein screening. Am J Obstet Gynecol 156:1501–1504, 1988

Evers-Kiebooms G, Swerts A, Van Den Berghe H: Psychological aspects of amniocentesis: anxiety feelings in three different risk groups. Clin Genet 33:196–206, 1988

Fajardo B: Parenting a damaged child: mourning, regression, and disappointment. Psychoanal Rev 74:19–43, 1987

Fava GA, Trombini G, Michelacci L, et al: Hostility in women before and after amniocentesis. J Reprod Med 28(1):29–34, 1983

Finley SC, Varner PD, Vinson PC, et al: Participants' reactions to amniocentesis and prenatal genetic studies. JAMA 238:2377–2379, 1977

Firth HV, Boyd PA, Chamberlain P, et al: Severe limb abnormalities after chorion villus sampling at 56–66 days gestation. Lancet 1:762–763, 1991

Fost N: Counselling families who have a child with a severe congenital anomaly. Pediatrics 67:321–324, 1981

Godmilow L, Weiner S, Dunn LK: Early genetic amniocentesis: experience with 600 consecutive procedures and comparison with chorionic villus sampling (abstract). Am J Hum Genet 43 (suppl 3):A234, 1988

Golbus MS, Conte FA, Schneider EL, et al: Intrauterine diagnosis of genetic defects: results, problems and follow up of one hundred cases in a prenatal genetic detection centre. Am J Obstet Gynecol 118:897–905, 1974

Green M, Solnit A: Reactions to the threatened loss of a child: a vulnerable child syndrome. Pediatrics 34:58–66, 1964

Harper PS: Genetic counselling and prenatal diagnosis. Br Med Bull 39(4):302–309, 1983

Hook EB, Cross PK, Schreinmachers DM: Chromosomal abnormality rates at amniocentesis and in live-born infants. JAMA 249:2034–2038, 1983

Jackson LG: Prenatal genetic counselling, in Psychosomatic Obstetrics and Gynecology. Edited by Youngs DD, Ehrhardt AA. New York, Appleton-Century-Crofts, 1980, pp 129–144

Johnson SR, Elkins TE: Ethical issues in prenatal diagnosis. Clin Obstet Gynecol 31(2):408–420, 1988

Kessler S, Kessler H, Ward P: Psychological aspects of genetic counselling, III: management of guilt and shame. Am J Med Genet 17:673–697, 1984

Knight GJ, Palomaki GE, Haddow JE: Use of maternal serum alpha-fetoprotein measurements to screen for Down's syndrome. Clin Obstet Gynecol 31:306–327, 1988

Langer M, Ringler M: Prospective counselling after prenatal diagnosis of fetal malformations and parental reactions. Acta Obstet Gynecol Scand 68:323–329, 1989

Leon IG: When a Baby Dies: Psychotherapy for Pregnancy and Newborn Loss. New Haven, CT, Yale University Press, 1990, pp 131–187

Lloyd J, Lawrence KM: Sequelae and support after termination of pregnancy for fetal malformation. BMJ 290:907–909, 1985

Lowe CU, Alexander D, Bryla D, et al (eds): The NICHD Amniocentesis Registry: the safety and accuracy of mid-trimester amniocentesis (DHEW Publ No NIH-78-190). Bethesda, MD, Department of Health, Education and Welfare, 1978

Lui LC, Lo FJ, Ho SC, et al: Early amniocentesis: complemented with in-situ amniocyte culture method. Am J Hum Genet 49(4) (suppl):223, 1991

Mack SA, Berman LC: A group for parents of children with fatal genetic illnesses. Am J Orthopsychiatry 58:397–404, 1988

Magyari PA, Wedehase BA, Ifft RD, et al: A supportive intervention protocol for couples terminating a pregnancy for genetic reasons, in Strategies in Genetic Counselling (March of Dimes Birth Defects: Original Articles Series, Vol 23.) Edited by Paul NW, Travers H. White Plains, NY, Alan R Liss, 1987, pp 75–83

Marteau TM, Johnston M, Plenicar M, et al: Development of a self-administered questionnaire to measure women's knowledge of prenatal screening and diagnostic tests. J Psychosom Res 32:403–408, 1988

McCormack MJ, Rylance ME, MacKenzie WE, et al: Patients' attitudes following chorionic villus sampling. Prenat Diagn 10:253–255, 1990

Naylor A: Premature mourning and failure to mourn: their relationship to conflict between mothers and intellectually normal children. Am J Orthopsychiatry 52:679–687, 1982

Nielson CC: An encounter with modern medical technology: women's experiences with amniocentesis. Women Health 6:109–124, 1981

Palomaki GE: Collaborative study of Down's syndrome screening using maternal serum alpha-fetoprotein and maternal age. Lancet 2:1460, 1986

Phipps S: Mourning response and intervention in stillbirth: an alternative genetic counselling approach. Soc Biol 28:1–13, 1981

Reading AE, Campbell S, Cox DN, et al: Health beliefs and health care behaviour in pregnancy. Psychol Med 12:1–5, 1982

Reading AE, Cox DN, Campbell S: A controlled prospective evaluation of the acceptability of ultrasound in prenatal care. Journal of Psychosomatic Obstetrics and Gynaecology 8:191–198, 1988

Robinson GE, Stewart DE: Motivation for motherhood and the experience of pregnancy. Can J Psychiatry 34:861–865, 1989

Robinson GE, Garner DM, Olmsted M, et al: Anxiety reduction following chorionic villus sampling and genetic amniocentesis. Am J Obstet Gynecol 159:953–956, 1988

Robinson GE, Carr M, Olmsted MP, et al: Psychological reactions to pregnancy loss after prenatal diagnostic testing: preliminary results. Journal of Psychosomatic Obstetrics and Gynaecology 12:181–192, 1991

Robinson J, Tennes K, Robinson A: Amniocentesis: its impact on mothers and infants: a one year follow-up study. Clin Genet 8:97–106, 1975

Robinson JO, Hibbard BM, Lawrence KM: Anxiety during a crisis: emotional effects of screening for neural tube defects. J Psychosom Res 28:163–169, 1984

Rooney DE, MacLachlan N, Smith J, et al: Early amniocentesis: a cytogenetic evaluation. BMJ 299:25, 1989

Shulman LP, Elias S, Simpson JL: Early amniocentesis: complications in initial 150 cases compared to complications in initial 150 cases of transabdominal chorionic villus sampling. Am J Hum Genet 49(4) (suppl):231, 1991

Solnit AJ, Stark MH: Mourning and the birth of a defective child. Psychoanal Study Child 16:523–537, 1961

Spencer JW, Cox DN: Emotional responses of pregnant women to chorionic villi sampling or amniocentesis. Am J Obstet Gynecol 157:1155–1160, 1987

Swerts A: Impact of genetic counselling and prenatal diagnosis for Down syndrome and neural tube defects. Birth Defects 23:61–83, 1987

Tabor A, Jonsson MH: Psychological impact of amniocentesis on low risk women. Prenat Diagn 7:443–449, 1987

Vlek C: Risk assessment, risk perception and decision making about courses of action involving genetic risk: an overview of concepts and methods, in Strategies in Genetic Counselling (March of Dimes Birth Defects: Original Articles Series, Vol 23). White Plains, NY, Alan R Liss, 1987, pp 171–207

Zaner RM, Boehm FH, Hill GA: Selective termination in multiple pregnancies: ethical considerations. Fertil Steril 54:203–205, 1990

Zuskar DM: The psychological impact of prenatal diagnosis of fetal abnormality: strategies for investigation and intervention. Women Health 12:91–103, 1987

Chapter 4

PSYCHIATRIC DISORDERS DURING PREGNANCY

Laura J. Miller, M.D.

❖ ❖ ❖ ❖ ❖ ❖ ❖ ❖ ❖ ❖ ❖ ❖ ❖ ❖

Since the time of Hippocrates, it has been a matter of controversy whether pregnancy is a time of increased or decreased vulnerability to psychiatric disturbance. Some theorists have conceptualized pregnancy as a period of maturational crisis, with concomitant emotional upheaval that may lead either to pathology or to a more mature developmental stage (Leifer 1977). The earliest major empirical study of the issue (Pugh et al. 1963), however, revealed that the incidence of first psychiatric admissions decreased during pregnancy, seeming to support the notion that pregnancy is a time of relative calm during which there is some protection against mental illness. Those data, in turn, have been questioned because they are confounded by the refusal of many psychiatric facilities to admit women who are pregnant.

More recent studies, taken as a whole, suggest that psychological correlates of pregnancy are highly individualized and are related to factors such as emotional stability, attitudes toward femininity, relationships with the husband and mother, cultural attitudes, preparation for parenthood (Leifer 1977), prior mental illness (Paffenbarger 1982), presence or absence of prior children and instrumental support (O'Hara 1986), prior induced abortion (Kumar and Robson 1978), marital status (Cox et al. 1982), life circumstances (Watson et al. 1984), and whether the pregnancy is medically high risk (Wohlreich 1986). Studies of severe psychiatric disorders, such as major depression and psychosis, have found either a decreased or an unchanged incidence during pregnancy, whereas others focusing on more minor distur-bances have reported a high incidence of symptoms such as depres-sion, anxiety, lability of mood, and suggestibility.

To the extent that generalizations can be made about normal psy-chological changes during pregnancy, the following observations have the most empirical support from the studies cited above and from oth-ers (extended references are available on request from the author). Increased anxiety seems typical, particularly if its content is focused more on the fetus than on the woman herself. Increased introspection and preoccupation with the pregnancy, with or without a correspond-ing decline in emotional investment in the external world, is com-mon. Heightened dependency needs may occur. A shift toward primary process thinking and "primitive" defenses has been noted by some (Condon 1987) but has been difficult to verify empirically.

The hormonal shifts occurring during pregnancy have led to spec-ulation about the contribution of psychoneuroendocrine factors to emotional disturbance. Several hormones that are thought to influ-ence mood states undergo marked, rapid changes during pregnancy, most notably estrogens, progesterone, and cortisol. In the case of the latter, the diurnal rhythm changes as well (Challis and Patrick 1983). Reproductive hormones may help regulate the metabolism of cate-cholamines; for example, progesterone may increase monoamine ox-idase activity (Sandler 1978). In turn, the mechanisms of action of estrogen and progesterone may depend on some of the biogenic amines most often associated with psychiatric disturbance (Jarrahi-Zadeh et al. 1969). Thus, although simple, direct causal connections among hormonal, neurotransmitter, and psychological changes are unlikely, the three are intimately linked and may influence one an-other in conjunction with other factors.

Regardless of its incidence or etiology, psychiatric disturbance during pregnancy remains an important focus because of its potential consequences. It is unclear whether emotional stress during preg-nancy directly affects obstetric outcome, but it has been implicated as a contributor to prematurity, low birth weight, subsequent child mor-bidity, and other complications. Symptoms of mental disorder may in-terfere with the normal progression of emotional attachment to the fetus (Cohen 1979), leading to difficulties in the mother-infant relationship. In addition, the occurrence or exacerbation of major psychiatric disorders during pregnancy may pose serious risks to both mother and fetus, as described in this chapter. Increases in fertility rates for chronically mentally ill women since the onset of deinstitutionalization (Burr et al. 1979) and the high incidence of unwanted, unplanned pregnancies among that population (Abernethy 1974; Coverdale and Aruffo 1989) pose complex challenges for clinicians attempting to understand and manage associated complications.

PSYCHIATRIC ILLNESS TEMPORALLY ASSOCIATED WITH PREGNANCY

Schizophrenia and Related Psychotic Disorders

Like all women, those with schizophrenia have varied reactions to pregnancy, ranging from a marked exacerbation of psychosis to a marked increase in well-being. Most demographic, situational, interpersonal, and attitudinal variables do not predict which women will worsen, improve, or stay the same, although younger age and perception of worse physical health may correlate with declining mental condition during pregnancy among schizophrenic women (McNeil et al. 1984).

A number of psychosocial factors complicate the experience of pregnancy for schizophrenic women. In comparison with matched control subjects, women with psychotic disorders are more likely to be unemployed, be impoverished, and have poor social support and poor relations with the baby's father. The pregnancy is more likely to be unplanned, with accompanying negative attitudes (McNeil et al. 1983). There is a high incidence of associated substance abuse (Rudolph et al. 1990).

Associated with these problems are a number of risks to both mother and baby, including the following:

❖ *Refusal of prenatal care.* This may stem from delusional beliefs about recommended procedures or from discomfort with the intrusive or intimate nature of prenatal care. Sometimes refusal stems from the perception that caregivers are more concerned about the fetus than about the woman.

❖ *Poor nutrition.* This may be based on delusions about food or about the baby, even when food and nutrition instruction are readily available.

❖ *Attempts at premature self-delivery.* Some schizophrenic women may attempt to pull their babies out or to induce others to do so. This may be motivated by fear of delivering in a hospital or difficulty managing the stress of waiting.

❖ *Fetal abuse or neonaticide.* This sometimes occurs in response to command hallucinations. It is likely to be based on difficulty accepting the pregnancy, which in its extreme form results in psychotic denial of pregnancy (Miller 1990).

❖ *Precipitous delivery.* Some schizophrenic women, even when closely observed and educated about labor, experience no symptoms of labor and show no warning signs until the baby emerges from the birth canal (Forcier 1990; Spielvogel and Wile 1986). For example, a woman may deliver an infant into the toilet, mistakenly believing she is passing feces.

The data on pregnancy outcome is unclear, but schizophrenia appears to be associated with more obstetric complications, more abnormal babies, shorter gestation, lower birth weight, and more miscarriages and neonatal deaths (Chang and Renshaw 1986). Although the evidence is complicated by methodological difficulties, these findings seem to be independent of psychotropic drug use during pregnancy.

Delusional material related to the pregnancy is a common trigger for bizarre or dangerous behavior. These delusions may be fueled by wrenching dilemmas, such as the strong desire to be a mother and nurture a baby despite a lack of the internal and external resources that are needed to do so.

Mood Disorders

The incidence of major depression does not appear to increase during pregnancy, although minor depressive reactions are common.

The causes of minor depression are probably multifactorial. Biological influences have been suggested: for example, the effects of progesterone on monoamine oxidase activity (Sandler 1978) and of vitamin B$_6$ deficiency and estrogen on tryptophan metabolism (Kaplan 1983). Psychosocial aspects have also been investigated: O'Hara (1986) found that women who became depressed during pregnancy differed from nondepressed women in having more children and less instrumental support.

When major depression does occur during pregnancy, two central concerns are the risk of inadequate nutrition and of suicide. Comparisons of pregnant to nonpregnant women who attempted suicide (D. Lester and Beck 1988; Whitlock 1968) found the two groups to be similar in most respects, but the attempts were directly related to the pregnancy in a large number of cases. Typical causes include the loss of prior children, potential loss of a partner, desire for abortion, and economic crises (Czeizel and Lendvay 1989; D. Lester and Beck 1988).

The evidence for exacerbation of mania during pregnancy is contradictory. When it does occur, the risks to the mother and fetus from both the illness and the pharmacologic treatment (see Chapter 5) warrant a careful risk-benefit analysis to determine the safest course.

Anxiety Disorders and Obsessive-Compulsive Disorder

Although data have been collected about the incidence and impact of anxiety during pregnancy, little is known about how pregnancy affects the course of specific anxiety disorders. Whereas puberty often triggers the onset of panic disorder (Hayward et al. 1992), cases of marked amelioration of panic disorder during pregnancy have been reported (Cowley and Roy-Byrne 1989; George et al. 1987; Villeponteaux et al. 1992). In addition to possible psychological explanations for this finding, biological hypotheses were suggested, including a blunting of sympathetic response to stimuli during pregnancy and barbiturate-like activity of progesterone metabolites. On the other hand, there may be some tendency for obsessive-compulsive disorder to worsen during pregnancy, and for pregnancy to be a common trigger for the onset of this disorder (Brandt and Mackenzie 1987; Neziroglu et al. 1992).

Personality Disorders

The effects of pregnancy on women with personality disorders have not been systematically studied, although pregnancy has been noted as a stressor that triggers brief psychoses in vulnerable characters. Individual psychodynamic features and social situation may heavily influence outcome. It is helpful, however, to be aware of common psychological themes activated by pregnancy. These include assumption of adult roles, revival of unresolved developmental conflicts and childhood affects, ambivalence toward the fetus, and changes in internal boundaries and body image (Notman and Lester 1988). Pregnancy may reactivate separation-individuation struggles and early experiences with the woman's own mother (E. P. Lester and Notman 1986). With preexisting character pathology, these and other conflicts may intensify during pregnancy. The availability of internal and external resources to resolve these conflicts is a major factor in the outcome. In a few individuals, pregnancy ameliorates the psychological distress associated with prior personality disorder by seeming to offer a solution to unresolved problems (Wenner et al. 1969). These solutions, however, often prove temporary or superficial (Loesch and Greenberg 1962).

Eating Disorders

Issues arising during pregnancy in women with eating disorders are reviewed in Chapter 21.

Sleep Disorders

Sleep disturbances are common during pregnancy. There is evidence suggesting that stage 4 sleep decreases during the latter part of pregnancy (Berlin 1988). Although there are few data about specific sleep disorders during pregnancy, disturbances related to stage 4 sleep, such as sleepwalking and sleep terror, may undergo marked exacerbations and remissions related to the various stages of pregnancy (Berlin 1988; Snyder 1986).

Factitious Disorders

Goodlin (1985) suggests that Munchausen syndrome is relatively common during pregnancy and may be a predictor of future child abuse. Feigned symptoms may include vaginal bleeding, hyperemesis, premature labor, premature rupture of membranes, seizures, and fetal distress.

Organic Disorders With Psychiatric Symptoms

Organic syndromes that may coexist with pregnancy can present with changes in mental status; these are discussed in Chapter 2.

OTHER PREGNANCY-RELATED DISORDERS

Pseudocyesis

Pseudocyesis is a syndrome in which an otherwise nonpsychotic woman firmly believes herself to be pregnant and develops symptoms and signs of pregnancy without actually being pregnant. Physical changes, including amenorrhea or hypomenorrhea, abdominal enlargement, inverted umbilicus, breast tenderness and enlargement, galactorrhea, "fetal" movements, and softened cervix, can be so striking that misdiagnosis on physical examination has frequently occurred. Pseudocyesis is differentiated from deliberate feigning of pregnancy, identifiable endocrinopathies incorrectly presumed to be pregnancy, and psychotic states accompanied by delusions of pregnancy (O'Grady and Rosenthal 1989). It also differs from associated phenomena in men, which include couvade syndrome (physical symptoms in association with a partner's pregnancy) and delusions of pregnancy in a male with underlying psychotic or organic disorders.

Correlates of pseudocyesis include psychological factors in virtually all cases and endocrine abnormalities in many cases. However, there is no uniform psychological or endocrinologic profile. Pseudo-cyesis has been seen in the context of major depression and borderline and histrionic personality disorders and as a prelude to schizophrenia. It most closely resembles a conversion disorder, with elements of primary and secondary gain and symptom modeling from familial or cultural sources. In some cases, there are histories of eating disorders, difficulties with separation, recent reproductive loss, infertility, sexual abuse, and troubled current relationships (O'Grady and Rosenthal 1989; Whelan and Stewart 1990). A desire for pregnancy, or its associated social role, may conflict with a fear of pregnancy (Murray and Abraham 1978).

Hormonal abnormalities associated with pseudocyesis may include high estrogen, low gonadotropin (Fried et al. 1951), high serum testosterone, abnormal growth hormone (Starkman et al. 1985), and high prolactin (O'Grady and Rosenthal 1989) levels. It is hypothesized that psychic factors may affect gonadotropin release, perhaps via the hypothalamus. In cases of major depression, disturbances in biogenic amines may trigger hormonal changes (Brown and Barglow 1971).

Effective treatment includes accurate diagnosis of pseudocyesis and its underlying psychiatric context and, where appropriate, intervention with significant others, psychotherapy, and pharmacotherapy. If ultrasound is performed, care must be taken to ensure that the patient does not misinterpret what she sees or overhears; for example, she may misinterpret shadows as fetal parts or misunderstand a technician's reference to a uterus being of "6-week size" (O'Grady and Rosenthal 1989). In some cases, administration of exogenous hormones may facilitate the return of normal menses. Collaboration between an obstetrician and a psychiatrist is essential for optimal management. Many women with this disorder are reluctant to undergo psychotherapy, and behavioral strategies are sometimes more successful. The woman is more likely to give up her belief that she is pregnant if a face-saving solution to her dilemma can be found.

Hyperemesis Gravidarum

Hyperemesis gravidarum is a condition of intractable vomiting during pregnancy that is of sufficient severity to result in electrolyte imbalance, significant weight loss, ketosis, acetonuria, and/or organ damage and is without a known organic cause other than pregnancy (Fairweather 1968). Although mild nausea and vomiting are experienced in over one-half of normal pregnancies, hyperemesis gravidarum is relatively rare and occurs in approximately 1 in 1,000 pregnancies (Gise 1985).

Various endocrinologic explanations for the etiology of hyperemesis gravidarum have been postulated, although none have been clearly proven. The etiologic role of psychogenic factors has been controversial. Belief in such factors arose because vomiting ceased in some cases with placebo treatments, hospital admission alone, or psychosocial interventions. This hypothesis was also supported by epidemiological data suggesting a lower incidence in wartime that was thought to be unrelated to food scarcity (Fairweather 1968). Psychodynamic explanations included the notion that vomiting represented an unconscious attempt to get rid of the fetus or reflected difficulties in the mother-daughter relationship (FitzGerald 1984).

Empirical studies have suffered from methodological difficulties, including a lack of adequate control subjects and a failure to differentiate the psychological causes of hyperemesis from its effects. One well-controlled follow-up study found no evidence of significant differences in long-term psychopathology between women with hyperemesis and control subjects, although acute psychiatric disturbance could not be excluded (Majerus et al. 1960). Other studies that employed different methods have found hyperemesis to be associated with factors such as hysterical personality; below-average intelligence (Fairweather 1968); poor mother-daughter relationships; unplanned, undesired pregnancies (FitzGerald 1984); and eating disorders (see Chapter 21).

The data suggest a spectrum of psychophysiological causation, with some cases heavily influenced by psychopathology, others apparently unrelated to psychological disturbance, and some having elements of both psychic and somatic determinants. A logical clinical approach, given current knowledge, would include screening for the presence of an underlying personality disorder, marital conflict, eating disorder, ambivalence about the pregnancy, disturbed maternal relationships, or low intelligence and considering, in each case, whether there are apparent connections between those factors and the symptoms.

Denial of Pregnancy

Normal adaptation to pregnancy is characterized by acceptance of the pregnant state, affiliation with the fetus, and preparatory behavior (Cohen 1979). This developmental process is impaired when the mother denies that she is pregnant. A spectrum of denial exists, ranging from subtle failures to adjust life-style, wardrobe, etc., to frank, psychotic denial that persists in the face of conclusive evidence of pregnancy. The consequences of denial can include lack of prenatal care, poor postpartum adjustment (Uddenberg and Nilsson 1975), and neonaticide (Resnick 1970).

Even in women who acknowledge that they are pregnant, denial mechanisms should be suspected in those who claim to feel absolutely no pregnancy symptoms (Uddenberg and Nilsson 1975) or who try to behave as though they were not pregnant (Loesch and Greenberg 1962). In extreme cases of nonpsychotic denial, women may suppress awareness of possible pregnancy. They are reported to have an unusually high incidence of continued cyclic vaginal bleeding, little change in abdominal girth, and no pregnancy-related symptoms. Family members and physicians are usually unaware of these pregnancies. The woman is typically astonished to give birth, often after a precipitous delivery in which labor pains are misinterpreted as indigestion or urges to defecate, amniotic fluid is misidentified as urine, and bloody show is thought to be menses. Psychological reasons for the denial noted in the above studies include fear of rejection by the mother, conflicts about sexuality, rejection of the fetus, or hostility toward the baby's father.

Psychotic denial of pregnancy, in contrast, is usually accompanied by the typical somatic changes of pregnancy. Signs and symptoms are misattributed by the pregnant woman, but other people are aware of the pregnancy. Sometimes ultrasound viewing of a live fetus will overcome denial (Cook and Howe 1984), but denial can persist in the face of any proof, including the birth of the baby. Psychotic denial is most common among women with schizophrenia and is significantly associated with prior or anticipated loss of custody of children (Miller 1990).

Violence

There is an increased incidence of physical abuse of women during pregnancy (Helton et al. 1987). This phenomenon is reviewed in Chapter 23.

ASSESSMENT

Prenatal obstetric and pediatric visits provide an opportunity for early identification of emotional disturbance. A study by Kumar and Robson (1984) suggested that this opportunity is often neglected; only a few of their sample of significantly depressed pregnant women received any attention for emotional problems, despite repeated health care contacts.

Cohen (1979) suggested that adequate psychosocial screening can be performed in about 15 minutes, without the need for experienced mental health personnel. A developmental framework can be used effectively for the detection of disorders ranging from subtle to severe: pregnant women can be considered normally to pass through stages of acceptance of the pregnancy and affiliative responses to the fetus. Difficulty in progressing through these stages can be detected by open-ended questions and behavioral observations. Relevant stressors include dislocating moves, loss of support from the baby's father, illness in the patient or significant others, death of significant others, career problems, a series of closely spaced pregnancies, prior induced abortions, periods of infertility, prior traumatic deliveries, or death of prior children.

The presence of warning signs suggests the need for more comprehensive psychiatric assessment. If the patient is unwilling to see a psychiatrist, psychiatric consultation to the obstetric staff may guide their interventions (see also Chapter 25).

For women with preexisting psychiatric disorders who wish to become pregnant or who become pregnant unexpectedly, assessment can focus on the patient's psychological readiness and ability for pregnancy and childrearing and the availability of external support. The motivation for pregnancy can be investigated, looking especially for cases in which the pregnancy is desired as a probably unrealistic solution to an intrapsychic or interpersonal problem. Counseling about the effects of illness, psychotropic drugs, and genetic factors on the baby should be given when indicated, and the mother's capacity to understand and to realistically evaluate these factors should be noted. Women with bipolar mood disorder or schizophrenia should be advised of the risk of postpartum psychosis (see Chapter 7).

Emergency assessment should focus on risk factors for both mother and fetus, including active psychosis (especially delusions about the fetus), malnutrition, denial of pregnancy, suicidal or homicidal ideation, fetal abuse, current or prior attempts at premature self-delivery, irrational fears about the pregnancy or fetus that persist despite explanations, and sudden loss of external support.

PRINCIPLES OF MANAGEMENT

Appropriate psychosocial management depends on the specific disorder and the individual situation, but some general principles apply:

❖ If obstetric personnel unrealistically idealize pregnancy, the patient may suppress or deny problems (Bibring and Valenstein 1976; Wohlreich 1986). In such cases, psychiatric consultation to the staff may promote a more communicative environment (see also Chapter 25).

❖ Psychosocial interventions, such as home visits by community nurses or midwives and 24-hour hot lines, have been shown to significantly improve pregnancy outcome in high-risk cases (Oakley et al. 1990). Scheduled times for telephone calls to the obstetrician are also helpful (Carnes 1983).

❖ Options such as prepared childbirth classes and rooming-in facilities in the hospital with the baby are beneficial for many women. In cases where a woman is not ready for the maternal role, however, these choices may increase her confusion (Bibring 1959).

❖ In women with severe psychiatric disorders, the risks of untreated illness must be carefully weighed against the risks of somatic therapies (see Chapter 5). Other treatment modalities can lessen or eliminate the need for pharmacotherapy, including psychotherapy, cognitive-behavior therapy, support groups, aggressive prenatal outreach, hospitalization, and mobilization of social support. In cases in which anxiety predominates, relaxation techniques and hypnotherapy may be useful adjuncts. Psychiatrists and obstetricians should coordinate care, ideally scheduling visits on the same day to facilitate attendance (Casiano and Hawkins 1987).

❖ Since the sudden loss of obstetric involvement after delivery may trigger problems, a prenatal pediatric visit is important (Wolfson and Bass 1979). Continued involvement of community nurses or mental health workers may ease the transition to parenthood.

❖ Clinicians treating pregnant women with psychiatric disorders are sometimes faced with ethical and medicolegal dilemmas stemming from conflicts in their duties to the pregnant woman versus those to the fetus. These issues are discussed in Chapter 24.

REFERENCES[1]

Abernethy V: Sexual knowledge, attitudes, and practices of young female psychiatric patients. Arch Gen Psychiatry 30:180–182, 1974

Berlin RM: Sleepwalking disorder during pregnancy: a case report. Sleep 11:298–300, 1988

Bibring GL: Some considerations of the psychological processes in pregnancy. Psychoanal Study Child 14:113–121, 1959

Bibring GL, Valenstein AF: Psychological aspects of pregnancy. Clin Obstet Gynecol 19:357–371, 1976

Brandt KR, Mackenzie TB: Obsessive-compulsive disorder exacerbated during pregnancy: a case report. Int J Psychiatry Med 17:361–366, 1987

Brown E, Barglow P: Pseudocyesis: a paradigm for psychophysiological interactions. Arch Gen Psychiatry 24:221–229, 1971

---

[1]Since space limitations preclude more extensive referencing, additional references are available on request from Laura J. Miller, M.D., Department of Psychiatry, University of Illinois, 912 S. Wood Street, MC913, Chicago, IL 60612.

Burr WA, Falek A, Strauss LT, et al: Fertility in psychiatric outpatients. Hosp Community Psychiatry 30:527–531, 1979

Carnes JW: Psychosocial disturbances during and after pregnancy. Postgrad Med 73:135–145, 1983

Casiano ME, Hawkins DR: Major mental illness and childbearing: a role for the consultation-liaison psychiatrist in obstetrics. Psychiatr Clin North Am 10:35–51, 1987

Challis JRG, Patrick JE: Changes in the diurnal rhythms of plasma cortisol in women during the third trimester of pregnancy. Gynecol Obstet Invest 16:27–32, 1983

Chang SS, Renshaw DC: Psychosis and pregnancy. Compr Ther 12:36–41, 1986

Cohen RL: Maladaptation to pregnancy. Semin Perinatol 3:15–24, 1979

Condon JT: Altered cognitive functioning in pregnant women: a shift towards primary process thinking. Br J Med Psychol 60:329–334, 1987

Cook PE, Howe B: Unusual use of ultrasound in a paranoid patient (letter). Can Med Assoc J 131:539, 1984

Coverdale JH, Aruffo JA: Family planning needs of female chronic psychiatric outpatients. Am J Psychiatry 146:1489–1491, 1989

Cowley DS, Roy-Byrne RP: Panic disorder during pregnancy. Journal of Psychosomatic Obstetrics and Gynaecology 10:193–210, 1989

Cox JL, Connor Y, Kendell RE: Prospective study of the psychiatric disorders of childbirth. Br J Psychiatry 140:111–117, 1982

Czeizel A, Lendvay A: Attempted suicide and pregnancy (letter). Am J Obstet Gynecol 161:497, 1989

Fairweather DVI: Nausea and vomiting in pregnancy. Am J Obstet Gynecol 102:135–175, 1968

FitzGerald CM: Nausea and vomiting in pregnancy. Br J Med Psychol 57:159–165, 1984

Forcier K: Management and care of the mentally disturbed pregnant patient. J Psychosoc Nurs Ment Health Serv 28:11–16, 1990

Fried PH, Rakoff AE, Schopbach RR, et al: Pseudocyesis: a psychosomatic study in gynecology. JAMA 145:1329–1335, 1951

George DT, Ladenheim JA, Nutt DJ: Effect of pregnancy on panic attacks. Am J Psychiatry 144:1078–1079, 1987

Gise LH: Psychiatric implications of pregnancy, in Rovinsky and Guttmacher's Medical, Surgical, and Gynecologic Complications of Pregnancy, 3rd Edition. Edited by Cherry SH, Berkowitz RL, Kase NG. Baltimore, MD, Williams & Wilkins, 1985, pp 614–654

Goodlin RC: Pregnant women with Münchausen syndrome. Am J Obstet Gynecol 153:207–210, 1985

Hayward C, Killen JD, Hammer LD, et al: Pubertal stage and panic attack history in sixth- and seventh-grade girls. Am J Psychiatry 149:1239–1243, 1992

Helton AS, McFarlane J, Anderson ET: Battered and pregnant: a prevalence study. Am J Public Health 77:1337–1339, 1987

Jarrahi-Zadeh A, Kane FJ, Van de Castlf RL, et al: Emotional and cognitive changes in pregnancy and early puerperium. Br J Psychiatry 115:797–805, 1969

Kaplan BJ: Causes and attributions of depression during pregnancy. Women Health 8:23–32, 1983

Kumar R, Robson K: Neurotic disturbance during pregnancy and the puerperium: preliminary report of a prospective survey of 119 primiparae, in Mental Illness in Pregnancy and the Puerperium. Edited by Sandler M. Oxford, UK, Oxford University Press, 1978, pp 40–51

Kumar R, Robson KM: A prospective study of emotional disorders in childbearing women. Br J Psychiatry 144:35–47, 1984

Leifer M: Psychological changes accompanying pregnancy and motherhood. Genetic Psychology Monographs 95:55–96, 1977

Lester D, Beck AT: Attempted suicide and pregnancy. Am J Obstet Gynecol 158:1084–1085, 1988

Lester EP, Notman MT: Pregnancy, developmental crisis and object relations: psychoanalytic considerations. Int J Psychoanal 67:357–366, 1986

Loesch JG, Greenberg NH: Some specific areas of conflicts observed during pregnancy: a comparative study of married and unmarried pregnant women. Am J Orthopsychiatry 32:624–636, 1962

Majerus PW, Guze SB, Delong WB, et al: Psychologic factors and psychiatric disease in hyperemesis gravidarum: a follow-up study of 69 vomiters and 66 controls. Am J Psychiatry 117:421–428, 1960

McNeil TF, Kaij L, Malmquist-Larsson A: Pregnant women with nonorganic psychosis: life situation and experience of pregnancy. Acta Psychiatr Scand 68:445–457, 1983

McNeil TF, Kaij L, Malmquist-Larsson A: Women with nonorganic psychosis: factors associated with pregnancy's effect on mental health. Acta Psychiatr Scand 70:209–219, 1984

Miller LJ: Psychotic denial of pregnancy: phenomenology and clinical management. Hosp Community Psychiatry 41:1233–1237, 1990

Murray JF, Abraham GE: Pseudocyesis: a review. Obstet Gynecol 51:627–631, 1978

Neziroglu F, Anemone R, Yaryura-Tobias JA: Onset of obsessive-compulsive disorder in pregnancy. Am J Psychiatry 149:947–950, 1992

Notman MT, Lester EP: Pregnancy: theoretical considerations. Psychoanalytic Inquiry 8:139–159, 1988

Oakley A, Rajan L, Grant A: Social support and pregnancy outcome. Br J Obstet Gynaecol 97:155–162, 1990

O'Grady JP, Rosenthal M: Pseudocyesis: a modern perspective on an old disorder. Obstet Gynecol Surv 44:500–511, 1989

O'Hara MW: Social support, life events, and depression during pregnancy and the puerperium. Arch Gen Psychiatry 43:569–573, 1986

Paffenbarger RS: Epidemiological aspects, in Motherhood and Mental Illness. Edited by Brockington IF, Kumar R. London, Academic Press, 1982, pp 21–36

Pugh TF, Jerath BK, Schmidt WM, et al: Rates of mental disease related to childbearing. N Engl J Med 268:1224–1228, 1963

Resnick PJ: Murder of the newborn: a psychiatric review of neonaticide. Am J Psychiatry 126:1414–1420, 1970

Rudolph B, Larson GL, Sweeny S, et al: Hospitalized pregnant psychotic women: characteristics and treatment issues. Hosp Community Psychiatry 41:159–163, 1990

Sandler M: Some biological correlates of mental illness in relation to childbirth, in Mental Illness in Pregnancy and the Puerperium. Edited by Sandler M. Oxford, UK, Oxford University Press, 1978, pp 9–24

Snyder S: Unusual case of sleep terror in a pregnant patient (letter). Am J Psychiatry 143:391, 1986

Spielvogel A, Wile J: Treatment of the psychotic pregnant patient. Psychosomatics 27:487–492, 1986

Starkman MN, Marshall JC, La Ferla J, et al: Pseudocyesis: psychologic and neuroendocrine interrelationships. Psychosom Med 47:46–57, 1985

Uddenberg N, Nilsson L: The longitudinal course of para-natal emotional disturbance. Acta Psychiatr Scand 52:160–169, 1975

Villeponteaux VA, Lydiard RB, Laraia MT, et al: The effects of pregnancy on pre-existing panic disorder. J Clin Psychiatry 53:201–203, 1992

Watson JP, Elliott SA, Rugg AJ, et al: Psychiatric disorder in pregnancy and the first postnatal year. Br J Psychiatry 144:453–462, 1984

Wenner NK, Cohen MB, Weigert EV, et al: Emotional problems in pregnancy. Psychiatry 32:389–410, 1969

Whelan CI, Stewart DE: Pseudocyesis—a review and report of six cases. Int J Psychiatry Med 20:97–108, 1990

Whitlock FA, Edwards JE: Pregnancy and attempted suicide. Compr Psychiatry 9:1–12, 1968

Wohlreich MM: Psychiatric aspects of high-risk pregnancy. Psychiatr Clin North Am 10:53–68, 1986

Wolfson JH, Bass LW: How the pediatrician can foster optimal parent-infant relationships. Semin Perinatol 3:101–105, 1979

Chapter 5

Psychotropic Drugs and Electroconvulsive Therapy During Pregnancy and Lactation

Donna E. Stewart, M.D., D.Psych., F.R.C.P.C.
Gail Erlick Robinson, M.D., F.R.C.P.C.

❖ ❖ ❖ ❖ ❖ ❖ ❖ ❖ ❖ ❖ ❖ ❖ ❖

Pregnant women may receive psychotropic drugs for a number of reasons. Some may be undergoing treatment with antidepressants, antipsychotics, mood stabilizers, or minor tranquilizers, either for an acute psychiatric illness or for maintenance therapy when they become pregnant. Other women may develop a psychiatric illness that requires treatment during pregnancy or lactation (Robinson et al. 1986). The potential benefits of pharmacotherapy in the pregnant or lactating woman must be carefully weighed against the possible risks to the woman and her developing fetus or infant. The risk side of the risk-benefit equation includes the risks of maternal and newborn toxicity, side effects and withdrawal, and fetal physical or behavioral teratogenicity (Cohen et al. 1989). Although the benefits of psychotropic drugs for the severely psychotic, depressed, or suicidal pregnant woman may outweigh the risks to the infant, a careful appraisal of current knowledge in this area is essential before a rational clinical decision can be reached (Robinson et al. 1986). This chapter contains current information on the use of antipsychotics, antidepressants, mood stabilizers, and anxiolytics during pregnancy and lactation. The use of electroconvulsive therapy in pregnancy is also discussed.

Despite much public education, drug use in pregnancy is still commonplace. Rayburn et al. (1982) showed that 90% or more of all pregnant women take one or more drugs in addition to dietary supplements during pregnancy. In a North American study, Heinonen et al. (1977) reported that 36% of pregnant women took sedatives, tranquilizers, or antidepressants at some time during their pregnancies.

Any discussion of the effects of psychotropic drugs in pregnancy must begin by stating the limits to our knowledge. Many studies have not considered confounding variables such as diagnosis; maternal age; use of alcohol, tobacco, or street drugs; gravidity; previous pregnancy loss; genetic history; use of multiple drugs; or timing of drug exposure and dosage. There are few prospective controlled studies of the treatment of psychiatric disorders in pregnant women. Moreover, drugs that consistently produce defects in other animals may not have similar effects in humans (Elia et al. 1987). It is wise to remember that the Food and Drug Administration (1979) has not approved a single psychotropic drug for administration during pregnancy and urges caution.

EFFECTS OF PREGNANCY ON DRUG METABOLISM, ACTION, AND SIDE EFFECTS

A number of physiologic changes in pregnancy alter the effects of drugs. Data on drug metabolism rates, dosages, and side effects in nonpregnant women may not apply to pregnant women.

The significant increases in total body water content that take place during pregnancy may result in lower drug serum concentrations than in nonpregnant women. Total protein is also reduced in pregnancy, thereby altering drug binding. A physiologic drop in blood pressure in the second trimester of pregnancy may result in orthostatic hypotension, causing significant problems in pregnant women treated with antipsychotic and antidepressant drugs. The emptying rate of the gastrointestinal tract is decreased by 30%–50%, and gastric acid is decreased, thus altering drug absorption. Constipation is another common problem in pregnancy that may be worsened by medications with anticholinergic side effects. Glomerular filtration rates are increased in pregnancy, causing some drugs, such as lithium, to be excreted more quickly and thereby requiring higher doses to achieve therapeutic serum levels. Hepatic hydroxylases involved in drug metabolism may be inhibited during pregnancy (Mortola 1989; Wisner and Perel 1988).

The physiologic changes of pregnancy necessitate careful monitoring of a woman's drug response, side effects, and toxicity throughout pregnancy and the early postpartum period (Wisner and Perel 1988). Higher doses are sometimes required in pregnancy to achieve therapeutic serum levels. After delivery, the doses may need to be decreased to prevent maternal toxicity (Koplan 1983; Stewart 1988).

All psychotropic drugs cross the placenta and enter the fetal circulation to some degree. The penetration to the fetal compartment is influenced by the characteristics of the drug, the dosage, and the stage of pregnancy (Mirkin 1976). When repeated doses of a psychotropic drug are administered to sustain plasma concentrations, the drug is usually distributed equally to mother and fetus (G. Levy 1981). Both the placenta and the fetus have enzyme systems involved in drug metabolism, but many details are as yet incompletely understood (Chao and Juchau 1983). It is also known that some enzyme systems are not mature at birth, impairing the ability of the newborn's liver to conjugate the metabolites of common drugs such as diazepam (Kanto 1982). Thus, fetal physiology must also be considered in prescribing psychotropic drugs in pregnancy.

GENERAL EFFECTS OF PSYCHOTROPIC DRUGS ON THE FETUS AND NEONATE

Morphologic Teratogenicity

During the first several cell divisions, the developing embryo is thought to be protected against the effects of drugs administered to the mother because the placenta has not yet formed. This period of protection is between conception (approximately day 14) and the first missed period (approximately day 28 of a 28-day cycle). After the first missed period, however, the placenta is sufficiently developed to transfer drugs in the maternal circulation to the developing fetus (Cohen 1992).

It is impossible to guarantee that any psychotropic drug is not teratogenic and able to cause fetal deformity (American Medical Association 1983). The baseline rate of birth defects in the Western world is approximately 3%, and the cause of the vast majority of them remains unknown (Beeley 1986). Although the incidence of birth defects caused by drugs is probably low, the low levels of teratogenicity due to drugs are extremely difficult to distinguish from the spontaneous occurrence of anomalies and require large exposure samples (American Medical Association 1983).

A number of factors, however, are known to increase the teratogenic risks of a drug:

1. Exposure to the drug during organogenesis: central nervous system, gestational days 10–25; limb development, days 24–26; cardiovascular system, days 20–40
2. Dosage and regularity of use: lack of maternal toxicity does not indicate lack of fetal toxicity
3. Interaction with other environmental factors, such as other drugs, alcohol, tobacco, and other toxins
4. Genetic constitution of the fetus

It is hypothesized that the continuum of abnormal development ranges from fetal death (resulting in miscarriage or stillbirth), to physical malformation, to growth retardation, or to functional deficits (behavioral teratogenicity) (J. G. Wilson 1977).

Behavioral Teratogenicity

The rapidly developing field of behavioral teratogenicity includes functional deficits such as delayed behavioral maturation, abnormal activity, and impaired problem solving and learning, all of which may develop following fetal exposure to teratogens (Vorhees and Butcher 1982). Research in animals has shown that most drugs that act on the central nervous system have a low potential for physical teratogenicity but a higher potential as behavioral teratogens, which probably arises from less-severe damage (Vorhees and Butcher 1982). Many behavioral teratogenic agents may not yet have been identified in humans because they are unaccompanied by physical malformation. There are few studies as yet on the long-term follow-up of children exposed to psychotropic drugs in utero. (See specific information on major tranquilizers and lithium in "Known Effects of Specific Psychotropic Drug Groups" in this chapter.) Other investigators have correctly criticized the available studies for their small sample sizes, lack of data on dosage and timing, circumscribed inquiry, lack of standardized psychometric instruments, and inadequate follow-up (Edlund and Craig 1984). It is therefore unwise to assume that any psychotropic agent is "safe" in pregnancy (Wisner and Perel 1988).

Effects of Psychotropic Drugs in the Second and Third Trimesters and During Labor

Psychotropic drugs appear to be safer during the second and third trimesters of pregnancy, although many clinicians recommend that the drug doses should be lowered or discontinued approximately 2 weeks prior to the expected date of delivery to reduce the possibility of side effects, toxicity, and withdrawal in the newborn (Kerns 1986; Robinson et al. 1986; Wisner and Perel 1988). Other clinicians do not discontinue psychotropic drugs before labor to reduce the risk of relapse of the psychiatric illness (Cohen 1992). Major malformations are not produced during the second and third trimesters, but drugs can affect the growth and functional development of the fetus. Effects on behavioral teratogenicity are unknown. In particular, the central nervous system continues to develop throughout pregnancy, and damage after the first trimester can produce microcephaly and mental retardation (Beeley 1986).

Both major and minor tranquilizers have long been used by obstetricians during labor to reduce anxiety, increase relaxation, or decrease nausea. Long-acting benzodiazepines, however, should be avoided in the third trimester because they adversely affect the neonate (Mandrelli et al. 1975).

Effects of Psychotropic Drugs on the Neonate

Antipsychotics, tricyclic antidepressants, and benzodiazepines are lipid soluble and largely protein bound and are therefore slowly eliminated from the newborn. Nahas and Goujard (1978) have stated that the neonate may be more susceptible to these drugs because liver enzymes are not fully developed; plasma protein concentrates are lower, leading to increased free drug available to act on the brain; the blood-brain barrier is incomplete; and the immature central nervous system may be more sensitive to these drugs.

Effects of Psychotropic Drugs During Lactation

Psychotropic drugs, like most medications, are excreted in breast milk. The concentration of the drug in breast milk depends on its solubility, protein binding, and drug pH compared with plasma (Robinson et al. 1986). There are wide variations among drugs, and concentrations may vary in breast milk samples taken at different times of the day.

The American Academy of Pediatrics Committee on Drugs (1989) has classified major and minor tranquilizers and antidepressants in the category of "drugs whose effects on nursing infants is unknown but may be of concern." A variety of case reports of toxic effects, drowsiness, impaired temperature regulation, and no ill effects have been described in breast-fed infants of mothers taking psychotropic or mood-stabilizing drugs (Gelenberg 1987). The effects of these drugs on the immature neurotransmitter system are unknown (Mortola 1989; Robinson et al. 1986).

KNOWN EFFECTS OF SPECIFIC PSYCHOTROPIC DRUG GROUPS

Major Tranquilizers

Teratogenicity. There are numerous reports in the literature describing individual or short series of cases in which the use of neuroleptics in the first trimester has coincided with the occurrence of congenital anomalies (Table 5–1). Results of larger studies are conflicting.

The French National Institute of Health and Medical Research conducted a retrospective study involving 12,764 births (Rumeau-Rouquette et al. 1977). Infants in the control group demonstrated congenital malformations not considered to be related to chromosomal abnormalities in 1.6% of cases. Of the 315 women who took phenothiazines during the first trimester, 3.5% gave birth to malformed infants. This was considered a statistically significant increase in malformations (especially following the use of aliphatic phenothiazines), but it is not clear that confounding variables such as dosage and maternal age were taken into account.

Slone et al. (1977) reported the results of the Collaborative Perinatal Project, a study of 5,282 gravidas and their children that included 1,309 cases of prenatal exposure to phenothiazines. They found no significant increase in the incidence of congenital malformations related to exposure in the first trimester, except for a questionable association with cardiovascular malformations. Perinatal mortality rate, birth weight, and IQ at age 4 were all found to be normal in this group.

The large California Child Health and Development Project, which took place from 1959 to 1966 and involved over 19,000 births, originally showed no increase in congenital anomalies following the use of phenothiazines in pregnancy (Milkovich and van den Berg 1976). On reanalyzing the data, Edlund and Craig (1984) demonstrated a trend toward increased congenital anomalies when the drugs were given after 4 weeks, the most critical period being from 6 to 10 weeks of gestation. The exposed samples yielded an incidence of congenital anomalies of 5.4% versus 3.2% in the control subjects.

Large studies to date have not revealed a significant increase in fetal abnormalities for women taking thioridazine, perphenazine, trifluoperazine, fluphenazine, or haloperidol (Ananth 1975; Goldberg and DiMascio 1978). There is no evidence of teratogenicity for the dibenzoxazepines, thioxanthenes, or diphenylbutylpiperidines; their safety in pregnancy, however, has not yet been established.

Caution must be exercised in drawing conclusions from these studies. Edlund and Craig (1984) and others have pointed out numerous confounding methodologic errors. Many studies may have minimized potential effects by looking at nonpsychotic populations using small amounts of drugs as antiemetics or anxiolytics rather than the

Table 5–1. Psychotropic drugs in pregnancy and lactation

Drugs	Teratogenicity	Effects on the neonate	Lactation
Major tranquilizers			
Phenothiazines (especially aliphatics)	Congenital anomalies increased if used weeks 6–10. Cardiovascular anomalies increased. Caution in first trimester. Appear to be fairly safe.	Third-trimester use of neuroleptics causes extrapyramidal symptoms in infant: excessive crying, motion, hypertonia, hyperreflexia, respiratory distress, vasomotor instability, slow early learning tasks. Possible jaundice, especially in premature infants.	Excreted in breast milk. No serious side effects reported as yet. Increased drowsiness. Use with caution.
Butyrophenones	No evidence at present for teratogenicity.		Haloperidol toxic in animal studies.
Antidepressants			
Tricyclics and heterocyclics	No link with fetal deformity or limb dysgenesis. Use with caution in first trimester. Appear to be fairly safe.	Withdrawal symptoms in infant include heart failure, tachycardia, myoclonus, seizures, respiratory distress, urinary retention, cyanosis, irritability, feeding difficulty. Discontinue 2 weeks before expected date of delivery.	Excreted in breast milk. Use with caution, as effect on developing neurotransmitter systems unknown.
Serotonin reuptake inhibitors	Insufficient data available.	Unknown.	Unknown.
MAOIs	Phenelzine teratogenic in animals. Avoid in first trimester.		Effects unknown.

Mood stabilizers			
Carbamazepine	Case reports of teratogenicity.		Effects unknown.
Lithium carbonate	Increased cardiovascular anomalies. Contraindicated in first trimester. Use small divided doses in late pregnancy.	Third-trimester use may cause hypotonia, lethargy, cyanosis, poor sucking, shallow respiration, low Apgar scores, arrhythmias, hypotension.	Excreted in breast milk. Severe toxic reactions. Contraindicated while breast-feeding.
Anxiolytics			
Benzodiazepines	Safety in first trimester not established. Controversial data on cleft lip/palate if used in first trimester.	Chronic use in pregnancy associated with withdrawal: tremor, hypertonia, hyperreflexia. High doses prior to delivery associated with low Apgar scores, hypothermia, neurological depression. "Floppy infant syndrome." Decreased sucking rate. Possible jaundice.	Excretion in breast milk associated with lethargy, jaundice, poor temperature regulation. Contraindicated while breast-feeding.
Meprobamate	Cleft lip, palate. Other severe congenital anomalies. Do not use in first trimester.		
Barbiturates	First-trimester use associated with growth retardation, facial dysmorphism, oral clefts, skeletal anomalies. Dose related.	Chronic use in pregnancy associated with withdrawal in infant 10–14 days after birth. Increased tone, tremor, irritability.	Long-term effects unknown.
Hydroxyzine	Teratogenic in animals.	Jitteriness, myoclonic jerks, hypotonia after large doses prior to delivery.	
Antiparkinsonian agents	No studies; usually given with neuroleptic. Amantadine teratogenic in animals. Possible cardiovascular malformations.	No studies.	No studies.

dosages typically used to treat psychoses. There is also some evidence that children of psychotic women have a higher risk of fetal damage independent of drug exposure (Stewart 1984; Wrede et al. 1980). Despite many years of widespread use of neuroleptics, however, there have been relatively few reports of malformations attributed to these drugs. In general, the higher-potency drugs appear to be safer.

Effects on the neonate.   The use of neuroleptics in the last trimester has been reported to cause extrapyramidal symptoms in the neonate, sometimes lasting up to 6 months (Levy and Wisniewski 1974; Tamer et al. 1969). Infants regularly exposed to neuroleptics in the third trimester may be especially difficult to care for because they may suffer from excessive motion, crying and sucking, hypertonicity, hyperreflexia, and vasomotor instability. Sobel (1960) studied 52 women who received chlorpromazine in pregnancy and found that 3 women who received higher doses (500–600 mg) had infants with respiratory distress and cyanosis, one of whom died. Brazelton (1970) found effects on neonatal weight, response to nursing, and early learning tasks, but these seemed to occur only in the immediate postnatal period. There has been debate over the use of phenothiazines and the possibility of their causing hyperbilirubinemia and neonatal jaundice. Scokel and Jones (1962), among others, found this to be a particular problem in premature infants.

Effects on breast-feeding infants.   The quantity of major tranquilizers excreted in breast milk is usually less than 30% of the maternal plasma concentration (Ananth 1978). An exception may be haloperidol excretion, which was reported in one case study to be approximately 60% (Whalley et al. 1981). Aside from some drowsiness with chlorpromazine and some galactorrhea with chlorpromazine and thioridazine, no significant human neonatal side effects have been reported, despite several large studies (Ananth 1978). Some studies in animals, however, have shown behavioral abnormalities in the offspring following the administration of haloperidol during lactation (Ananth 1978). Infants who are breast-fed while their mothers are taking major tranquilizers should be carefully clinically monitored. Serum levels in the infant may be helpful in assessing risk and drowsiness. Breast milk drug concentrations done on milk expressed over a 24-hour period may also be useful in assessing the drug dose obtained by the infant.

Long-term effects on children exposed in utero.   Slone et al. (1977) looked at 4-year-old children whose mothers had taken phenothiazines in pregnancy and found their IQ scores to be the same as those of a control population. Kris (1965) followed a small sample of children exposed to 50–150 mg of chlorpromazine throughout pregnancy and found the children to be "healthy" with "normal behavior." The flaws of these studies are described in the section "Behavioral Teratogenicity" earlier in this chapter.

Antidepressants

Teratogenicity.   Crombie et al. (1975) looked at 10,000 pregnancies in England and Wales, and Kuenssberg and Knox (1972) reviewed another 15,000 pregnancies in Scotland. The Finnish Register of Congenital Malformations for 1964–1972 was used by Idanpaan-Heikkila and Saxen (1973) to analyze 2,784 cases of birth defects and an equal number of matched control births. No link was found between fetal deformities, including limb dysgenesis, and the use of tricyclics in pregnancy. The Collaborative Perinatal Project (Heinonen et al. 1977) prospectively examined the relationship of antidepressants to pregnancy outcome. Twenty-one pregnant women were exposed to amitriptyline during the first trimester, and no infant malformations were noted at birth. Twenty pregnant women were exposed to either imipramine or nortriptyline; although malformations in two infants were found, the numbers are too small to justify generalizations.

Postmarketing data available from the manufacturer of fluoxetine as of June 1990 reveal 226 prospective spontaneous reports of exposure during pregnancy. Of the 112 outcomes available, 64 women had normal births, 8 had premature births, 18 underwent therapeutic abortions, 16 had spontaneous abortions, 3 had twins, 2 had multiple categories, and 1 had transposition of the great arteries after exposure in the second trimester. The population of patients treated with fluoxetine through this date was estimated to be 2,382,000 (Eli Lilly

Company, personal communication, February 5, 1991). An important consideration, however, is the long elimination half-life (6–8 weeks) of the metabolite norfluoxetine, which persists after discontinuation of the drug.

Inadequate data are available to evaluate new antidepressants such as sertraline, fluvoxamine, bupropion, trazodone, or buspirone.

Phenelzine is the only monoamine oxidase inhibitor shown to have teratogenic properties in animals, an effect that is possibly related to its ability to deactivate DNA (Poulson and Robson 1964). Twenty-one pregnant women taking monoamine oxidase inhibitors were monitored in the Collaborative Perinatal Project, and 3 of their infants had malformations (Heinonen et al. 1977). Although the numbers in this study were small, it is probably wise to use other antidepressants in pregnancy.

Effects on the neonate.   Withdrawal symptoms in the neonate have been reported following the use of desipramine, imipramine, and nortriptyline during pregnancy (Shearer et al. 1972; Webster 1973). There have been case reports of infants born with heart failure, tachycardia, myoclonus, respiratory distress, and urinary retention. Signs of toxicity in the infants of mothers taking large amounts of these medications just before delivery may include breathlessness, cyanosis, tachypnea, irritability, seizures, and feeding difficulties (Ananth 1976; Eggermont et al. 1972).

Effects on breast-feeding infants.   There is controversy concerning the effects of antidepressants on breast-feeding infants. Ananth (1978) and Goldberg and DiMascio (1978) stated that therapeutic levels of tricyclic antidepressants do not reach breast milk in sufficient amounts to harm the baby. Sovner and Orsulak (1979) suggested that amounts of imipramine and desipramine in samples of breast milk are similar to those found in plasma and recommended that women do not breast-feed while taking antidepressants because of concern about subtle effects on neurologic or behavioral maturation of the infant. Current information does not warrant an absolute recommendation on the use of tricyclics in women who are breast-feeding, because the risk-benefit ratio must be assessed on an individual basis. Infants who are breast-fed while their mothers are taking antidepressants, however, should be carefully clinically monitored, and infant serum levels of antidepressants should be measured in cases of extended drug exposure (Wisner and Perel 1988). Breast milk drug levels can also be obtained to determine infant drug exposure levels.

Lithium, Carbamazepine, and Valproic Acid

Teratogenicity. Weinstein (1980) reviewed the records of the International Register of Lithium Babies and found an 11% rate of malformations in 225 exposed infants. Eight percent of these malformations were Ebstein's anomaly or other major cardiovascular malformations. Subsequent investigators (Kallen and Tandberg 1983) also reported that exposure to lithium is linked to cardiovascular anomalies, resulting in a contraindication for lithium in the first trimester. Although two recent studies (Jacobson et al. 1992; Zalzstein et al. 1990) suggested that the link to Ebstein's anomaly is much weaker than previously reported, it is our opinion that lithium should be avoided when possible in the first trimester. However, in unstable bipolar women or women with a recent severe affective illness, it may be reasonable to continue lithium and screen for cardiovascular effects with a targeted ultrasound at week 18 of gestation. The use of lithium in the second and third trimesters occasionally causes a large fetal goiter that may necessitate a cesarean section (Nars and Girard 1977).

Carbamazepine, previously considered to be safe in pregnancy, has recently been associated with fetal craniofacial defects, developmental delay, and nail hypoplasia (Jones et al. 1989). Caution should be exercised until further data are available.

Valproic acid, another mood stabilizer used in bipolar affective disorder, has been associated with spina bifida in the offspring of mothers treated during the first trimester. The risks of valproic acid are even greater than lithium for teratogenic potential, and its use is contraindicated in pregnancy in our opinion and that of others (Cohen 1992).

Effects on the neonate. Life-threatening toxicity from lithium has been noted in some newborns of mothers taking lithium in the third trimester, particularly when maternal lithium levels exceed therapeutic levels (Morrell et al. 1983). Affected babies may show hypotonia, lethargy, cyanosis, depressed Apgar scores, hypotension, cardiac arrhythmias, poor sucking reflex, and shallow respiration (Ananth 1976; N. Wilson et al. 1983). Lithium levels may remain high for over a week; the serum half-life in infants has been estimated at 96 hours (MacKay et al. 1976).

Effects on breast-feeding infants.   Levels of lithium in breast milk average 40%–50% of those in maternal serum, and levels in infant serum are approximately equal to those in breast milk (Schou and Amdisen 1973). Lithium in breast milk has been associated with cyanotic episodes, lethargy, hypothermia, and hypotonia in the neonate (Tunnessen and Hertz 1972). Because the long-term effects of lithium on neonates are unknown, mothers taking lithium are advised not to breast-feed (Ananth 1978; Robinson et al. 1986; Wisner and Perel 1988). If a woman insists on breast-feeding while taking lithium, her infant should be carefully monitored.

Long-term effects on children exposed in utero.   Schou (1976) discovered no significant differences in physical or mental anomalies at age 5 between children exposed to lithium in utero and their non-exposed siblings. This study is too poorly designed, however, to draw definitive conclusions.

Anxiolytics

Teratogenicity.   A number of studies have yielded conflicting evidence concerning the relationship between the use of benzodiazepines during pregnancy and the occurrence of fetal malformations, especially cleft lip with or without cleft palate. Milkovich and van den Berg (1974) reviewed 19,044 live births and found that infants of women who used meprobamate in the first trimester had a significantly increased incidence of severe congenital anomalies.

In a retrospective study of 30 mothers of children with cleft palate, Aarskog (1975) found that 6.3% of mothers whose babies had oral cleft palate had used diazepam in the first trimester, versus 1.1% of the control subjects. Safra and Oakley (1975) found a 4:1 relative risk that mothers of babies with cleft lip and/or cleft palate had used diazepam in the first trimester compared to mothers of infants with other birth defects. These authors cautioned, however, that this finding indicates a risk of only 4%, versus an overall risk of birth defects of 2%. In a case-control study carried out in Boston, Toronto, and Philadelphia, 445 children with cleft lip, with or without cleft palate, or with cleft palate alone were compared with a control group of 498 children with other birth defects; no evidence was found that diazepam played an etiological role (Rosenberg et al. 1983). Unfortunately, all of these studies had design problems (Gelenberg 1983). The better designed and more recent studies from Europe find no evidence that diazepam causes oral cleft problems. Despite a large increase in the use of diazepam over the last several years, there has not been a concomitant increase in the occurrence of cleft lip and/or cleft palate (Jick 1988).

Effects on the neonate.   Benzodiazepines, which are lipid soluble and have a low molecular weight, can easily cross the placenta, especially late in pregnancy (Kanto 1982). The long half-lives of these drugs may result in their marked accumulation in the mother and fetus when they are regularly administered (Mirkin 1976). The chronic use of diazepam throughout pregnancy has been reported to lead to withdrawal symptoms, including tremor, hypertonia, and hyperreflexia, lasting up to 8 weeks in the neonate (Volpe 1981). These irritable infants are difficult for anxious mothers to manage. Mandrelli et al. (1975) reported hypotonia, low Apgar scores, hypothermia, impaired response to cold, and neurological depression in infants whose mothers had received high doses of diazepam prior to delivery. The muscular hypotonia sometimes found in these infants has been labeled the "floppy infant syndrome" (Gillberg 1977). The use of injectable diazepam at delivery has been linked to kernicterus due to competition between bilirubin and the preservative sodium benzoate (Schiff et al. 1971). Long-acting benzodiazepines should be avoided in the third trimester, as they may inhibit newborn respiration and diminish responsiveness immediately after birth. Moreover, the immature fetal liver has difficulty metabolizing these drugs (Kanto 1982). Larger doses of diazepam may result in low Apgar scores at birth, apneic spells, hypotonia, and poor sucking (Cree et al. 1973).

All sedative drugs have been associated with decreased newborn sucking rates (Kanto 1982).

The chronic use of barbiturates prior to delivery can lead to withdrawal symptoms in the newborn that may not occur until 10–14 days after birth. Symptoms may include tremulousness, crying, irritability, hyperphagia, and increased tone (Hill and Stern 1979).

Effects on the breast-feeding infant.   The benzodiazepines constitute a risk to nursing newborns by producing lethargy and impaired temperature regulation. They are not metabolized in the fetal liver or gut, and from days 1 to 4 the infant is unable to conjugate them with glucuronic acid, which may result in newborn jaundice (Kanto 1982). If a mother uses benzodiazepines on a prolonged basis, breast-feeding is contraindicated because of the possibility of accumulation and lack of data on the effects of long-term exposure through breast milk (Mortola 1989; Robinson et al. 1986). When given to the nursing mother in therapeutic doses, phenobarbital appears to have little or no demonstrable effect on the infant, but long-term effects are unknown (Ananth 1978).

Antiparkinsonian Agents

There are few studies investigating the teratogenicity of antiparkinsonian agents in the first trimester. These drugs are often coadministered with neuroleptics. Some reports link diphenhydramine to congenital anomalies (Heinonen et al. 1977), and cardiovascular malformation has been reported in an infant exposed to amantadine during the first trimester (Nora et al. 1975).

GUIDELINES FOR CLINICAL USE

The goals for treating psychiatric disorders in pregnancy may be altered to achieve control of symptoms rather than complete remission. Nonpharmacologic strategies, such as cognitive-behavior therapy, psychotherapy, family or marital therapy, environmental support, and sometimes hospitalization, may be preferable to the use of drugs, particularly in the first trimester (Mortola 1989; Nurnberg and Prudic 1984). Despite these strategies, psychotropic drugs are sometimes required, particularly if the woman is so severely depressed or psychotic that her well-being or that of her fetus is in jeopardy. A severely ill woman may fail to eat properly, may not attend appointments for prenatal care, and may respond to command hallucinations to harm herself or her fetus. Such women should certainly be treated. The American Medical Association (1983) recommends the following guidelines for physicians when prescribing drugs to women of childbearing age or to those who are already pregnant: 1) avoid unnecessary exposure to drugs and select those drugs with the most favorable risk-benefit ratios; 2) inform patients of the implications of drug exposures in pregnancy; 3) when drugs are necessary, advise patients of the need for contraceptive measures when indicated; and 4) identify and report any birth defects.

In general, psychotropic drugs should be used in pregnancy only when they are clearly indicated for the prophylaxis or treatment of psychiatric illness, and then only in the lowest effective doses. It is generally believed that divided maternal doses have less effect on the fetus than once-daily dosage schedules. New drugs should be avoided until safety and side effects have been well established by use in nonpregnant women (Wisner and Perel 1988).

Antipsychotics

There are few data to support the choice of one antipsychotic over another during pregnancy. The halogenated phenothiazines, however, appear to slightly increase teratogenicity (Rumeau-Rouquette et al. 1977). We favor high-potency agents because they cause fewer autonomic, anticholinergic, and cardiovascular effects and less hypotension and sedation, and a lower dose is possible. We currently prescribe haloperidol during pregnancy and lactation in the lowest effective divided dose and try to avoid its use in the first trimester when possible.

Antidepressants

Because dose-response curves and therapeutic efficacy of any antidepressant have not yet been established in pregnancy, the choice of which of these drugs to use is primarily based on side effects and safety. We tend to favor nortriptyline or desipramine in pregnancy and lactation because of their lower anticholinergic side effects and the correlation between serum levels and therapeutic effect. Because nortriptyline is a high-potency tricyclic, a lower dose may be effective, thus reducing the risk of teratogenic effects. The lowest effective divided dose is given, and we try to avoid exposure in the first trimester. We avoid maprotiline, as there have been reports of maternal seizures (Edwards 1979), and monoamine oxidase inhibitors, as they may be teratogenic (Heinonen et al. 1977). There are still insufficient data to evaluate the serotonin reuptake inhibitors or the reversible monoamine oxidase inhibitors in pregnancy.

Lithium and Carbamazepine

General recommendations for the use of lithium in women of childbearing age include the following: 1) the drug should be given only for unequivocal indications, 2) patients should be warned of the possible teratogenic and toxic effects on the fetus, 3) effective contraception should be encouraged, 4) the drug should be withdrawn in the first trimester in cases of unexpected pregnancy (unless the bipolar illness is unstable), and 5) referral for a targeted ultrasound examination to detect fetal cardiovascular malformations should be considered (Gelenberg 1983; Weinstein 1980).

We avoid both lithium and carbamazepine in the first trimester (when possible) and during lactation and withdraw them 2 weeks before the expected due date to reduce the risk of fetal toxicity. However, recent studies suggest that lithium may be less teratogenic than previously thought (Jacobson et al. 1992; Zalzstein et al. 1990). Unstable bipolar patients may be maintained on lithium with close monitoring and targeted ultrasound at week 18 of gestation to rule out cardiovascular malformation. Weinstein (1980) has suggested that, when lithium is used in pregnancy, sodium-depleting diuretics and low-salt diets should be avoided, serum lithium levels should be closely monitored (at least once per month in early pregnancy and weekly toward the end), care should be taken to distinguish nausea and vomiting of pregnancy from effects of lithium toxicity, serum levels should be kept at the lowest effective level, and lithium should be given in three to five equal doses not exceeding 300 mg per dose. Lithium levels should be carefully monitored after delivery to avoid toxicity, as physiologic fluid shifts occur.

Anxiolytics

Nonpharmacologic interventions should be the main strategy for the management of anxiety or insomnia during pregnancy and lactation. These interventions include relaxation techniques, cognitive-behavior therapy, psychotherapy, and environmental changes and support. No anxiolytic can be regarded as completely safe in pregnancy or lactation, but if circumstances dictate (such as in panic disorder), lorazepam may be the best choice because of its lack of active metabolites, glucuronide metabolism, high potency, and good absorption (Wisner and Perel 1988). There are few data on the effects of this drug in pregnancy, however, and it appears to be conjugated slowly in the neonate. The drug should be given in the lowest effective dose for the briefest possible time and avoided if possible in the first trimester and near term, bearing in mind that sleep disturbance and anxiety are common in late pregnancy and that risk-benefit considerations seldom warrant hypnotics or anxiolytics at this time except for the treatment of severe anxiety and panic disorder.

ELECTROCONVULSIVE THERAPY IN PREGNANCY

Indications

Electroconvulsive therapy (ECT) is generally regarded as a safe and effective treatment for specific psychiatric diagnoses in pregnancy and the puerperium (National Institutes of Health Consensus Conference 1985). ECT is an underused treatment modality in treating pregnant women with psychiatric illnesses. It is primarily useful for severe depression, psychosis with affective features, and catatonia. ECT may be prescribed in the following situations: 1) on an emergency basis when the psychiatric status of the mother presents a hazard to herself or the fetus, 2) as a backup for failure of other treatments in severe psychiatric conditions, and 3) to avoid the risk of exposure to potential teratogens in the first trimester (Fink 1981; Sobel 1960). It may also be used in pregnant patients who have a history of previous successful treatment with ECT. It is an effective treatment for postpartum psychosis and also allows continuation of breast-feeding.

Clinical Guidelines

Other clinicians (Remick and Maurice 1978; Wise et al. 1984) have commented on the lack of conclusive data on the use of ECT in pregnancy and have suggested the following guidelines:

1. Thorough physical examination
2. Involvement of an obstetrician who is present at the procedure
3. Consideration of high-risk pregnancy as a relative contraindication
4. External fetal monitoring for several hours before and after ECT
5. Endotracheal intubation
6. Low-voltage, nondominant ECT with electroencephalographic monitoring
7. Electrocardiographic monitoring of the mother
8. Oxygen pretreatment and assisted ventilation until the return of spontaneous respiration in the mother
9. Evaluation of maternal arterial blood gases during or after ECT
10. Doppler ultrasonography of the fetal heart rate
11. Tocodynamometer recording of uterine tone
12. Glycopyrrolate as anticholinergic of choice
13. Screening for pseudocholinesterase deficiency if using succinylcholine
14. Weekly nonstress tests of fetal well-being
15. Careful monitoring and control of maternal blood pressure

The patient should be positioned in the left lateral position by the placement of a wedge under the right hip to ensure that the gravid uterus does not obstruct blood flow through the inferior vena cava. It is our opinion that these extremely cautious recommendations should be taken only as general guidelines, and the advice of an obstetrician and an anesthesiologist should be obtained for the individual patient.

CONCLUSIONS

The clinician who is presented with a psychiatrically ill pregnant or lactating patient must make important clinical decisions about the use of psychotropic drugs and ECT in the face of some uncertainty. Careful attention to the most recent and reliable information available and consideration of the unique features of each patient's circumstances will assist in weighing the risk-benefit ratio and determining the best clinical strategy. Written documentation of the factors considered, the patient's informed consent, and careful, ongoing monitoring are vital in the optimal management of this difficult clinical dilemma.

REFERENCES

Aarskog D: Association between maternal intake of diazepam and oral clefts (letter). Lancet 2:921, 1975

American Academy of Pediatrics Committee on Drugs: Transfer of drugs and other chemicals into human milk. Pediatrics 184:924–935, 1989

American Medical Association: Drug interactions and adverse drug reaction, in AMA Drug Evaluations. Edited by Bennett DR. Chicago, IL, American Medical Association, 1983, pp 31–44

Ananth J: Congenital malformations with psychopharmacologic agents. Compr Psychiatry 16:437–445, 1975

Ananth J: Side effects on fetus and infant of psychotropic drug use during pregnancy. International Pharmacopsychiatry 11:246–260, 1976

Ananth J: Side effects in the neonate from psychotropic agents excreted through breast-feeding. Am J Psychiatry 135:801–805, 1978

Beeley L: Adverse effects of drugs in the first trimester of pregnancy. Clin Obstet Gynecol 13:177–195, 1986

Brazelton TB: Effect of prenatal drugs on the behavior of the neonate. Am J Psychiatry 126:1261–1266, 1970

Chao ST, Juchau MR: Placental drug metabolism, in Teratogenesis and Reproductive Toxicology. Edited by Johnson EM, Kochhar DM. New York, Springer-Verlag, 1983, pp 31–48

Cohen L: The use of psychotropic drugs during pregnancy and the puerperium. Currents in Affective Illness 11(9):5–13, 1992

Cohen LS, Heller VL, Rosenbaum JF: Treatment guidelines for psychotropic drug use in pregnancy. Psychosomatics 30:25–33, 1989

Cree JE, Meyer J, Hailey DM: Diazepam in labour: its metabolism and effect on the clinical condition and thermogenesis of the newborn. BMJ 4:251–255, 1973

Crombie DL, Pinsent RJ, Fleming DM, et al: Fetal effects of tranquilizers in pregnancy. N Engl J Med 293:198–199, 1975

Edlund MJ, Craig TJ: Antipsychotic drug use and birth defects: an epidemiologic reassessment. Compr Psychiatry 25:32–37, 1984

Edwards JG: Antidepressants and convulsions. Lancet 2:1368–1369, 1979

Eggermont E, Raveschot J, Deneve V, et al: The adverse influence of imipramine on the adaptation of the newborn infant to extrauterine life. Acta Paediatrica Belgica 26:197–204, 1972

Elia J, Katz IR, Simpson GM: Teratogenicity of psychotherapeutic medications. Psychopharmacol Bull 23:531–586, 1987

Fink M: Convulsive and drug therapies in depression. Annu Rev Med 32:405–412, 1981

Food and Drug Administration: Drug Bulletin. Washington, DC, September 1979, pp 22–23

Gelenberg AJ: When a woman taking lithium wants to have a baby. Biological Therapies in Psychiatry 6:19–20, 1983

Gelenberg AJ: Antidepressants in milk. Biological Therapies in Psychiatry 10:1, 1987

Gillberg C: "Floppy infant syndrome" and maternal diazepam (letter). Lancet 2:244, 1977

Goldberg HL, DiMascio A: Psychotropic drugs in pregnancy, in Psychopharmacology: A Generation of Progress. Edited by Lipton MA, DiMascio A, Killam KF. New York, Raven, 1978, pp 1047–1055

Heinonen OP, Slone D, Shapiro S: Birth Defects and Drugs in Pregnancy. Littleton, MA, Publishing Sciences Group, 1977

Hill RM, Stern L: Drugs in pregnancy: effects on the fetus and newborn. Drugs 17:182–197, 1979

Idanpaan-Heikkila J, Saxen L: Possible teratogenicity of imipramine-chloropyramine. Lancet 2:282–284, 1973

Jacobson J, Jones K, Johnson K, et al: Prospective multicentre study of pregnancy outcome after lithium exposure during first trimester. Lancet 339:530–533, 1992

Jick H: Early pregnancy and benzodiazepines (editorial). J Clin Psychopharmacol 8:159–160, 1988

Jones KL, Lacro RV, Johnson KA, et al: Pattern of malformations in the children of women treated with carbamazepine during pregnancy. N Engl J Med 320:1661–1666, 1989

Kallen B, Tandberg A: Lithium and pregnancy: a cohort study on manic depressive women. Acta Psychiatr Scand 68:134–139, 1983

Kanto JH: Use of benzodiazepines during pregnancy, labour, and lactation with particular reference to pharmacokinetic considerations. Drugs 23:354–380, 1982

Kerns LL: Treatment of mental disorders in pregnancy. J Nerv Ment Dis 174:652–659, 1986

Koplan CR: The use of psychotropic drugs during pregnancy and nursing, in The Practitioner's Guide to Psychiatric Drugs, 2nd Edition. Edited by Bassuk EL, Schoonover SC, Gelenberg AJ. New York, Plenum, 1983, pp 353–372

Kris EB: Children of mothers maintained on pharmacotherapy during pregnancy and postpartum. Current Therapeutic Research 7:785–789, 1965

Kuenssberg EV, Knox JD: Imipramine in pregnancy (letter). BMJ 2:292, 1972

Levy G: Pharmacokinetics of fetal and neonatal exposure to drugs. Obstet Gynecol 58(5) (suppl):9S–16S, 1981

Levy W, Wisniewski K: Chlorpromazine causing extrapyramidal dysfunction in newborn infants of psychotic mothers. N Y State J Med 74:684–685, 1974

MacKay AV, Loose R, Glen AI: Labour on lithium (letter). BMJ 1:878, 1976

Mandrelli M, Morselli P, Nordic S, et al: Placental transfer of diazepam and its deposition in the newborn. Clin Pharmacol Ther 17:564–572, 1975

Milkovich L, van den Berg BJ: Effects of prenatal meprobamate and chlordiazepoxide hydrochloride on human embryonic and fetal development. N Engl J Med 291:1268–1271, 1974

Milkovich L, van den Berg BJ: An evaluation of the teratogenicity of certain antinauseant drugs. Am J Obstet Gynecol 125:244–248, 1976

Mirkin BL: Drug disposition and therapy in the developing human being. Pediatr Ann 5:542–557, 1976

Morrell P, Sutherland GR, Buamah PK, et al: Lithium toxicity in a neonate. Arch Dis Child 58:538–539, 1983

Mortola JF: The use of psychotropic agents in pregnancy and lactation. Psychiatr Clin North Am 12:69–87, 1989

Nahas C, Goujard J: Phenothiazines, benzodiazepines and the fetus, in Reviews in Perinatal Medicine. Edited by Scarpelli EM, Cosini EV. New York, Raven, 1978, pp 243–280

Nars PW, Girard J: Lithium carbonate intake during pregnancy leading to large goiter in a premature infant. Am J Dis Child 131:924–925, 1977

National Institutes of Health Consensus Conference: Electroconvulsive therapy. JAMA 254:2103–2108, 1985

Nora JJ, Nora AH, Way GL: Cardiovascular maldevelopment associated with maternal exposure to amantadine (letter). Lancet 2:607, 1975

Nurnberg GH, Prudic J: Guidelines for treatment of psychosis during pregnancy. Hosp Community Psychiatry 35:67–71, 1984

Poulson E, Robson JM: Effect of phenelzine and some related compounds on pregnancy. J Endocrinol 30:205–215, 1964

Rayburn W, Wible-Kant J, Bledsoe J: Changing trends in drug use during pregnancy. J Reprod Med 27:569–575, 1982

Remick RA, Maurice WL: ECT in pregnancy. Am J Psychiatry 135:761–762, 1978

Robinson GE, Stewart DE, Flak E: The rational use of psychotropic drugs in pregnancy and postpartum. Can J Psychiatry 31:183–190, 1986

Rosenberg L, Mitchell AA, Parsells JL, et al: Lack of relation of oral clefts to diazepam use during pregnancy. N Engl J Med 309:1282–1285, 1983

Rumeau-Rouquette C, Goujard J, Huel C: Possible teratogenic effects of phenothiazines in human beings. Teratology 15:57–64, 1977

Safra MD, Oakley GP: Association between cleft lip with or without cleft palate and prenatal exposure to diazepam. Lancet 2:478–540, 1975

Schiff D, Chan G, Stern L: Fixed drug combinations and the displacement of bilirubin from albumin. Pediatrics 8:139–141, 1971

Schou M: What happened later to the lithium babies? follow-up study of children born without malformations. Acta Psychiatr Scand 54:193–197, 1976

Schou M, Amdisen A: Lithium and pregnancy: lithium ingestion by children breast-fed by women on lithium treatment. BMJ 2:138, 1973

Scokel PW, Jones WD: Infant jaundice after phenothiazine drugs for labor: an enigma. Obstet Gynecol 20:124–127, 1962

Shearer WT, Schreiner RL, Marshall RE: Urinary retention in a neonate secondary to maternal ingestion of nortriptyline. J Pediatr 81:570–572, 1972

Slone D, Suskind V, Heinonen OP, et al: Antenatal exposure to the phenothiazines in relation to congenital malformations, perinatal mortality, birth weight and intelligence quotient score. Am J Obstet Gynecol 128:486–488, 1977

Sobel DE: Fetal damage due to ECT, insulin coma, chlorpromazine or reserpine. Arch Gen Psychiatry 2:606–611, 1960

Sovner R, Orsulak PJ: Excretion of imipramine and desipramine in human breast milk. Am J Psychiatry 136:451–452, 1979

Stewart DE: Schizophrenia and pregnancy. Canadian Family Physician 30:1537–1542, 1984

Stewart DE: Prophylactic lithium in postpartum affective psychosis. J Nerv Ment Dis 176:485–489, 1988

Tamer A, McKay R, Arias D, et al: Phenothiazine induced extrapyramidal dysfunction in the neonate. J Pediatr 7:479–480, 1969

Tunnessen WW Jr, Hertz CG: Toxic effects of lithium in newborn infants: a commentary. J Pediatr 81:804–807, 1972

Volpe JJ: Teratogenic effects of drugs and passive addiction, in Neurology of the Newborn. Edited by Volpe JJ. Philadelphia, PA, WB Saunders, 1981, pp 601–635

Vorhees CV, Butcher RE: Behavioral teratogenicity, in Developmental Toxicology. Edited by Snell K. New York, Praeger, 1982, pp 249–298

Webster PAC: Withdrawal symptoms in neonates associated with maternal antidepressant therapy. Lancet 2:318–319, 1973

Weinstein MR: Lithium treatment of women during pregnancy and in the post-delivery period, in Handbook of Lithium Therapy. Edited by Johnson FN. Lancaster, UK, MTP Press, 1980, pp 421–429

Whalley LJ, Blain PG, Prime JK: Haloperidol secreted in breast milk. BMJ 282:1746–1747, 1981

Wilson JG: Current status of teratology: general principles and mechanisms derived from animal studies, in Handbook of Teratology: General Principles and Etiology, Vol 1. Edited by Wilson JG, Fraser FC. New York, Plenum, 1977, pp 47–74

Wilson N, Forfar JC, Godman MJ: Atrial flutter in the newborn resulting from maternal lithium ingestion. Arch Dis Child 58:538–549, 1983

Wise MG, Ward SC, Townsend-Parchman W, et al: Case report of ECT during high-risk pregnancy. Am J Psychiatry 141:99–101, 1984

Wisner KL, Perel JM: Psychopharmacologic agents and electroconvulsive therapy during pregnancy and the puerperium, in Psychiatric Consultation in Childbirth Settings. Edited by Cohen RL. New York, Plenum, 1988, pp 165–206

Wrede G, Mednick SA, Huttenen MO, et al: Pregnancy and delivery complications in the births of an unselected series of Finnish children with schizophrenic mothers. Acta Psychiatr Scand 62:369–381, 1980

Zalzstein E, Koren G, Einarson T, et al: A case-control study on the association between first trimester exposure to lithium and Epstein's anomaly. Am J Cardiol 65:817–818, 1990

Chapter 6

ADOLESCENT PREGNANCY

Miriam B. Rosenthal, M.D.

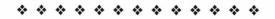

Paris
  But now, my Lord, what say you to my suit?
Capulet
  But saying o'er what I have said before:
  My child is yet a stranger in the world,
  She hath not seen the change of fourteen years;
  Let two more summers wither in their pride,
  Ere we may think her ripe to be a bride.
Paris
  Younger than she are happy mothers made.
Capulet
  And too soon marr'd are those so early made.

The Tragedy of Romeo and Juliet, Act I, Scene ii
William Shakespeare

Adolescent pregnancy is a complex subject reaching far beyond the elaborate statistics and extensive media campaigns that exhort teenagers to say "no" to sexual activity, even while such behaviors are promoted on television and in advertising. The pregnancy rate for young women age 19 years and younger in the United States is one of the highest among the industrialized nations of the world. The costs on personal, social, and economic levels are immense, because most of these pregnancies are consciously unplanned and unintended. Adolescent pregnancy constitutes a major

97

health dilemma as well as a challenge to mental health professionals to join with their obstetric colleagues and others in an effort to help young people enhance their control over their reproductive lives.

During adolescence, or perhaps more precisely the "teenage years" from ages 13–19, puberty occurs, representing one of the three major biologically determined maturational crises in women, along with pregnancy and menopause (Bibring et al. 1961; Nadelson et al. 1978). Pregnant girls, especially the younger ones, face two of these major developmental milestones at the same time that they are struggling to separate from parents and to find their way in the adult world. Although they have these circumstances in common, they bring to them other particular biopsychosocial individualities. Spurlock and Robinowitz (1986, p. 401) pointed out that adolescents "don't live in a vacuum, but some live in stable families, some have been adopted at birth or abandoned, some have experienced good health and good fortune, while others have been subjected to abuse and illness." They vary greatly in size, shape, personal interactions, and the social systems in which they exist.

Historians believe that pregnancy did not occur despite high levels of sexual activity among young people in many primitive societies because these were years of subfertility (Konner and Shostak 1986). There have been debates over whether adolescence as a developmental stage was recognized in the past as it is today. Some scholars of family development believe that this stage is a concept of the late 19th and 20th centuries as the life span was lengthening, puberty was occurring earlier, and agricultural societies were evolving into industrial ones, where adolescents had a more ambiguous role (Vinovskis 1986). This age group, representing the bridge between childhood and adulthood, was often defined by social and economic status rather than chronological age.

A major problem in looking over the vast literature on adolescence is that females ages 13–19 years are often grouped together despite considerable biological, psychological, and social variations. Hamburg (1986) emphasized that there are three societal constructs and definitions of age. *Chronological age* is the number of years from birth, on which many major life events, such as entering school, voting, getting a driver's license, and entering military service, are based.

Biological age refers to the degree of physical maturity and the changes of puberty, growth, and development. Finally, *social age* is the time when "cultural milestones are achieved" for societal norms, such as leaving home, marrying, and assuming adult work roles.

This chapter addresses some of the issues surrounding adolescent pregnancy and childbearing, the scope of the problem, precursors and consequences for the mother, effects on the offspring, adolescent fathers, and finally, strategies for prevention.

SCOPE OF THE PROBLEM

Each year in the United States, approximately 1 million teenagers ages 15–19 become pregnant, a figure that remained fairly constant since the 1970s, but began to rise in the late 1980s. The births to teens under age 15 was 10,169 in 1980 and 10,588 in 1988. In 1985, there were 477,710 live births and 416,170 induced abortions; the rest of these pregnancies ended in miscarriages or stillbirths. Young women under age 20 accounted for 26% of all induced abortions and 13% of all births (Henshaw and Van Vort 1989; National Center for Health Statistics 1985). In 1987, 18% of pregnancies to women under age 20 resulted in planned births, 40% in unplanned births, and 42% in induced abortions (National Center for Health Statistics 1985, 1987, 1988, 1989).

The rates of teenage pregnancy, childbearing, and induced abortion are higher in the United States than in most industrialized nations, including Canada, England, Wales, Sweden, the Netherlands, and France. This is especially surprising because the best estimates indicate that there are similar rates of sexual activity among teenagers in those countries. Sex education and contraceptives are more widely available to youth in those countries than in the United States. These measures presumably have had a distinct influence on lowering rates of teenage pregnancy and induced abortion as well as sexually transmitted diseases (Jones 1986). In 1985, costs for public assistance to families begun by a teenage parent totaled $16.65 billion (aid to families of dependent children, Medicaid, and food stamps) (Federman 1990).

PUBERTY

Puberty is a major developmental transition from childhood to adulthood in the life cycle. It is the period during which males and females experience a growth spurt, the appearance of secondary sex characteristics, the beginning of the ability to reproduce, and major psychological changes. The hypothalamic-pituitary-gonadotropin axis is developed and functional during fetal life and earliest infancy. It remains suppressed until the onset of puberty. In girls, the axis becomes reactivated with the secretion of gonadotropin-releasing hormone. Levels of follicle-stimulating hormone and luteinizing hormone begin to rise, accompanied by an increase in estradiol. With rising amounts of gonadal estrogens, breast development starts and female fat distribution occurs, along with vaginal and uterine growth. Skeletal growth occurs in response to estrogens. *Adrenarche* refers to adrenal androgens that, along with gonadal androgens, cause pubic and axillary hair growth. At midpuberty, estrogen levels are high enough to bring about endometrial proliferation, and the first menses occur. The first periods after menarche are usually anovulatory (Speroff et al. 1989).

The average age at puberty and menarche in the general population has been declining over the past several years, a trend that is thought to be due to overall improvements in socioeconomic conditions, nutrition, and general health. In the United States, the median age at menarche is 12.8 years, and fertility occurs about 1 year later. The normal pubertal age range in girls is 9.1–17.7 years. Although anovulation can last 12–18 months after menarche, pregnancies have been reported even before the onset of menses. The average age of first conscious ejaculation in boys is reported as 14.3 years (Laron et al. 1980), although this has not been well studied.

The onset of menses is a dramatic event for girls. The timing of pubertal events varies widely; girls who perceive that they have been "on time" in terms of pubertal events and physical maturation have a more positive body image and feel more physically attractive than early or late maturers. The early-maturing girls often have the least positive view of their bodies, whereas many girls of all ages have been found to feel positive about having breast development. Girls value being thin or of average weight. Another contribution to positive self-image and self-esteem in girls is the acceptance of pubertal change and sexuality within the family. The father is especially important in helping a girl to establish a feminine sense of self, and the mother is influential in offering sex education (Hamburg 1986). The changes of puberty require complex adjustments that may be accompanied by considerable stress and demand a whole new set of behaviors. Deferment of sexual behaviors has been correlated with better cognitive development (Offer 1986). It is essential for the clinician working with adolescent pregnant girls and their infants to be aware of their physical and psychological stage of development in relation to norms.

ETIOLOGY OF ADOLESCENT PREGNANCY

Lack of knowledge about and lack of use of contraceptives are not the only factors contributing to the high rates of adolescent pregnancy, although they are certainly major ones. Because menarche is occurring earlier in the general population, a much longer time span elapses between the onset of biological maturity and the assumption of adult roles, such as finishing school and marrying. Coital activity among young people is steadily increasing. In 1970, 28% of girls ages 15–19 years had had sexual intercourse. This number rose to 51% by 1988 (Centers for Disease Control 1991). Children are exposed daily to sexual encounters by attractive people on television, in magazines, and in advertising generally. A study by Louis Harris and associates found that 65,000 sexual references were broadcast each year during afternoon and prime-time evening hours on television, although there were virtually no examples of references to contraceptive use ("A Study Has Found a Barrage of Sex on TV" 1988).

Although much of the literature stresses the level of sexual activity and the absent or erratic use of contraception among teenagers, much less has been published about some of the psychological aspects of what motivates them to become pregnant. For many girls, living in poverty with relatively few future-oriented goals related to education or career, the bringing of a baby into the home usually occasions a great deal of joy. Sex education courses in junior high schools usually emphasize the physiology of sex and include very little discussion of the responsibilities of sexuality, what it is like to raise a child, or practicing family planning through the use of birth control and induced abortion. When first starting their sexual lives, many adolescents do not consider themselves as sexual persons and do not believe that they will become pregnant. Their first sexual encounters are usually unplanned and unprotected.

Psychodynamic theory has contributed to our thinking about teenagers' motivations for becoming pregnant, yet this body of knowledge is not often cited. The wish for a pregnancy is not the same as the wish for a baby or a child. A pregnancy may be desired to ensure that one's body works correctly and that one has a female identity with a functioning reproductive system. Having such a sense can enhance self-esteem, as may be the case for some young women with chronic illnesses who have been warned that pregnancy would be dangerous to their health:

> M. is a 16-year-old, single, high school student who has had diabetes since age 8. She is now 12 weeks pregnant. Because many of her friends were having babies, she needed to be reassured that she could do what they could do. She did not have any counseling regarding the use of contraception or sexual activity. Her clinic doctor told her, "Don't get pregnant; your diabetes will get much worse." She has chosen to continue her pregnancy.

These young women need good counseling regarding sexuality. In addition to the wish for a pregnancy, there may be the conscious wish for a baby and the pleasure it may bring to the family. Some girls may be unconsciously fulfilling the desire of their mothers for more children. This is sometimes seen after the mother has had a hysterectomy or has undergone menopause. Other conscious or unconscious motivations may be rebellion against parents, a response to the loss of a close person or of some important aspect of their lives (Rosenthal and Rothchild 1975), or a response to loneliness, with the idea that the baby will "love me." There can be identification with the fantasied child or concerns about retaining a partner and maintaining a relationship. Pregnancy may be the way to separate from one's parents or to resolve competitive feelings with parents. The possible reasons are many; this is an area needing a great deal more research, with considerable emphasis on the psychodynamics of pregnancy motivations, not just on the biology of contraceptive use (Nadelson et al. 1978).

Some pregnancies occur as a result of incest, sexual abuse, or rape. Patients and their families are often reluctant to discuss these issues or to reveal the true state of affairs to clinical staff. Those who work with adolescents are well aware that these are not rare occurrences. There is a need for better identification of these girls, and even more to determine what kind of sensitive interventions can help them.

Experiences in European countries and Canada have shown that, if adolescents are informed and counseled regarding contraception, many will use it. Five million teenagers were sexually active in the United States in 1981. Of the 57% who received family planning services, 30% went to clinics and 21% went to private doctors (Federman 1990). Access to clinics where teenagers can get birth control services is limited. There is considerable controversy about school-based health clinics and storefront family planning clinics. Physicians may not accept Medicaid patients or may not treat teenagers without parental consent. Many adolescents believe that birth control pills are harmful to health, and in addition, oral contraceptives require a visit to a doctor, a prescription, and money to buy them. In actuality, morbidity associated with adolescent pregnancy is higher than that of pill use. A very successful experiment in providing health services for adolescents in high schools was piloted in Baltimore, Maryland, at Johns Hopkins University. Services included contraceptives. The pregnancy rate was reduced considerably, but the programs were discontinued (Zabin et al. 1988). The challenge here is to be able to provide access to medical services that include protection from unwanted pregnancy and sexually transmitted diseases for sexually active teenagers (Goldstein 1980; Hatcher 1986; Miller 1986).

An important feature in understanding the medical care and treatment of adolescents is that those under age 18 are minors and, as such, are not legally able to consent to medical treatments except in special circumstances. These exceptions include 1) being emancipated, which means that they are married or self-supporting, and 2) special circumstances, including treatment for sexually transmitted

diseases, intervention for drug or alcohol abuse or conditions resulting from such abuse, or examinations if sexual assault or abuse is suspected, as in Ohio. Parenthood alone does not legally entitle a minor
to consent to her own treatment.

THE PREGNANT ADOLESCENT: ANTENATAL PSYCHIATRIC CONSIDERATIONS

Hamburg (1986) has suggested that pregnant adolescents can be classified into three subsets. The first group are *problem prone*. These girls
have a number of problems and may abuse alcohol and drugs, drop
out of school, or run away from home. They are at highest risk for
pregnancy because of their personalities, risk-taking behaviors, and
environmental situation. Some of the behaviors may help them
achieve otherwise unobtainable goals, to act as a learned way of coping with frustrations and repeated failures, to oppose conventional societal norms, to get through the developmental transitions of early
life, and to belong to a peer group that gives them support and suste-
nance. Hamburg believes that problem proneness and school-age
pregnancy ought to be combined into a syndrome recognized by psychiatrists and mental health workers.

The second subset of adolescent mothers are called *adequate copers*.
These girls have been moving through adolescence steadily and manage to keep their lives going. Their mothers may also have experienced early childbearing. They continue in school and continue to
have future goals. They take care of the children they have or arrange
for their care. They may belong to a culture where early childbearing
is a viable and accepted alternative. An urban black mother, for instance, may have children in her teens, finish school and build a career in her 20s, and consolidate career and family in her 30s.

The third subset of adolescent mothers are *depressed*. This subset
has not been well studied and is often not recognized, because the
pregnancy may mask the depression. The usual signs and symptoms of
depression, such as mood and vegetative changes, may not be evident.
Depressive mood is often the start of drug use or other adolescent
risk-taking behaviors. Cutrona (1982) noted that in about 8%–9% of

pregnant adolescents, severe depressive symptoms were noted prior to the pregnancy. These symptoms included feeling very unhappy, worthless, guilty, and occasionally suicidal, as well as having disturbances of sleep, eating, energy, and concentration. She considers these adolescents to be severely depressed and believes many more to have milder degrees of mood disturbances. For adolescents, pregnancy may be one way of dealing with depression.

Other special populations of pregnant teenagers, including those with mental disorders such as schizophrenia or psychotic disorders, as well as those who are mentally retarded, require specialized study and clinical attention.

DECISION MAKING IN ADOLESCENT PREGNANCY

When an adolescent first suspects that she is pregnant, she often feels denial and disbelief. She may avoid telling anyone or may be very dependent on her family or a boyfriend. The father, who is likely to be an adolescent male unprepared to deal with parenthood, often withdraws from her at this time. The parents may have emotional, financial, and social resources to help her or may be absent, unavailable, overwhelmed, angry, punitive, or abusive.

Pregnant adolescents often present for prenatal care later in pregnancy. They may deny their pregnancies, either consciously or unconsciously (Milden et al. 1985), until the second or third trimester or even until labor and delivery. This delay is associated with increased obstetric and perinatal morbidity. Good prenatal care often leads to outcomes for adolescents and their babies that are equally as good as those for older women. Early recognition is also essential, though often lacking, to give the young woman a chance to make a decision about whether to continue the pregnancy, to give the baby up for adoption, or to terminate the pregnancy by induced abortion. About half the pregnancies in the United States to teenagers ages 19 years and younger end in induced abortion. Teenagers who have chosen abortion do not appear to have any increase in psychological morbidity and may feel more in control of their lives (Adler et al. 1990). The pregnant adolescent should have an opportunity to discuss her options, including abortion (Luker 1975), with a nonjudgmental counselor, physician, or nurse who can talk to her alone and with the father of the baby, or with a parent or guardian if the adolescent agrees. Decision making in general is often difficult enough for the adolescent, but a decision concerning whether to keep or to end a pregnancy is especially troublesome, because ambivalence about the pregnancy is normal. Adolescents, in particular, do not have very mature cognitive processes with which to handle such a decision. Janis (1982) described five patterns of coping with decisions:

1. Unconflicting inertia in which all new information is ignored
2. Unconflicted change in which any new course of action is undertaken without careful consideration; panic may replace thought
3. Defensive avoidance in which decision making is avoided altogether; someone else may make the decisions
4. Hypervigilance, when there is even more panic than with unconflicted change
5. Vigilance and logic, where adequate knowledge and consideration are used to come to a conclusion

The last pattern, although the most desirable, is often the least likely to be seen in most adolescents, particularly young ones. Girls in junior high school still use fairly concrete reasoning and have a narrowed ability to perceive alternatives. They often overlook long-term consequences and distort expected outcomes. They may make quick decisions because they take the advice of friends without thinking critically. They also generalize about what they think everyone else is doing, often with considerable error. They may be very egocentric and feel they are invulnerable. Despite their biologically mature appearance, they may be socially very immature (Hamburg 1986).

Some of the areas to be covered in interviewing adolescents considering abortion are as follows (Rosenthal and Rothchild 1975):

❖ Pregnancy
   1. Was there a conscious wish to be pregnant?
   2. Have there been any recent life events that may have played a role?
   3. Have there been previous pregnancies or induced abortions?

4. What emotional and physical symptoms have been experienced during this pregnancy?
5. What is her attitude about this pregnancy?
6. What is the attitude of the father and of her parents?
7. Is there a history of losses, psychiatric problems, or family difficulties?
8. Has she used contraception?
9. What is her relationship to the baby's father?

❖ Induced abortion
1. What are reasons that might support it—or oppose it?
2. Who wants it (i.e., patient, partner, mother, father)?
3. How were her decisions reached?
4. What are the alternatives?
5. What will be done if abortion is unavailable?
6. How well does she understand what is involved in induced abortion?
7. Are there religious feelings about abortion?

❖ Adoption: Has she considered this as an option?

❖ General functioning
1. How is present functioning at home and school, and what are school grades?
2. Does she have friends?
3. Is there a need for further counseling?

It is helpful to have the patient consider each option and go over it in careful detail as if she had chosen that alternative. If abortion is chosen, some time should be allowed for consideration before the procedure is done. It may be helpful to have her write down the pros and cons to look back on at a later time.

Because induced abortion requires surgical intervention, and reproductive decision making is of major importance, there are those who strongly advocate parental involvement when minors are to undergo such procedures. At this time, 10 states require parental consent for minors to receive abortions, and 5 require parents to be notified.

Federal courts have upheld the mandatory notification of parents provided that a judicial bypass is available. Minnesota requires both parents of a minor requesting abortion to be notified, even if the parents are divorced or have never married. They must be told by certified mail, unless the minor wishes to go to court instead (Blum et al. 1990).

Younger pregnant minors are more likely to involve their parents than older ones. Mothers of pregnant minors are the most likely of the two parents to be involved in the decision-making process. Some of the reasons for avoiding parental notification are absent fathers, severe family stresses other than the minor's pregnancy, family violence, drug or alcohol abuse in the family, and feelings of having "betrayed" the family by becoming pregnant. When states with and without parental notification laws were compared, there seemed to be no difference in the number of adolescents who told their parents. One of the major problems with the law in Minnesota is that it undermines the authority of the one parent who may be most involved with the minor, since the other parent must be found and informed, even in single-parent homes (Blum et al. 1990; Melton et al. 1987).

In Ohio, parental notification laws for minors requesting abortion were passed in 1985 with a judicial bypass mechanism. Under these laws, the judge must hear the case within 5 working days and decide whether the adolescent is mature enough to make the decision and that the procedure is in her best interest. Although the law was passed in 1985, it did not go into effect until October 5, 1990, because of reviews in the U.S. Supreme Court. The term "maturity" is not defined in the statutes and has presented difficulties for the courts, although the Ohio Valley Chapter of the Society for Adolescent Medicine has suggested that characteristics of maturity include a minor who is age 15 years or older, a minor who understands the risks and benefits of the procedure and of carrying the pregnancy to term, the abortion is consistent with good medical judgment, and a minor who has accepted responsibility in other aspects of her life (Rauh 1991).

Prenatal Care

Good prenatal care reduces morbidity and mortality for mother and infant: "a review of more than 55 studies by OTA revealed that the weight of evidence supports the contention that two key birth outcomes—low birth weight and neonatal mortality—can be improved with earlier and more comprehensive prenatal care, especially in high-risk groups such as adolescents and poor women" (Klerman 1990, p. 105). In 1987 in the United States, 10 out of every 1,000 newborns died. The neonatal death rate was 8.6 per 1,000 births for whites and 18 per 1,000 births for blacks. This high rate is largely due to the birth of low–birth-weight babies. Adolescents are at extremely high risk for having low–birth-weight infants unless they receive good, early care. Fourteen percent of low–birth-weight infants in the United States are born to adolescents under age 15 years, and another 9.3% are born to girls ages 15–19 years. Some of the other risks for adolescents during pregnancy are toxemia, anemia, premature labor, and more obstetric complications. Prenatal care with good medical intervention and the ability to encourage good nutrition and healthy behaviors can reverse the poor outcomes (Klerman 1990). At University MacDonald Women's Hospital in Cleveland, Ohio, there has been success with special prenatal clinics for pregnant teenagers, with hours after school and groups for the prospective fathers led by a social worker who enjoys working with adolescents.

The obstacles to prenatal care include the inability to pay, a shortage of clinics, doctors who do not accept Medicaid patients, restriction of nurse-midwives, lack of transportation to clinics, inconvenient clinic hours (during school hours), long waiting times, and staff attitudes. Some reasons patients give for not obtaining prenatal care are cultural inhibitions and fear. Some women who use drugs or alcohol fear they will get into trouble with the law or have their babies taken from them if they come to prenatal clinics and their substance abuse is discovered. Further research on how to improve prenatal care and make it more widely available is desperately needed (Klerman 1990).

There should be a liaison psychiatrist available in prenatal clinics to consult with staff, to see patients referred to them by the staff, and to participate in discussions about how to help teenagers with problem behaviors, difficulty with family and boyfriends, mental symptoms, and fears. The prevention of further psychological difficulties could be begun in such a setting. Groups for adolescent parents, for adolescent fathers, and for grandmothers raising children of adolescent parents are often very helpful. The mental health professionals in such settings should have some expertise in adolescent psychiatry and family systems, as well as general consultation-liaison psychiatry.

CHILDREN OF TEENAGE PARENTS

Although there are some general data concerning the outcomes for offspring of teenage mothers, considerable differences exist among this group, depending on culture, socioeconomic status, and the nature of the family rearing the children. In some studies, infants raised in homes with a single parent, with a nuclear family, and with extended families have been compared. It is not clear whether grandmothers' care leads to better outcomes.

Overall, babies of adolescent mothers have poorer health (Federman 1990), less verbal stimulation (Field et al. 1986; Osofsky and Osofsky 1970), and developmental delays. Preschoolers do less well, and school-age children have more school problems and more cognitive difficulties (Field et al. 1986). As adolescents, they have more problems with anger control, fearfulness, feelings of inferiority, behavior problems in school, substance abuse, and early sexual activity. One study found that one-third of daughters of adolescent mothers had become pregnant themselves before age 20 years (Furstenberg 1976). Adolescent mothers are often poor and poorly educated, conditions that affect their offspring. When adolescent mothers are helped to find some financial security, complete their educations, and see their way to a productive future, the children fare much better.

PREVENTION OF ADOLESCENT PREGNANCY

All pregnancies should be wanted and planned, but this goal is obviously unrealistic and does not take into account the many psychological features of reproductive life. For teenagers, sexual activity and subsequent pregnancies may indeed alter their goals, their relationships, and their chances for taking control of their futures. For their offspring, the outcome varies. Psychological variables must be considered along with biological and social factors in addressing this subject. This is a field rich in research possibilities.

To make more reasonable social policy to reduce the pregnancy rate among adolescents, an Alan Guttmacher Institute study (Jones 1986) recommends that some of the first steps should be to dispel the myths surrounding teenage childbearing in this country. It is not true that the high rate of teenage pregnancy in the United States is due only to high pregnancy rates among minority teenagers. American adolescents do not start sexual activity earlier or have more sexual activity than do their counterparts in other developed nations. Not all adolescents are too immature to use contraception effectively. Single mothers are rarely motivated to have babies in order to get public assistance. The provision of contraceptive and abortion services has not been shown to increase promiscuity among young people; rather, it has been shown to decrease the pregnancy rate (Zabin et al. 1988).

Some of the major strategies proposed by interdisciplinary conferences and the literature consist of providing accessible, affordable, and high-quality health services to adolescents; providing sex education that includes the psychological aspects of sexuality, contraception, and pregnancy (Marsiglio and Mott 1986; Roberts 1980); and improving the responsibility of the media in providing adolescents with proper information in regard to sex and contraception and the consequences of early childbearing. For the young woman who is already pregnant, good prenatal care should be available. Adolescent fathers need to be included and should take part in the health care plan during the pregnancy and afterward (Elster and Lamb 1986).

Some of the areas that need further research are adolescent behaviors, including sexuality and use of contraception; relationships in the family, communication regarding sexuality, the enhancement of self-esteem, and creation of future goals; the behaviors and concerns of young men regarding relationships and sexuality; and the influence of school performance. Studies of the offspring of adolescent mothers and parenting issues are of importance. A major area to be emphasized is the influence of incest, sexual abuse, and domestic violence on children and adolescents and how these affect early childbearing. Adolescent pregnancy is a major policy issue—medically, psychiatrically, and socially—in the United States.

REFERENCES

A study has found a barrage of sex on TV. New York Times, January 27, 1988

Adler NE, David HP, Major BN, et al: Psychological response after abortion. Science 248:41–43, 1990

Bibring G, Dwyer T, Huntington D, et al: A study of the earliest mother/child relationship. Psychoanal Study Child 16:9–72, 1961

Blum RW, Resnick MD, Stark T: Factors associated with the use of court bypass by minors to obtain abortions. Fam Plann Perspect 22:158–160, 1990

Centers for Disease Control: Premarital sexual experience among adolescent women—United States, 1970–1988. MMWR 39:929–932, 1991

Cutrona C: Non-psychotic postpartum depression: a review of recent research. Clinical Psychology Review 2:487–503, 1982

Elster AB, Lamb M: Adolescent fathers: the understudied side of adolescent pregnancy, in School-Age Pregnancy and Parenthood: Biosocial Dimensions. Edited by Lancaster JB, Hamburg BA. New York, Aldine De Gruyter, 1986, pp 177–190

Federman D: The dilemma of teenage parenthood, in Science and Babies: Private Decisions, Public Dilemmas. Washington, DC, Institute of Medicine, National Academy Press, 1990

Field T, Widmayer S, Stoller S, et al: School-age parenthood in different ethnic groups and family constellations: effects on infant development, in School-Age Pregnancy and Parenthood: Biosocial Dimensions. Edited by Lancaster JB, Hamburg BA. New York, Aldine De Gruyter, 1986, pp 263–272

Furstenberg F: The social consequences of teenage pregnancy. Fam Plann Perspect 8:148–164, 1976

Goldstein D: Contraceptive counseling for teenagers. Medical Aspects of Human Sexuality 14:23–24, 1980

Hamburg B: Subsets of adolescent mothers: developmental, biomedical, and psychosocial issues, in School-Age Pregnancy and Parenthood. Edited by Lancaster JB, Hamburg BA. New York, Aldine De Gruyter, 1986, pp 115–145

Hatcher R: Contraceptive Technology: 1986–1987. New York, Irvington, 1986

Henshaw SK, Van Vort J: Teenage abortion, birth and pregnancy statistics: an update. Fam Plann Perspect 21:85–88, 1989

Janis IL: Decision making under stress, in Handbook of Stress: Theoretical and Clinical Aspects. Edited by Goldberger L, Breznitz S. New York, Free Press, 1982, pp 69–87

Jones E: Teenage Pregnancy in Industrialized Countries: A Study Sponsored by the Alan Guttmacher Institute. New Haven, CT, Yale University Press, 1986

Klerman L: Prenatal care, in Science and Babies: Private Decisions, Public Dilemmas. Edited by Wymelenberg S. Washington, DC, Institute of Medicine, National Academy Press, 1990, pp 96–125

Konner M, Shostak M: Adolescent pregnancy and childbearing: an anthropological perspective, in School-Age Pregnancy and Parenthood: Biosocial Dimensions. Edited by Lancaster JB, Hamburg BA. New York, Aldine De Gruyter, 1986, pp 325–345

Laron Z, Arad J, Gurewitz R, et al: Age at first conscious ejaculation: milestones in male puberty. Helvetica Paediatrica Acta 35:13–20, 1980

Luker K: Taking chances. Berkeley, University of California Press, 1975

Marsiglio W, Mott F: The impact of sex education on sexual activity, contraceptive use and premarital pregnancy among American teenagers. Fam Plann Perspect 18:151–162, 1986

Melton G, Adler N, David HP, et al: Adolescent abortion: psychological and legal issues. Am Psychol 42:73–78, 1987

Milden R, Rosenthal M, Winegardner J, et al: Denial of pregnancy: an exploratory investigation. Journal of Psychosomatic Obstetrics and Gynaecology 4:255–261, 1985

Miller W: Why some women fail to use their contraceptive method: a psychological investigation. Fam Plann Perspect 18:27–32, 1986

Nadelson C, Notman M, Gillon J: Adolescent sexuality and pregnancy, in The Woman Patient, Vol 1: Sexual and Reproductive Aspects of Women's Health Care. Edited by Notman M, Nadelson C. New York, Plenum, 1978, pp 123–130

National Center for Health Statistics: Advance report of final natality statistics, 1985. Monthly Vital Statistics Report. Hyattsville, MD, National Center for Health Statistics

National Center for Health Statistics: Advance report of final natality statistics, 1987. Monthly Vital Statistics Report, Vol 36. Hyattsville, MD, National Center for Health Statistics

National Center for Health Statistics: Advance report of final natality statistics, 1988. Monthly Vital Statistics Report, Vol 37. Hyattsville, MD, National Center for Health Statistics

National Center for Health Statistics: Advance report of final natality statistics, 1989. Monthly Vital Statistics Report, Vol 40, suppl 8. Hyattsville, MD, Public Health Service, 1991, pp 20–21 (Table 4)

Offer D: Adolescent development: a normative perspective, in Psychiatry Update: American Psychiatric Association Annual Review, Vol 5. Edited by Frances AJ, Hales RE. Washington, DC, American Psychiatric Press, 1986, pp 404–419

Osofsky H, Osofsky J: Adolescents as mother: results of a program for low income pregnant teenagers with some emphasis upon infants' development. Am J Orthopsychiatry 40:825–834, 1970

Rauh JL: Ohio's parental notification of abortion law: one doctor's experience. Ohio Valley Chapter of the Society for Adolescent Medicine, February/March, 1991

Roberts EJ: Sex education versus sexual learning, in Women's Sexual Development: Explorations of Inner Space. Edited by Kirkpatrick M. New York, Plenum, 1980, pp 239–250

Rosenthal M, Rothchild E: Some psychological considerations in adolescent pregnancy and abortion. Advances in Planned Parenthood 9:3–4, 60–69, 1975

Speroff L, Glass H, Kase N: Clinical Gynecology, Endocrinology, and Infertility. Baltimore, MD, Williams & Wilkins, 1989

Spurlock J, Robinowitz CB: Foreword to Section IV: adolescent psychiatry, in Psychiatry Update: American Psychiatric Association Annual Review, Vol 5. Edited by Francis AJ, Hales RE. Washington, DC, American Psychiatric Press, 1986, pp 401–403

Vinovskis M: Adolescent sexuality, pregnancy and childbearing in early America: some preliminary speculations, in School-Age Pregnancy and Parenthood: Biosocial Dimensions. Edited by Lancaster JB, Hamburg BA. New York, Aldine De Gruyter, 1986, pp 303–322

Zabin LS, Hirsch MB, Street MR, et al: The Baltimore pregnancy prevention program for urban teenagers, I: how did it work? II: what did it cost? Fam Plann Perspect 20:182–192, 1988

Chapter 7

Postpartum Disorders

Gail Erlick Robinson, M.D., F.R.C.P.C.
Donna E. Stewart, M.D., D.Psych., F.R.C.P.C.

❖ ❖ ❖ ❖ ❖ ❖ ❖ ❖ ❖ ❖ ❖ ❖ ❖ ❖

Mental disturbance following childbirth was first mentioned by Hippocrates, but the first good clinical description of postpartum psychosis was written by a French psychiatrist, Louis Marcé, in 1858. There was little interest in this disorder until Paffenberger (1961) showed that admission to mental hospitals was enormously increased during the first month postpartum and Hamilton (1962) argued that puerperal psychosis was a distinct disorder. Psychological disturbances can occur in the postpartum period in the form of maternity ("baby") blues, postnatal depression, or psychosis. Although any psychiatric disorder may present or recur in the postpartum period, it is clear that affective disorders are most common. Not uncommonly seen after delivery, however, are adjustment and attachment disorders, schizophrenia, obsessive-compulsive disorder, and anxiety disorders.

Postpartum Adaptation

The postpartum period involves numerous physiological, psychological, and sociocultural changes. All of these have been investigated as possible etiologic factors in postpartum disorders.

Biological Factors

Dramatic changes in hormone and electrolyte balance and fluid volume occur during labor and the postpartum period. After birth, levels of both progesterone and estriol rapidly fall, returning to prepregnancy levels by 3 days after delivery. When estrogen levels fall after birth, prolactin, levels of which have risen during pregnancy, is no longer blocked and lactation is initiated. Suckling by the infant stimulates the secretion of oxytocin. The usual cyclic variation of androgens is absent during both pregnancy and lactation. Plasma corticosteroid levels reach a peak during labor and decrease significantly within 4 hours postpartum. Thyroid function returns to prepregnancy levels approximately 4 weeks after delivery. Beta-endorphin levels rise during labor, reaching a peak immediately before delivery and declining after parturition. Plasma renin levels fall after childbirth. Several days after birth, a rapid weight loss occurs. Sodium excretion rises, and calcium excretion falls.

Various methodologic problems have hampered studies of the biologic basis of postpartum disorders. Early researchers could not accurately assay hormones, particularly free, unbound plasma concentrations. Rating scales used in various studies differed; some, confounded by the normal physical symptoms of the puerperium, were obviously inappropriate measures of maternal mental illness. Blood sampling often took place at inappropriate times, ignoring activities such as breast-feeding, which can alter levels of some hormones. Seasonal variations in hormones and circadian rhythmicity were often overlooked. Studies that examined one particular hormone in isolation were also inadequate because of complex endocrine interrelationships.

Psychosocial Factors

The transition to parenthood has a significant impact on both men and women, their relationship as a couple, and their daily activities, including work and social contacts. New conflicts may arise and old ones resurface. Problems in the relationship between the woman and her own mother may increase her difficulties in the development of her new identity as a mother. She must also come to terms with her own femininity.

A woman's postpartum adaptation is intimately linked to the quality of the relationship with her partner (Andersen 1984). A supportive relationship with the child's father can help mitigate the stresses of being a new mother. In many cases, the family system must be reorganized, and thus many couples adopt more traditional roles. Couples with reasonably egalitarian relationships often have more difficulty adjusting to new parenthood, because regardless of previous philosophies, it is usually the mother who accepts the major share of parenting tasks. The parents must decide how their new roles will affect their previous work patterns and assess the necessary changes. With the added burden of child care, the relationship between the couple often suffers, and there is less time for socializing. Groups of other new parents can be very supportive in helping couples work through these normal adjustments. Age, parity, culture, expectations, financial problems, and housing difficulties may all affect normal postpartum reactions and the developing relationship between the mother and her new baby.

Infant Feeding

It is generally agreed that breast-feeding is best for young infants, for both nutritional and health reasons. It may also facilitate mother-child bonding. Although 65% of mothers start off breast-feeding, only 25% continue for 4 months. Although they are aware of the benefits of breast-feeding, many mothers prefer bottle-feeding for various reasons (Wollett 1987), including modesty, discomfort, an unsupportive environment, difficulty in initiating breast-feeding, or uncertainty about the amount of breast milk that should be provided. The father's attitude toward breast-feeding often plays a vital role. Either partner's beliefs about the effect of breast-feeding on contraception or breast size and shape can also influence its acceptance. In addition, women who are returning to the workplace shortly after the birth may find it impossible to continue breast-feeding, whereas women on a demand schedule may feel overburdened by the responsibility of being available every few hours. Some women think their husbands will become more involved if they choose bottle-feeding. A woman's attitude toward breast-feeding is greatly improved with support from her physician, hospital staff, and other health care providers. Information and support about breast-feeding is valuable in helping women to weather the difficult first few weeks after birth. It is vital, however, that the woman not be made to feel guilty, whatever her informed choice.

MATERNITY BLUES

Maternity blues is a common, benign, transitory condition occurring in the first 10 days postpartum. Its incidence ranges from 50% (Pitt 1973) to 70% (Harris 1980).

Clinical Presentation

Maternity blues typically begin 3–4 days after delivery (Stein 1982) and peak on days 4–5. The most frequently reported symptom is weeping. In the first few hours after delivery, crying may be accompanied by happy feelings. Handley et al. (1980) felt that depressed mood is characteristic of maternity blues, whereas Kennerley and Gath (1986) found that, although women described themselves as "low spirited," they did not consider themselves to be depressed. Emotional lability seems to be a characteristic feature. Elation ("postpartum pinks") may also occur, most commonly on day 1.

Researchers have also described irritability, lack of affection for the baby, hostility toward the husband, sleep disturbance, headaches, feelings of unreality, depersonalization, exhaustion, and restlessness in women suffering from maternity blues. Although many mothers describe themselves as being absentminded, distracted, and lacking in concentration, these cognitive deficits are usually not verified by psychological testing.

Etiology

Psychosocial factors.   No clear correlations have been established between maternity blues and various psychosocial factors. Maternity blues have been reported in all social classes (Ballinger et al. 1979; Stein 1980) and in many different cultures (Davidson 1972; Harris 1980). The condition is unrelated to marital status (Davidson 1972), although associations have been reported with poor marital relationships (Ballinger et al. 1979; Cutrona 1984). No positive association has been reported between the blues and other external stressors (Paykel et al. 1980; Pitt 1973). Hospitalization does not appear to be a causal factor, as there is an equal incidence in home deliveries (Yalom et al. 1968).

Contradictory findings have been reported for the association of maternity blues and personality factors (Kendell et al. 1984; Nott et al. 1976; Pitt 1973), the primiparous state (Ballinger et al. 1979; Nott et al. 1976; Stein 1980), ambivalent attitudes to pregnancy (Nilsson and Almgren 1970), fear of labor (Ballinger et al. 1979; Kennerley and Gath 1986), and anxiety and depression during pregnancy (Davidson 1972; Handley et al. 1980). O'Hara et al. (1991) recently reported a history of personal and family depression, more problems with social adjustment, and stressful life events in women who get postnatal blues compared with women who do not.

Biological factors. The high incidence of maternity blues, the typical onset at 3 days postpartum, the fluctuating course, and the lack of clear psychosocial causation have led many researchers to suspect a biological cause. However, no consistent correlations have been found for maternity blues and progesterone, estrogen, prolactin, cortisol, thyroid hormones, beta-endorphins, norepinephrine, 5-hydroxytryptamine, cyclic adenosine monophosphate (cAMP), electrolytes, or pyridoxine (George and Sandler 1988). O'Hara et al. (1991) recently reported higher levels of free and total estriol before and after delivery in women who develop blues compared with those who do not.

Obstetric and gynecologic factors. Yalom et al. (1968) noted a higher incidence of obstetric anomalies or subjective discomfort during pregnancy in women with maternity blues, whereas Pitt (1973) and Ballinger et al. (1979) did not. No link was found between maternity blues and physiological monitoring during pregnancy (Long Blumberg 1980), cesarean delivery (Kendell et al. 1981), or breastfeeding versus bottle-feeding (Ballinger et al. 1979; Cox et al. 1982). Researchers have reported that women who experience maternity blues were of a younger age at menarche (Yalom et al. 1968) and have a shorter menstrual flow (Yalom et al. 1968), more menstrual irregularities (Handley et al. 1980), and a history of premenstrual tension (Ballinger et al. 1979). Davidson and Robertson (1985), however, failed to find any association with previous menstrual difficulties.

Treatment

Women with maternity blues require reassurance that the symptoms are common and will disappear quickly. Emotional support and instruction on newborn care may also be helpful. Women should be advised to seek help if symptoms persist for more than 2 weeks.

Prognosis

Most women completely recover from maternity blues in a few days to 2 weeks. In a small number, however, the symptoms seem to merge into a more serious condition known as postnatal depression. Many women experience maternity blues after each pregnancy.

DISORDERS OF MOTHER-INFANT RELATIONSHIP

Disorders of the mother-infant relationship range from delayed attachment to infanticide. Studies of these disorders suffer from problems in methodology, including the difficulty of measuring maternal-infant attachment.

Incidence

Delayed attachment is reported in approximately 10% of mothers. Rejection of the infant and obsessive, hostile thoughts about the baby are seen in 1% of mothers. Estimates of child abuse vary greatly and depend on the criteria used and cultural norms. Infanticide occurs in 1/50,000 births (Brockington and Cox-Roper 1988).

Clinical Presentation

Approximately 40% of primiparous women appear to experience mild detachment or negative feelings in the immediate postnatal period and a gradual increase in the strength of maternal feelings over the ensuing few weeks (Robson and Powell 1982). In more severe, persistent disorders of attachment, the mother expresses disinterest, neglect, and failure to protect, nurture, or interact with the infant. Delayed attachment can be primary or can occur secondary to another psychiatric disorder, such as an adjustment disorder, depression, mania, psychosis, anxiety, obsessive-compulsive disorder, or personality disorders. Margison (1982) has described infant rejection in which the mother shows persistent hostility, often wishes the child had never been born, and is determined to avoid the maternal role. Other women may feel normally loving toward the infant but afraid of contact because of obsessional intrusive and distressing thoughts about the baby, including impulses to harm it (Brockington and Cox-Roper 1988).

Etiology

Cultural factors and social class influence the way a woman first relates to her child (Robson and Powell 1982). The role of maternal personality factors in facilitating or interfering with attachment is still being studied. Women who have had disrupted or inadequate mothering themselves (Frommer and O'Shea 1973), as well as single teenage mothers without social supports, should be considered at special risk for attachment disorder. Painful and difficult childbirth experiences have also been linked to early maternal detachment (Robson and Kumar 1980). Congenital defects or prematurity may result in a lack of attachment out of rejection or fear of subsequent loss. Problems with obsessional hostile feelings toward the newborn may be a manifestation of obsessive-compulsive illness or depression. Socioeconomic or environmental stresses tend to exacerbate difficulties in attachment. Rejection of the newborn is found most frequently in unwanted pregnancies.

Management

Most delays in attachment resolve spontaneously within the first few days or weeks postpartum. Prenatal education about delayed attachment may alleviate the mother's guilt. Although it has not been clearly established that brief separation leads to attachment disorders, it is important to maintain close contact if either the mother or the baby requires hospitalization. Mothers who suffer from continued bonding problems may benefit from practical advice and support concerning infant care, exploratory psychotherapy to understand the relationship to previous conflicts, behavioral approaches designed to decrease anxiety when coping with the baby, and occasionally, joint admission to a mother-infant unit. Obsessional thoughts of hostility toward the baby may respond to psychotherapy often combined with pharmacotherapy with an antidepressant such as clomipramine or fluoxetine. Women with attachment difficulties secondary to other psychiatric disorders should be reassessed after the primary disorder has been treated.

Effects on the Neonate

Delayed attachment or early temporary separation from the mother has not been proven to have significant long-term effects on the baby (Robson and Powell 1982). Children who suffer from ongoing lack of bonding, however, may show failure to thrive, stunted emotional and cognitive development, and difficulty in developing peer relationships. These infants are also at increased risk of being abused and rejected. A comprehensive review of infanticide (Resnick 1970) found that neonaticide (murder of the newborn within 24 hours of birth) was seen most often in mothers who were young, unmarried, and without evidence of psychosis or depression, but by whom the child was unwanted.

POSTNATAL DEPRESSION

Postnatal depression is an affective disorder lasting more than 2 weeks, the severity of which falls between maternity blues and puerperal psychosis (O'Hara and Zekoski 1988; Robinson and Stewart 1986). Recent research has cast doubt on the existence of postnatal depression as a distinct entity (O'Hara and Zekoski 1988). In a group of pregnant women and matched, nonpregnant control women, rates of depression were 10.6% for postpartum women and 10.0% for control subjects during the first 9 weeks after delivery. O'Hara and Zekoski (1988) concluded that there was no evidence that the postpartum subjects were at greater risk for depression than were the control subjects. Regardless of whether there is a distinct illness, the frequent lack of detection of postnatal depression and the subsequent negative consequences for the mother, her marital relationship, and her child make this an important condition to diagnose and treat.

Prevalence and Epidemiology

Prevalence rates of postnatal depression in studies using the same diagnostic standards range from 8.2% (Cutrona 1983) to 14.9% (Kumar and Robson 1984). Most studies have failed to find any consistent relationship between postnatal depression and socioeconomic status, age, or parity (O'Hara and Zekoski 1988). Only one study (Fegetter and Gath 1981) found single parenthood to be associated with a higher risk of depression.

Clinical Presentation

Postnatal depression usually begins within 3–6 months after delivery. In some women, maternity blues simply continue and become more severe. In others, there is a period of well-being followed by the gradual onset of depression, which is characterized by tearfulness, despondency, emotional lability, guilty feelings, anorexia, and sleep disturbances, as well as feelings of inadequacy in coping with the infant, poor concentration and memory, fatigue, and irritability (Robinson and Stewart 1986). Some women may worry excessively about the baby's health or feeding habits and see themselves as "bad," inadequate, or unloving mothers.

Etiology

Psychosocial factors. Studies of postnatal depression have been handicapped by methodologic errors and the inability to identify it as a distinct disorder. A relationship has been reported, however, between measurable anxiety during pregnancy and the level of postpartum depressive symptomatology (Hayworth et al. 1980; Watson et al. 1984). Kumar and Robson (1984) found no increase in previous psychiatric diagnoses in women with postpartum depression, in contrast to O'Hara (1986) and O'Hara et al. (1983). O'Hara (1986) also found that a higher percentage of depressed subjects (66.7%) had a family history of depression than did nondepressed women (20.7%).

Several well-designed studies (Braverman and Roux 1978; Kumar and Robson 1984) have reported an increased risk of postpartum depression in women who experienced marital problems during pregnancy. Hopkins et al. (1986), however, failed to confirm this finding. Women with postnatal depression perceive their husbands to be less supportive than women who are not depressed, but these differences were apparent only postpartum, not during pregnancy (O'Hara 1986; O'Hara et al. 1983). Cutrona (1984) found that the availability of companionship and a feeling of belonging to a group were more important predictors of good adjustment than was intimacy with the husband. Only a few studies (Hopkins et al. 1986) found no association between measures of social support and the occurrence of postnatal depression. No relationship has been demonstrated between various obstetric variables and postnatal depression.

Contradictory findings have been reported concerning the contribution of a poor relationship between the woman and her mother to postnatal depression (Kumar and Robson 1984; Nilsson and Almgren 1970; Paykel et al. 1980; Watson et al. 1984). Although O'Hara et al. (1984) and Cutrona (1983) found a relationship between external stressors and higher levels of postpartum depressive symptoms, Hopkins et al. (1986) found a relationship only with having a baby who is difficult to care for or a baby with neonatal complications. Similarly, Kumar and Robson (1984) found no association between stressful life events and postnatal depression.

Biological factors.   Although it has been suggested that postnatal depression is due to low levels of progesterone or estrogen or to high levels of prolactin (Steiner 1979), no significant relationships have been found (Gard et al. 1986). Alder and Cox (1983) found that women who were breast-feeding their infants and taking oral contraceptives postpartum had a higher risk of depression 3–5 months postnatally than did women who were breast-feeding exclusively but not taking oral contraceptives. No conclusive evidence relating free or total tryptophan levels (Gard et al. 1986) or cortisol levels (Handley et al. 1980) and postnatal depressive symptoms has been demonstrated. However, Harris et al. (1989) showed a minor association of postnatal depression and thyroid dysfunction.

Summary of Etiologic Factors

The most relevant etiological factors for postnatal depression are those found in association with depression in general: a personal or family psychiatric history of depression; lack of support, especially from the spouse; and the occurrence of a number of negative life events around the time of delivery.

Treatment

Postnatal depression is treated on both a psychosocial and a biological basis. Identification and acknowledgment of the depression itself may be a helpful feature, dispelling the woman's fears of physical disease and personal inadequacy. Individual or group psychotherapy may help the woman to resolve conflicts about mothering or her new role. Joint counseling is indicated if there are conflicts or a lack of support from her partner. Information about newborn care, social assistance, and practical supports such as homemaking may also be beneficial. Antidepressant medication, such as nortriptyline, 30–100 mg/day; desipramine, 150–300 mg/day; or fluoxetine, 20–60 mg/day, may be required. The use of minor tranquilizers to reduce anxiety should be limited to brief or adjunctive therapy in order to reduce the risk of dependency. Chapter 5 discusses the use of drugs in the breast-feeding mother.

Prevention

Gordon and Gordon (1960) found that patients with postnatal depression who received active social intervention as well as dynamic psychotherapy required briefer treatment and were less likely to require hospitalization. The women attending these groups, especially those accompanied by their husbands, experienced fewer emotional problems than the control group. Halonen and Passman (1985), Shereshefsky and Lockman (1973), and Broussard (1976) found that either prenatal counseling or relaxation training could decrease the level of the woman's distress and improve the marital relationship postpartum.

Prognosis

Postpartum depression usually lasts several months (Kumar and Robson 1984; Watson et al. 1984). Women may have difficulties in bonding to their infants and may express feelings of rejection, dislike, or indifference (Margison 1982; Robson and Kumar 1980). Women with postpartum depression are also more likely to experience future episodes of depression (Caplan et al. 1989). Their children may also develop behavioral, cognitive, and social problems (Cogill et al. 1986).

PUERPERAL PSYCHOSES

Puerperal psychoses are psychotic disorders arising after childbirth. Controversy exists over the specificity and timing of these disorders, as early research suffered from confounding variables such as differences in case definitions and the time period to be allowed for the occurrence of such disorders (Brockington et al. 1982). Consequently, some authors consider these disorders to be distinct entities with specific etiologies, clinical presentations, and prognoses (Brockington et al. 1982; Hamilton 1962), whereas others believe that they are simply episodes of affective psychotic illness triggered by the stresses of pregnancy and delivery (Kendell et al. 1987). Although women with schizophrenia frequently suffer from psychotic relapses within weeks after delivery, most authorities now agree that the majority of postpartum psychoses are affective illnesses (Kendell et al. 1987).

Brockington et al. (1982) found that early postpartum psychosis could be blindly differentiated from nonpuerperal psychosis. McNeil (1986) found that manic postpartum disturbances were characterized by more confusion and disorganized speech than were nonpuerperal episodes, and postpartum psychoses were generally characterized by more disorganized behavior. Other distinctive characteristics include a symptom-free phase between delivery and the onset of the psychosis, marked confusion, changeability and unpredictability in clinical features, and distinguishing psychological characteristics related to concerns about motherhood (Hamilton 1982). Clouding of consciousness (Protheroe 1969) and an excess of Schneiderian symptoms (Kadrmas et al. 1979) are also characteristic features.

Incidence and Prevalence

The incidence of psychiatric admission for postpartum psychosis is 1–2 per 1,000 postpartum women. The relative risk of admission for psychosis within the first 30 days following childbirth is 21.7, decreasing to 12.7 in the first 90 days. Despite this decrease over time, the relative risk remains elevated for 2 years following delivery. Women with a history of bipolar affective disorder appear to be particularly vulnerable (Kendell et al. 1987).

Epidemiology

Primiparous women constitute 54% of all patients exhibiting psychoses (Thomas and Gordon 1959). There is no significant relationship to maternal age (Kendell et al. 1987), class, or culture. Although Kendell et al. (1987) found an increased number of admissions in single women, this may be related to a lack of spousal support (Paffenberger 1964).

Early Versus Late Onset

McNeil (1986, 1987, 1988a, 1988b) found a number of significant differences between women who had early-onset (within 3 weeks of delivery) and late-onset postpartum illness. Women with early-onset psychoses tended to have affective illnesses; to be primiparous, younger at the time of onset, and younger during any previous illness; and to have had an emotional disturbance during pregnancy. Women with late-onset illnesses tended to have schizophreniform illnesses; to be older, of lower socioeconomic class, and single; and to have had premorbid mental problems and more emotional disturbances before pregnancy, but fewer during pregnancy.

Clinical Presentation

Most postpartum psychoses begin within the first 3 weeks following delivery. There is nearly always an asymptomatic period of 2–3 days after delivery. Prodromal symptoms include sleep disturbances, fatigue, depression, irritability, and emotional lability. The mother often has difficulty caring for her infant. Characteristically, she feels confused, perplexed, bewildered, and dreamy and may complain of poor memory, although performance on formal mental tests is often normal (Brockington et al. 1982). The clinical presentation may be an atypical or brief reactive psychosis, a major affective disorder, a schizophreniform disorder, or an organic brain syndrome.

The most common presentation of puerperal psychosis is an affective disorder. In psychotic depression, the woman is tearful, has psychomotor retardation, has sleep and appetite disturbances, and is preoccupied with feelings of guilt and worthlessness. She may have delusions about the infant being dead or defective. She may deny having given birth or may have hallucinations commanding her to harm the baby. These typical depressive features are often accompanied by a sense of confusion.

A woman with postpartum mania is excited, euphoric, grandiose, irritable, and hyperactive. She requires little sleep, and her appetite may be markedly reduced or exaggerated. She may have grandiose delusions about her baby. Insight is usually lacking.

A woman with a schizophreniform presentation demonstrates thought disorder, delusions, inappropriate affect, hallucinations, agitation, motor retardation, bizarre delusional ideas about herself or her child, and lack of insight.

Women who present with an "organic brain syndrome" have prominent symptoms of confusion, bewilderment, and memory loss.

This syndrome may be due to medical conditions such as encephalitis, autoimmune disorders, endocrine and electrolyte disturbances, or sepsis, but it can occur in the absence of any recognizable medical disorder (Robinson and Stewart 1986; Welner 1982).

Etiology

Researchers have been unable to confirm a link between puerperal psychosis and levels of prolactin, thyroxine, estrogen, progesterone, adrenocorticoids, follicle-stimulating hormone, or beta-endorphins (Brockington et al. 1982; Steiner 1979; Stewart et al. 1988). An increased incidence of puerperal psychosis is seen after cesarean delivery (20% versus 8% in vaginally delivered control subjects) (Kendell et al. 1981). Other obstetric variables have not been found to increase risk.

Studies by Protheroe (1969) and Winokur et al. (1978) suggest that, although there is an inherited predisposition to psychotic illness, there is no specific inherited predisposition to puerperal illness. There is, however, a strong link between bipolar disorder and puerperal psychosis with affective symptoms: women with a history of bipolar affective disorder have a 50% chance of developing postpartum psychosis (McNeil 1987). Women with a history of manic episodes are especially at risk for developing postpartum psychosis (Brockington et al. 1982). Moreover, the severity of past psychiatric illness appears to be significantly related to the occurrence of postpartum psychosis (McNeil 1987). First-degree relatives of women with bipolar disorders also have an increased incidence (20%) of postpartum psychosis (Uddenberg and Englesson 1978). No evidence has been found for a relationship between postpartum disorders and unipolar disorders (Winokur and Ruangtrakool 1966). Women with a history of schizophrenia have a 24% chance of developing postpartum psychosis.

Treatment

Treatment of puerperal psychosis usually requires admission to a hospital, particularly if the mother appears to be in any danger of harming herself or her child through neglect, abuse, or acting on delusions or hallucinations. Mothers may be admitted independently or, preferably, together with their infants, if feasible. The woman's partner should be involved in the ongoing treatment from the beginning. Puerperal psychosis requires both psychosocial and drug therapy.

Specific drug treatments vary with the presentation. For depressive psychosis, an antidepressant such as nortriptyline, desipramine, or a serotonin reuptake inhibitor, combined with a major tranquilizer such as haloperidol, 4–10 mg per day, usually controls the psychotic symptoms as well as the depression. If the woman does not respond to these medications, electroconvulsive therapy is often effective, usually providing complete remission after six to eight treatments.

Hypomanic or manic presentations are treated with lithium carbonate in daily doses of 600–1,200 mg until a therapeutic serum level of 0.8–1.2 mg/L is reached. Patients who are unresponsive to lithium carbonate may be treated with other mood stabilizers such as carbamazepine. A major tranquilizer may be necessary to control acute symptoms until an adequate serum level of lithium or another mood stabilizer is obtained.

Women who present with a schizophreniform disorder should be treated with a major tranquilizer such as haloperidol, 4–10 mg/day. Those who do not respond adequately sometimes benefit from a trial of electroconvulsive therapy, particularly if affective or catatonic symptoms are present.

Individual or marital therapy may be indicated. Conflicts about mothering, career, marital problems, issues relating to the woman's own mother, and concerns about femininity may require attention. Overidealistic expectations of parenthood often need to be explored. The woman requires both practical and emotional support from her spouse, family, and friends, sometimes including education about child care. Community social services may be extremely helpful for the mother and infant after discharge.

Prognosis

Prior to the development of psychotropic drugs, untreated puerperal psychosis required an average of 5–8 months of hospitalization, many women continuing to have symptoms for 2–4 years (Brockington et al.

1982). Current treatments have substantially shortened the psychotic episodes: 95% of adequately treated women improve within 2–3 months.

Reviewing the results of a number of studies, Brockington et al. (1982) found that 31% of women suffered a further puerperal episode and that psychosis complicated 21% of future pregnancies. They estimated the risk for each succeeding pregnancy to be 1/5 and postulated that there was a higher risk in women with more severe psychosis and multiple risk factors. Prophylactic lithium given immediately after delivery to women with a history of postpartum affective psychosis appears to reduce the recurrence risk to 10% (Stewart et al. 1991). Careful follow-up is indicated after subsequent deliveries, both for support and early case identification and treatment.

Schopf et al. (1984) found that 65% of women studied had at least one nonpuerperal relapse and only 25% remained free of later psychopathology. Of those who had nonpuerperal relapses, 43% had been diagnosed as suffering from affective psychosis, 38% from schizoaffective psychosis, and only 19% from schizophrenia. They found that nonpuerperal relapses were strongly related to a family history of psychosis and the occurrence of a psychotic episode before the index episodes. Davidson and Robertson (1985) looked specifically at women in whom the puerperal illness was the first onset of illness. Overall, 56% had at least one recurrent illness during follow-up. Of those women diagnosed as having unipolar depression, 40% had a nonpuerperal illness, whereas 30% had another puerperal disorder. Those diagnosed as having bipolar affective disorders had a 66% recurrence of nonpuerperal disorders and a 50% occurrence of subsequent puerperal psychosis. All the schizophrenic women developed a chronic illness with frequent exacerbations.

Effect on the Mother-Child Relationship

Conflicting evidence exists about the long-term effects on children of mothers with puerperal psychosis. The psychiatric history, premorbid personality, nature and timing of the puerperal psychosis, current marital and environmental circumstances, degree of life stress, access to support, and the health and temperament of the baby may all play a role. In the United Kingdom, many women are admitted to the hospital with their babies, either to a specialized mother-infant unit or to a general psychiatric ward. Although it is difficult to perform randomized, controlled studies of the effectiveness of mother-infant admissions, there appears to be a beneficial effect on the parent-child relationship and on parenting competence measured at 2 years (Stewart 1989).

It is difficult to predict which infants may be at risk of harm from their mothers. Most women who commit neonaticide are not psychotic at the time (Resnick 1970). Filicide (the murder of a child by its parent more than 24 hours after birth), however, is most often associated with mental illness as part of a suicide attempt, as a response to hallucinations or delusions, as a delusional attempt to prevent the child from suffering, or as an accidental result of a violent outburst. Women with manic, depressed, or schizophrenic illnesses may also place their children at risk through neglect, and careful supervision is required while the mother is ill and recovering.

POSTPARTUM ANXIETY DISORDERS

Anxiety disorders, with or without panic attacks, may develop in the postpartum period, or a previous anxiety disorder may be exacerbated at this time (Cowley and Roy-Byrne 1989). Metz et al. (1988) have reported panic disorder presenting for the first time in the postpartum period in the absence of major depression. The panic attacks were typical in nature and responded to the usual pharmacological treatments. Further work on anxiety and panic disorders in pregnancy and the puerperium is required.

POSTPARTUM OBSESSIVE-COMPULSIVE DISORDERS

The development of obsessive-compulsive disorders and obsessive-compulsive symptoms is not uncommon in the early postpartum period. Such women usually experience unwanted intrusive thoughts about harming their babies and may avoid situations in which they feel they are at risk of acting on their thoughts (e.g., bathing or sleeping with the infants, preparing food with sharp knives). Not infrequently, women with postpartum depression may also develop obsessive-compulsive symptoms. These women usually recover promptly when treated with serotonin reuptake inhibitor antidepressants or clomipramine combined with supportive psychotherapy. However, some postpartum women appear to have a pure obsessive-compulsive disorder without affective changes. These women are more treatment resistant, although some success has recently been experienced by using higher doses of serotonin reuptake inhibitor antidepressants (e.g., fluoxetine 80 mg/day) with cognitive-behavior therapy over several months. Further work is in progress studying postpartum obsessive-compulsive disorder (Doyle et al. 1992; Sichel et al. 1992).

CONCLUSIONS

Postpartum psychiatric disorders have a major impact on the woman, her child, and her family. It is important for physicians to be aware of the possibility that a woman will develop an emotional disorder during this time. Frequently, the woman is isolated at home and does not see a health care provider until her 6-week postpartum follow-up visit, when it may be discovered that she has been ill for many weeks. Women who may be particularly vulnerable to developing a postpartum disorder include those who have a history of psychiatric disorders, especially a bipolar affective disorder; are anxious or depressed during pregnancy; are younger mothers; lack a support network; have had difficult deliveries; or are under other current stresses. All women, however, should be considered to be at risk. There is a great need for physicians and community-based groups to provide information, support, and reassurance to new mothers and to participate in detecting and treating postpartum illness at an early stage.

REFERENCES

Alder EM, Cox JL: Breast feeding and postnatal depression. J Psychosom Res 27:139–144, 1983

Andersen I: Transition to parenthood research. Journal of Psychosomatic Obstetrics and Gynaecology 3:3–16, 1984

Ballinger CB, Buckley DE, Naylor GJ, et al: Emotional disturbance following childbirth: clinical findings and urinary excretion of cyclic AMP. Psychol Med 9:293–300, 1979

Braverman J, Roux JF: Screening for the patient at risk for postpartum depression. Obstet Gynecol 52:731–736, 1978

Brockington IF, Cox-Roper A: The nosology of puerperal mental illness, in Motherhood and Mental Illness, Vol 2: Causes and Consequences. Edited by Kumar R, Brockington IF. London, Wright, 1988, pp 1–16

Brockington IF, Winokur G, Dean C: Puerperal psychosis, in Motherhood and Mental Illness, Vol 1. Edited by Kumar R, Brockington IF. London, Academic Press, 1982, pp 37–70

Broussard ER: Evaluation of televised anticipatory guidance to primiparae. Community Ment Health J 12:203–210, 1976

Caplan HL, Cogill SR, Alexandra H, et al: Maternal depression and the emotional development of the child. Br J Psychiatry 154:818–822, 1989

Cogill SR, Caplan HL, Alexandra H, et al: Impact of maternal postnatal depression on cognitive development of young children. BMJ 292:1165–1167, 1986

Cowley D, Roy-Byrne PP: Panic disorders during pregnancy. Journal of Psychosomatic Obstetrics and Gynaecology 10:193–210, 1989

Cox JL, Connor Y, Kendell RE: Prospective study of the psychiatric disorders of childbirth. Br J Psychiatry 140:111–117, 1982

Cutrona CE: Casual attributions and perinatal depression. J Abnorm Psychol 92:161–172, 1983

Cutrona CE: Social support and stress in the transition of parenthood. J Abnorm Psychol 93:378–390, 1984

Davidson JRT: Postpartum change in Jamaican women: a description and discussion of its significance. Br J Psychiatry 121:659–663, 1972

Davidson J, Robertson E: A follow-up study of postpartum illness 1946–1978. Acta Psychiatr Scand 71:451–459, 1985

Doyle W, Fairman M, Scordino K, et al: Postpartum obsessive compulsive disorders. Marcé Society Annual Meeting Abstracts, Edinburgh, Scotland, September 1992, p 49

Fegetter P, Gath D: Non-psychotic psychiatric disorders in women one year after childbirth. J Psychosom Res 25:369–372, 1981

Frommer EA, O'Shea G: Antenatal identification of women liable to have problems in managing their infants. Br J Psychiatry 123:149–156, 1973

Gard PR, Handley SL, Parsons AD, et al: A multivariate investigation of postpartum mood disturbance. Br J Psychiatry 148:567–575, 1986

George A, Sandler M: Endocrine and biochemical studies in puerperal mental disorders, in Motherhood and Mental Illness, Vol 2: Causes and Consequences. Edited by Kumar R, Brockington IF. London, Wright, 1988, pp 78–112

Gordon RE, Gordon KK: Social factors in the prevention of postpartum emotional problems. Obstet Gynecol 15:433–438, 1960

Halonen JS, Passman RH: Relaxation training and expectation in the treatment of postpartum distress. J Consult Clin Psychol 53:839–845, 1985

Hamilton JA: Postpartum Psychiatric Problems. St. Louis, MO, CV Mosby, 1962

Hamilton JA: The identity of postpartum psychosis, in Motherhood and Mental Illness, Vol 1. Edited by Brockington IF, Kumar R. London, Academic Press, 1982, pp 1–20

Handley SL, Dunn TL, Waldron G, et al: Tryptophan, cortisol and puerperal mood. Br J Psychiatry 136:498–508, 1980

Harris B: Maternity blues. Br J Psychiatry 136:520–521, 1980

Harris B, Fung H, Johns S, et al: Transient post-partum thyroid dysfunction and postnatal depression. J Affective Disord 17:243–249, 1989

Hayworth J, Little BC, Carter SB, et al: A predictive study of postpartum depression: some predisposing characteristics. Br J Med Psychol 53:161–167, 1980

Hopkins J, Campbell SB, Marcus M: The role of infant-related stressors in postpartum depression. J Abnorm Psychol 96:237–241, 1986

Kadrmas A, Winokur G, Crowe R: Postpartum mania. Br J Psychiatry 135:551–554, 1979

Kendell RE, Rennie D, Clarke JA, et al: The social and obstetrics correlates of psychiatric admission in the puerperium. Psychol Med 11:341–350, 1981

Kendell RE, MacKenzie WE, West C, et al: Day to day mood changes after childbirth: further data. Br J Psychiatry 145:620–625, 1984

Kendell RE, Chalmers JC, Platz C: Epidemiology of puerperal psychoses. Br J Psychiatry 150:662–673, 1987

Kennerley H, Gath D: Maternity blues reassessed. Psychiatr Dev 1:1–17, 1986

Kumar R, Robson KM: A prospective study of emotional disorders in childbearing women. Br J Psychiatry 144:35–47, 1984

Long Blumberg N: Effects of neonatal risk, maternal attitude and cognitive style on early postpartum adjustment. J Abnorm Psychol 89:139–150, 1980

Marce LV: Traite de la Folie des Femmes Enceintes, des Nouvelles Accouchees et des Nourrices. Paris, Balliere, 1858

Margison F: The pathology of the mother-child relationship, in Motherhood and Mental Illness, Vol 1. Edited by Brockington IF, Kumar R. London, Academic Press, 1982, pp 191–232

McNeil TF: A prospective study of postpartum psychoses in a high risk group, I: clinical characteristics of the current postpartum episodes. Acta Psychiatr Scand 74:205–216, 1986

McNeil TF: A prospective study of postpartum psychoses in a high risk group, II: relationships to demographic and psychiatric history characteristics. Acta Psychiatr Scand 75:35–43, 1987

McNeil TF: A prospective study of postpartum psychoses in a high risk group, III: relationship to mental health characteristics during pregnancy. Acta Psychiatr Scand 77:604–610, 1988a

McNeil TF: A prospective study of postpartum psychoses in a high risk group, IV: relationship to life situation and experience of pregnancy. Acta Psychiatr Scand 77:645–653, 1988b

Metz A, Sichel DA, Goff DC: Postpartum panic disorder. J Clin Psychiatry 49:278–279, 1988

Nilsson A, Almgren P: Perinatal emotional adjustment: a prospective investigation of 165 women. Acta Psychiatr Scand Suppl 220, 1970

Nott PN, Franklin M, Armitage C, et al: Hormonal changes and mood in the puerperium. Br J Psychiatry 128:379–383, 1976

O'Hara MW: Social support, life events and depression during pregnancy and the puerperium. Arch Gen Psychiatry 43:569–573, 1986

O'Hara MW, Zekoski EM: Postpartum depression: a comprehensive review, in Motherhood and Mental Illness, Vol 2: Causes and Consequences. Edited by Kumar R, Brockington IF. London, Wright, 1988, pp 17–63

O'Hara MW, Rehm LP, Campbell SB: Postpartum depression: a role for social network and life stress variables. J Nerv Ment Dis 171:336–341, 1983

O'Hara MW, Neunaber DJ, Zekoski EM: A prospective study of postpartum depression: prevalence, course and predictive factors. J Abnorm Psychol 93:158–171, 1984

O'Hara MW, Schlechte JA, Lewis DA, et al: Prospective study of postpartum blues: biologic and psychosocial factors. Arch Gen Psychiatry 48:801–806, 1991

Paffenberger RS: The picture puzzle of postpartum psychosis. J Chronic Dis 13:161–173, 1961

Paffenberger RS Jr: Epidemiological aspects of postpartum mental illness. British Journal of Preventive and Social Medicine 18:189–195, 1964

Paykel ES, Emms EM, Fletcher J, et al: Life events and social support in puerperal depression. Br J Psychiatry 136:339–346, 1980

Pitt B: Maternity blues. Br J Psychiatry 122:431–435, 1973

Protheroe C: Puerperal psychoses: a long term study 1927–1961. Br J Psychiatry 115:9–30, 1969

Resnick PJ: Murder of the newborn: a psychiatric review of neonaticide. Am J Psychiatry 126:1414–1420, 1970

Robinson GE, Stewart DE: Postpartum psychiatric disorders. Can Med Assoc J 134:31–37, 1986

Robson KM, Kumar R: Delayed onset of maternal affection after childbirth. Br J Psychiatry 136:347–353, 1980

Robson KM, Powell E: Early maternal attachment, in Motherhood and Mental Illness, Vol 1. Edited by Brockington IF, Kumar R. London, Academic Press, 1982, pp 155–190

Schopf J, Bryois C, Jonquiere M, et al: On the nosology of severe psychiatric postpartum disorders. European Archives of Psychiatry and Neurological Sciences 234:54–63, 1984

Shereshefsky PM, Lockman RF: Comparison of counselled and non-counselled groups, in Psychological Aspects of a First Pregnancy. Edited by Shereshefsky PM, Yarrow LJ. New York, Raven, 1973, pp 151–163

Sichel D, Cohen L, Dimmock J, et al: Postpartum obsessive compulsive disorders: a case series. Marcé Society Annual Meeting Abstracts, Edinburgh, Scotland, September 1992, p 44

Stein GS: The pattern of mental change and body weight change in the first postpartum week. J Psychosom Res 24:165–171, 1980

Stein G: The maternity blues, in Motherhood and Mental Illness, Vol 1. Edited by Brockington IF, Kumar R. London, Academic Press, 1982, pp 119–154

Steiner M: Psychobiology of mental disorders associated with childbearing: an overview. Acta Psychiatr Scand 60:449–464, 1979

Stewart DE: Psychiatric admission of mentally ill mothers with their infants. Can J Psychiatry 34:34–38, 1989

Stewart DE, Addison AM, Robinson GE, et al: Thyroid function in psychosis following childbirth. Am J Psychiatry 145:1579–1581, 1988

Stewart DE, Klompenhouwer JL, Kendell RE, et al: Prophylactic lithium in postpartum affective psychosis—3 centres' experience. Br J Psychiatry 158:393–397, 1991

Thomas CL, Gordon JE: Psychosis after childbirth: etiological aspects of a single impact stress. Am J Med Sci 238:363–388, 1959

Uddenberg N, Englesson I: Prognosis of postpartum disturbance. Acta Psychiatr Scand 58:201–212, 1978

Watson JP, Elliott SA, Rugg AJ, et al: Psychiatric disorder in pregnancy and the first postnatal year. Br J Psychiatry 144:453–462, 1984

Welner A: Childbirth-related psychiatric illness. Compr Psychiatry 23:143–154, 1982

Winokur G, Ruangtrakool S: Postpartum impact on patients with independently diagnosed affect disorder. JAMA 197:83–88, 1966

Winokur G, Behar D, Vanvalkenburg C, et al: Is a familial definition of depression both feasible and valid? J Nerv Ment Dis 166:764–768, 1978

Wollett A: Who breastfeeds? the family and cultural context. Journal of Reproductive and Infant Psychology 5:127–131, 1987

Yalom I, Lunde DT, Moos RH, et al: Postpartum blues syndrome: a description and related variables. Arch Gen Psychiatry 18:16–27, 1968

Chapter 8

PERINATAL LOSS

Elisabeth K. Herz, M.D.

❖ ❖ ❖ ❖ ❖ ❖ ❖ ❖ ❖ ❖ ❖ ❖ ❖ ❖

"Mourning is treated as if it were a weakness, a self indulgence, a reprehensible bad habit instead of as a psychological necessity," writes the British anthropologist Geoffrey Gorer (1965) in *Death, Grief, and Mourning* about the current attitudes toward bereavement in Western cultures. The phrase "life must go on" epitomizes the attitude of stoic composure expected of the bereaved. This death-denying conspiracy of silence becomes deafening in the case of the loss of a child never born. More sympathy goes to parents with a late fetal or neonatal loss, but relatives or friends have difficulty acknowledging the parental attachment to this nascent life that had never been an integrated part of the family or community. In the prevailing perception, the loss is "replaceable." It has taken societal changes to break the taboo against recognizing perinatal loss.

In the 1970s, women began to speak out about their pain after pregnancy loss. Medical advances incorporated and promoted a greater emphasis on perinatal care, making perinatal death appear more preventable. Women requested more emotional understanding from health professionals. Publications by women who had gone through the experience (Berg 1981; Borg and Lasker 1981; Friedman and Gladstein 1982) and by clinicians in professional journals caught the attention of the mass media.

Descriptive studies uncovered the unique features of grief after pregnancy loss: complex intrapsychic, interpersonal, and social ramifications are superimposed on the previously known stages of mourn-

139

ing. These studies were augmented by research publications, but the results conflicted, especially when attempts were made to quantify grief by using nonspecific depression scales. Recent research has applied clinical observations about the specifics of this grief process; for instance, a Perinatal Grief Scale has been developed for the prediction of complicated grief (Toedter et al. 1988).

In a monumental review of accumulated literature and clinical material, Leon (1990) conceptualized the psychodynamic impact of perinatal loss and outlined psychotherapeutic interventions. His book is a milestone on the road to understanding perinatal loss and preventing or resolving long-lasting maladaptive responses (Leon 1990). The profusion of literature on this subject allows the inclusion of only selected publications in the reference list at the end of this chapter.

DEFINITION

Perinatal loss refers to stillbirth as well as neonatal death, two variably defined terms. Commonly, stillbirth is interpreted as the delivery of a dead fetus beyond 20 weeks of gestation or weighing more than 500 g. By another definition, only late fetal deaths beyond 28 weeks qualify as stillbirths. A loss in an earlier stage of fetal development is referred to as spontaneous abortion or miscarriage. Neonatal death is variously defined as the loss of an infant during the first 3, 7, or even 28 days postpartum. For a meaningful comparison of statistical and research data to be made, a consensus about definitions needs to be established.

Regardless of the length of gestation or the number of days an infant lived, any prenatal or postnatal loss has emotional, psychosocial, and behavioral consequences. It therefore appears justified to use the loosely defined term *perinatal loss* in an even wider sense to include the grief experienced after spontaneous abortion, ectopic pregnancy, partial fetal loss in a multiple pregnancy, and sudden infant death syndrome (SIDS) (Gardner and Merenstein 1986).

EPIDEMIOLOGY

The perinatal mortality rate in 1987 was 10.0/1,000 live births, including fetal deaths after 28 weeks of gestation and neonatal deaths within

7 days of life, according to the National Center for Health Statistics (U.S. Department of Health and Human Services 1990). The rate of neonatal deaths within 28 days of life and stillbirths beyond 20 weeks of gestation is 14.1/1,000 deliveries. The perinatal mortality rate for blacks is nearly twice that of whites. Prematurity—the prime factor for the higher loss rate in the black population—cannot be explained by lower socioeconomic status alone, because it does not play the same role in developing countries.

Enormous progress has been made in saving fetal and neonatal lives in recent decades. The perinatal mortality rate in the United States in 1950 was 32.5–38.9/1,000 depending on the definition used. In the past, the difference in perinatal mortality rates between developed countries and developing countries was very slight, but since then it has consistently grown. In 1987, in the least-developed countries, 125 infants/1,000 live births died by age 1 year, compared with 10.1/1,000 in the United States (World Health Organization 1989). Other industrialized countries have considerably lower counts than the United States: Japan's was half the rate of the United States in 1989. Clearly, much can still be done to reduce the rates of perinatal loss.

Other unsuccessful reproductive outcomes also need to be considered. The rate of miscarriages is estimated to be 15%–20% of all recognized pregnancies, and the number of undetected spontaneous abortions is probably much higher. Chronic spontaneous or habitual abortions, defined as three or more successive miscarriages, make up about 1% of spontaneous abortions and carry a higher risk for subsequent losses.

The incidence of ectopic pregnancies has increased in the last 20 years. There are several reasons for this increase, including the increased incidence of pelvic inflammatory disease, in utero exposure to diethylstilbestrol, and in vitro fertilization. In 1985, about two-thirds of all pregnancies were ectopic. The number of multiple pregnancies, which carry a higher risk of fetal wastage, has also increased with the use of new reproductive technologies. In the United States, SIDS occurs in 1 of every 350 live births. This leading cause of death remains unpredictable and unpreventable. Behind all these "cold" figures are many grieving parents.

ETIOLOGY AND MEDICAL INTERVENTIONS

Spontaneous abortion may be caused by genetic, environmental, anatomical, infectious, metabolic, endocrine, or immunologic factors. Although the possibility has been raised that psychogenic factors may contribute to spontaneous abortions, particularly repeated ones (Rock and Zacur 1983; Stray-Pedersen and Stray-Pedersen 1984), no definitive evidence of this relationship exists. No etiologic factor can be identified in 40%–50% of patients with spontaneous abortion, but new research in immune factors may further reduce these numbers (Naor et al. 1983).

A large-scale collaborative perinatal project identified 80% of the causes of perinatal deaths by using detailed clinical information, autopsy, and thorough investigation of the placenta. Of the diagnostically identified perinatal deaths in that study, 73% resulted from disorders that are not preventable by current medical knowledge (Naeye 1977). Many deaths are due to congenital malformations, which can be caused by chromosomal disorders or by polyfactorial syndromes. Most of these losses will remain nonpreventable for the foreseeable future, despite hopes for genetic therapy and some success with corrective prenatal and neonatal surgery.

The most significant obstetric cause for perinatal loss is preterm delivery associated with complications such as preterm labor, premature rupture of membranes, and cervical incompetence. Tocolysis, the drug-induced inhibition of preterm contractions, combined with supervised restriction of activity, often can prolong pregnancy until fetal viability. Given the uncertainty of the outcome and the length of confinement usually required, however, this treatment can be very taxing for the patient and her family. After premature rupture of membranes has occurred, labor ensues in most cases within 1 week. Attempts to delay delivery are often unsuccessful and can even add to complications. Cervical incompetence—one cause for premature rupture of membranes—may be prevented in a subsequent pregnancy by surgical cerclage in the midtrimester. For the woman, it means a long, anxiety-filled time until fetal viability, but up to 85% of ensuing pregnancies have been saved by this procedure.

Maternal disorders, such as hypertension, collagen vascular disease or, rarely, primary placental failure, may cause uteroplacental insufficiency with subsequent intrauterine growth retardation and fetal demise. Many placental disorders are still poorly understood, and drug treatment (except in the case of hypertension) is often experimental. Until recently, a previous stillbirth was a significant risk factor for the need for premature medical intervention and respiratory distress of the neonate in the subsequent pregnancy (Freeman et al. 1985). Sophisticated biophysical testing makes this increasingly preventable. Pregnancy complications such as diabetes, preeclampsia, and rhesus erythroblastosis fetalis have also become much more amenable to treatment.

Fetal deaths due to intrapartum events such as umbilical cord accidents, hemorrhage from placenta or vasa previa, uterine rupture, or abruptio placentae have been and may be still more reduced by prompt interventions (Cruikshank and Linyear 1987). All these benefits for fetal survival depend on accessibility to health care and the active cooperation of informed pregnant women. Social changes have yet to catch up with medical advances to facilitate the downward trend in fetal mortality.

SOCIAL CONTEXTS AND BELIEFS

Until early in the 20th century, the high rate of reproductive losses was an inevitable part of life and was possibly accepted by some bereaved parents as God's inscrutable will. In the Middle Ages, Christian funerals were disallowed for unbaptized and stillborn infants, who were buried with other outcasts, such as excommunicates. According to church doctrine, the souls of these infants were blemished for eternity by original sin and remained in limbo on the border of Hell, never to be reunited with their mothers in Heaven (Lovell 1983a). It is difficult to imagine how intensely religious women who had experienced perinatal loss were able to reconcile their pain with their faith. It is not uncommon for a woman to feel like the biblical Job after a perinatal loss. Even now, despite the Church's broadened views, she may rage against God at the time of her greatest need for her faith. Restricted reproduction, planned parenthood, and presumed medical omnipotence contribute to the expectation of a perfect, healthy child as well as to the profound disappointment about a negative outcome (Stotland 1988).

For Moslems, the rituals for stillborn infants are the same as for other deceased persons and follow a time-honored tradition (Bourne 1983). Relatives and friends surround the bereaved for a number of days, participating in their grief and regathering according to long-standing rituals. Grief is shared as a community, and all have a part in it on a very personal level.

In the Western world, particularly in Anglo Saxon–Protestant cultures, the "stiff upper lip" approach has become a virtue that precludes sharing. "If one can deny one's own grief, how much more easily can one deny the grief of others" (Gorer 1965, p. 131). Often, the fear of being intrusive prevents personal contact just when the bereaved needs support and intimate sharing. The detrimental effects of missing social supports are further complicated in the specific circumstances of perinatal loss. What remains is a sense of bewilderment, awkwardness, and greatly inhibited expression of feelings by all concerned.

STAGES OF BEREAVEMENT

After the loss of a loved one, the grieving person experiences several stages of the mourning process, as described by various investigators (Bowlby 1969, 1973, 1980; Kubler-Ross 1969; Lindemann 1944). The initial reactions of shock and denial gradually give way to a chaotic stage of emotional and somatic distress with cognitive lapses and behavioral changes while the full weight of the grief sinks in. The emotional turmoil includes agonizing preoccupation with the deceased, guilt, anger, and despair. At best, working through the grief leads to gradual resolution of the attachment to the love object, with ultimate resolution and acceptance of the loss. The duration of this process varies considerably, and resolution may never be effectively accomplished. Unresolved grief can present in many forms, such as delayed, chronic, or other presentations of pathological grief with persistent impairment.

SPECIAL ASPECTS OF PERINATAL GRIEF

Bereaved parents experience additional specific aspects of grief. These can be understood within the context of the unique circumstances of pregnancy and prospective parenthood and the special relationship to the nascent child (Leon 1986). (The psychology of pregnancy is described in Chapter 2.) The ability to provide with her body the indispensable means for the child to grow enhances the pregnant woman's self-worth. She generally assumes responsibility for the progress of the gestation by creating the best possible conditions for the fetus. Infantile and maternal identification during pregnancy bring three phases of a woman's life cycle together (Benedek 1970). This may explain why so many women profess to feel "whole" during this time.

The prospective father proceeds more slowly through a process of growing attachment and anticipation (Condon 1985). His sense of masculinity may be enhanced by his ability to impregnate and by his protective feelings for the woman who carries their baby. Friends and relatives, medical contacts, and society treat the expectant couple— especially the pregnant woman—with friendly attention and more than usual consideration. (Special issues for men are also discussed in Chapter 19.)

Suddenly, without warning, this process may get interrupted by ominous signs and—sometimes after a nightmare of frantic activity to rescue the pregnancy—it is over. The ominous signs may wax and wane over an extended period. Delivery may ensue and, despite all efforts, the extrauterine life of the premature infant may be unsustainable. Whatever the scenario of the individual perinatal loss, one can understand the specific nature of the subsequent grief only against the unique background of that pregnancy.

Maternal Intrapsychic Consequences of Perinatal Loss

"Empty" is the adjective women use most often to describe their feelings after perinatal loss. Many variables determine how long it takes before numbness gives way to pain. For instance, after a life-threatening delivery, the woman's depleted physical and psychological condition may render her emotionally unresponsive for some time. Eventually, however, the pain takes over and is often associated with a relentless preoccupation with questions of "why?" and "why me?" Feelings of guilt, self-blame, anger, and overwhelming envy of reproductively successful women can be so intense that at times they may overshadow the sadness (Peppers and Knapp 1980a).

Perinatal loss is a severe narcissistic blow. The woman's inability to carry the child to term often makes her feel like a failure and undermines her female identity. She may search relentlessly for an explanation, both to absolve herself from guilt and to gain a sense of control. Once the cause is known, she hopes the effect can be prevented in the future. Many women experience self-blame, which is almost always unfounded. They castigate themselves with self-recriminations: "If I had stopped working . . . "; "If I hadn't gone on the trip. . . . " However painful these self-accusations, they also carry the hope for future control: "If I don't repeat this behavior next time, it won't happen again."

Much more devastating is self-blame accentuated by guilt when the loss is perceived as deserved punishment for some moral deviation in the past. It can best be illustrated with a case example:

> M., a 34-year-old woman, sought therapy 6 months after her second miscarriage. She was distressed after she lost her first pregnancy early on, but devastated by the second miscarriage at a later stage of gestation. She tried to cope with her grief by immersing herself in work, but gradually her depression became so severe that she could barely function. She suffered from severe sleep disturbance, appetite loss, and emotional outbreaks. Communication with her husband had practically ceased, despite his repeated efforts to comfort her. His only child in a previous marriage died of a genetic defect at birth.
>
> The couple wanted very much to have a child, but M. could not bring herself to make another attempt. She was convinced the miscarriage was her fault, but could not come up with any behavior to blame for the loss. In therapy, the irrationality of her guilt was confronted and childhood experiences were searched for clues. She was an only child until she was 12 years old, when her mother had two more children in short succession and developed severe postpartum depression. She remained chronically depressed. After a happy childhood with all of her parents'

attention centered on her, the patient suddenly had to shoulder adult responsibilities for her infant siblings. She hated them and, although she took compulsively good care of them, wished only for their deaths. She was raised strictly Catholic, and for her, a wrongful thought was as much a sin as a wrongful deed. She lived in fear of eventual punishment for each sin she committed.

Finally, she uncovered her irrational belief that she caused the demise of her two babies as a deserved punishment for her "sin" of wishing deaths on her two infant siblings.

A woman's perception of herself as a reproductive failure can produce intense shame. "My body killed my perfectly healthy baby" is a recurring regressive defense against the perceived inadequacy dissociating the "bad body" from the "good, loving self." This body-mind split can have grievous long-term effects on her mature femininity. Sometimes she may project this shame and feel she has lost value in the eyes of those whose expectations she had disappointed, such as the expectant grandparents.

Envy of women who succeed where she failed is inevitable and may be most pronounced toward relatives and friends. Consequently, the grieving woman often withdraws, depriving herself from compassionate support. She may also fear ostracism because some pregnant women avoid contact with reminders of their own precarious condition and the "evil eye" of envy. Magical thinking and superstition are an inherent part of reproduction.

Anger is a common reaction to the narcissistic blow, the disappointment of joyful anticipation, the helplessness and uncertainty, the perceived devaluation by others, the envy, the sense of injustice, and the frustration surrounding perinatal loss. Medical caregivers are often the target for this rage, which undermines trust in subsequent care. (Awareness of this dynamic is important for those involved in the care of a women who has experienced pregnancy loss.) Some of the woman's anger may also turn against herself and those close to her. Alienation and self-perpetuating anger can result in a vicious cycle that prevents her from dealing with the underlying pain.

Physical and emotional components are inseparably intertwined in the psychobiological process of mourning. Physical factors such as anemia or thyroid dysfunction may contribute to a lack of energy and inability to cope. Somatic symptoms typically associated with general grief are accentuated by the concomitant physical aspects of the puerperium. The rapid shifts of hormones back to the prepregnant state exacerbate emotional lability. The discomfort of lactating breasts aggravates the emotional pain. Her arms ache to hold a baby. These factors are specific to perinatal grief.

Paternal Intrapsychic Consequences of Perinatal Loss

The bereaved prospective father seldom experiences and expresses his grief with the same intensity as his female partner, however much he was emotionally invested in the pregnancy (Wilson et al. 1985). Furthermore, his first concern is for the health of his partner. He feels relieved when the danger for her has passed, and the loss assumes secondary importance for him. Often his protectiveness leads him to suppress his pain out of fear of burdening her further. Commonly, he deals with his feelings by seeking distraction through various activities to avoid the full impact of the sadness and to build security for the future. His primary goal is for both partners to leave behind what happened and to move on. This reaction—and his future-oriented male response to perinatal loss—is especially pronounced after early pregnancy loss and can conflict with the slower grief process of the woman (LaRoche et al. 1984). The prospective father's grief seems to be a function of the length of time he has had for developing an attachment and becomes more intense the later in pregnancy that the loss occurs.

For the prospective mother, this "hierarchy of sadness" does not exist (Peppers and Knapp 1980b), but subtle differences in the quality of her grief relate to the stages of fetal development. Although she cannot feel that the earlier the pregnancy fails, the "lesser" is the loss (Seibel and Graves 1980), the emphasis shifts from losing part of herself early in gestation to the loss of a separate, living entity later in pregnancy.

An ectopic pregnancy accentuates the loss of "part of self" and adds anxiety or grief for all children planned for the future. The mourning process is also complicated when joy and grief are felt simultaneously, as after the loss of one twin. The concurrent process of attachment and detachment may be impossible to accomplish, causing attachment problems with the living child or unresolved grief for the lost one (Wilson et al. 1982).

The catastrophic circumstances of SIDS intensify the torture of unfounded guilt over the infant's death. The totally unexpected nature of the loss of the healthy baby makes the mourning process particularly difficult (Nicholas and Lewin 86).

Interpersonal Consequences of Perinatal Loss

For many couples, pregnancy loss is a crisis, a turning point that can bring a couple closer but that often splits them apart or festers as an unresolved conflict. Although a healthy marriage usually pulls a couple closer together during a crisis and in the immediate aftermath, working through the grief becomes a major test for many couples. Grieving aggravates preexisting problems and creates new ones.

The impact of an early pregnancy loss must not be underestimated (Herz 1984, 1985). Each of the partners goes through the process of mourning differently (Wijmak 1983), and each partner's needs can interfere with the response to the needs of the other. Since these needs are often not directly expressed, resentment builds when the partner cannot identify and respond intuitively to them.

Often the woman wants to talk about her feelings over and over again, craves unlimited compassion and emotional sharing, looks for reassurance from her partner to bolster her diminished sense of self-worth, and above all needs confirmation of his continued love for her. He, on the other hand, often resists dwelling on the painful memories and gets annoyed when she does not respond favorably to the distractions he tries to promote. He may feel that it may be an additional burden for her to hear about his disappointment. His lack of emotional expression makes her feel that he was not equally invested in their child, resolves his grief too easily, and lacks understanding for what she is going through. The more she becomes resentful, the more she withdraws; the isolation worsens her depression. Alternatively, the resentment may lead to angry outbursts, hurtful accusations, and destructive arguments that separate them even more. His feeling of helplessness leads to frustration and anger, either overtly or covertly expressed. He often withdraws into work, sports, or other distractions. The result is mutual hurt and complete breakdown of communication.

Tension is often heightened by the diminished sexual responsiveness on the part of the woman. Libido is wiped out by depression, resentment toward her partner, fear of another pregnancy, negative feelings about her own body, and doubts about her femininity. All of these feelings stifle sexual desire. Often she wants only to be held and cuddled, but she avoids even this contact for fear it might lead to sexual demands. She feels guilty about not responding, but angry if she does. In response, her partner feels rejected and frustrated and becomes increasingly angry himself.

In many cases, even the most well-meaning family is not perceived as a helpful support. Siblings who are successful in parenting may be envied, reinvoking buried rivalries. The mother who is compassionate to her daughter's pain may want to talk her out of her grief or advise against another pregnancy altogether. The in-laws may be felt to have found ultimate proof of her not being the best wife for their son. She may perceive remarks that are meant to give comfort, such as "it might have been for the best" or "next time it will be all right," as a trivialization of her pain.

These common problems during the mourning period present in countless permutations depending on the innumerable variables influencing the grieving process. At best, both partners will support each other and gradually detach from their acute grief. The aim is to free their feelings to deal with the living, despite the "shadow grief" that may persist (Peppers and Knapp 1980b).

ROLE OF CAREGIVERS

The Obstetric Team

Benfield et al. (1978) found that "a parent's grief response to neonatal death is highly individualized and may depend more on compassionate concern of caregivers than any other single factor" (p. 176; also Knapp and Peppers 1979; Murray and Callan 1988). One-third of bereaved women perceive their obstetrician as unresponsive to their emotional needs. The physician frequently becomes the target of the patient's anger. This reaction may be partly displaced anger toward the bearer of bad news who was not able to prevent or even explain the loss. Some obstetricians elicit the anger, however, by distancing themselves to avoid discomfiting emotions or because they perceive the loss as personal defeat (Costello et al. 1988; Turco 1981). Others are afraid that whatever they say may be used against them in a potential lawsuit.

Furthermore, many physicians find themselves inadequately trained to act as counselors and consolers. (Bourne 1968; Costello et al. 1988; Cullberg 1972; Stirtzinger and Robinson 1989). All that bereaved parents want, however, is empathy for their feelings, available information about their baby, and the offer of continued support. The responses offered or missed by the obstetrician in the crucial time prior and subsequent to the death are strong determinants of the couple's emotional outcome and the future doctor-patient relationship (Condon 1987).

The Support Team

A hospital-based perinatal bereavement team and a protocol for the care of the grieving parents have proven to be of great value (Condon 1987; Hutti 1988a, 1988b; Kellner et al. 1984; Lake et al. 1983; Leppert and Phalka 1984). The team includes perinatally trained obstetric nurses, a social worker, the obstetrician, a neonatologist, and a psychiatric consultation-liaison. The objective of the team is to facilitate the grief process by encouraging emotional expression and by validating the couple's feelings through empathic listening. A room offering privacy—possibly on a floor of the woman's choice—needs an inconspicuous, prearranged sign on the door to alert the hospital staff. The team members provide comfort and support while helping the couple to make the loss real—for example, by seeing and holding the baby if so desired, choosing further arrangements for the fetus's or infant's remains, discussing how to share grief with children at home, and preparing to face the outside world. Seeing and touching the dead baby underscores the finality of the loss. Mementos such as photos, footprints, or the baby's bracelet can be kept for later.

Continued communication about the loss needs to be encouraged, with the caveat that the partners' reactions to the grief may be incongruent and additional support may be desired (Lovell 1983b). Local perinatal bereavement groups can be of great help, particularly for women or couples without a social network. An experienced team will call the psychiatric consultant for uncommon bereavement reactions or preexisting problems such as psychopathology, marital discord, and other risk factors predisposing the woman to emotional decompensation under the impact of grief. This psychiatric assessment will determine whether work with a mental health professional is to be recommended after discharge.

Under ordinary circumstances, a follow-up visit 4–6 weeks postpartum serves to evaluate the progress of each partner and their interaction. The autopsy report may be available at this time and usually evokes intense emotions. Problems with incongruent grieving, isolation, and lack of social support are easily uncovered and may be addressed before they become rigidified.

Many couples ask about the timing of a subsequent pregnancy. The general consensus is that conception within 6 months of the loss can complicate the grief, intensify anxiety in the next pregnancy, and distort the attachment to the next child (Bourne and Lewis 1984; Kennell and Trause 1978; Lewis and Page 1978). The intent of such a pregnancy may be to avoid pain, but the "replacement child" can interfere with the process of mourning and may never be able to live up to the idealized sibling (Poznanski 1972). How long it takes for a couple to detach sufficiently from the lost child and to be ready for the next attempt is highly individual. Furthermore, other factors such as maternal age and fertility also need to be considered (Davis et al. 1989; Mandell and Wolfe 1975).

"Anniversary reactions" at 1 year following the expected due date are common but can also occur at other milestones of the lost pregnancy and are often relived in a subsequent one. A reassessment at the prior expected date for delivery or 4–6 months after the loss may uncover warning signs for pathological developments that warrant a psychiatric referral. Controlled follow-up studies show considerably enhanced adjustment for women who are supported by a grief team (Lake et al. 1987; Murray and Callan 1988), which ought to be established, at the least, in every tertiary obstetric center.

RISK FACTORS FOR COMPLICATED GRIEF

Twenty to thirty percent of grieving women experience significant psychiatric morbidity in the first year after perinatal loss, but symptoms may persist much longer (Cullberg 1972; LaRoche et al. 1984; Nicol et al. 1986; Tudehope et al. 1986). The initial intensity of the grief is no predictor for the duration, nor is the adjustment related only to the length of time that has passed since the loss. Many investigators have tried to define the normative range of a grief reaction and have examined predictive factors for subsequent psychopathology or interpersonal impairment. The findings were often conflicting or returned counterintuitive results (Zeanah 1989). One predictor for complications that persistently emerges, however, is the perceived lack of social support and concern by caregivers (Lake et al. 1987).

Psychological measures also show repeatedly that the mother's grief reaction is more intense than the father's, although large individual differences exist (Klaus and Kennell 1982; Wilson et al. 1982). Significant life stresses in pregnancy, a poor marital relationship, certain personality characteristics, and antecedent mental and physical health problems can also play a role as risk factors for the aggravation of grief (Toedter et al. 1988). It has yet to be determined to what extent these factors constitute dependent or independent variables.

Conflicting evidence remains about potential vulnerability predictors such as fetal gestational age at the time of the loss, previous reproductive failure, living children, maternal age, socioeconomic class, ambivalence toward pregnancy, fertility problems, and many more (LaRoche et al. 1984; Peppers and Knapp 1980; Theut et al. 1989; Toedter et al. 1988; Tudehope et al. 1986). It seems evident that the importance of each factor will depend on its perceived meaning within the context of an individual's life situation and cannot have identical predictive value for each person's grief. Furthermore, accumulation of factors will potentiate the risk for a complicated mourning process. We cannot yet quantify grief so as to have a reliable predictor for subsequent psychopathology.

PATHOLOGICAL GRIEF

Pathological grief—also called morbid, disordered, or complicated grief—has never been clearly defined. Its recognition was expanded by bereavement research based on the classic studies of Lindemann (1944) and Parkes (1965). Pathognomonic for complicated grief is a significant deterioration in mental or physical health as well as in social adjustment, which persists or replaces the predictable symptomatology and characteristics of the normal mourning process (Bowlby 1980; Raphael and Middleton 1990; Volkan 1970, 1972).

The manifestations of pathological grief include chronic, delayed, absent, or distorted grief. Characteristics of distorted grief include irritability, furious hostility, social isolation or aimless overactivity, and an inability to let go of the lost one. So far, little, if any, research has addressed the differences between pathological mourning after perinatal bereavement and the loss of an adult love object (Hutti 1984). Furthermore, the lack of a consensus about normative behavior after perinatal loss makes conclusions tentative at best (Zeanah 1989). Clinicians note a variety of idiosyncratic manifestations (Corney and Horton 1974). Here is one example:

L., a 32-year-old married woman was referred for evaluation by an in vitro fertilization team because she insisted on continuing her attempts to become pregnant despite 16 unsuccessful embryo transfers to various surrogate gestational mothers. She had drained her inheritance, and her marriage had become severely strained.

The couple had lost a premature infant 4 years previously, and L. conceived again very shortly thereafter. This pregnancy was complicated by a cesarean section close to term, and an unremitting hemorrhage mandated an emergency hysterectomy.

The couple's life plan had included a large family, and L.'s joy with the newborn concurred with a profound grief about the loss of her firstborn and the loss of her ability to have all the children she had anticipated in her dreams. Her husband and friends admonished her whenever she mourned until she felt her grief was selfish and a betrayal of her son. She defied her grief by holding tenaciously to hope by producing embryos for transfer into her womb substitutes.

Hutti (1984) suggests that it is very possible that the families themselves would be capable of describing many of the risk factors involved in pathological grieving, if a different approach and method of analysis were used.

PSYCHIATRIC INTERVENTION

Psychiatric intervention after a recent perinatal loss has two major functions: 1) to facilitate the mourning process and 2) to assess concurrently for potential risk factors that could interfere with the resolution of grief. Gentle encouragement and empathic listening to a detailed account of the traumatic events and their emotional repercussions will fulfill the first task. Open-ended questions about the surrounding circumstances and the meaning of the loss within the context of the woman's or the couple's life may uncover potential vulnerability factors. As in any crisis, latent intrapsychic and interpersonal conflicts are revived and become interwoven with the ongoing emotional turmoil. These unresolved conflicts can then become the obstacles for the resolution of grief.

The first case example outlined in this chapter is an example of an unresolved intrapsychic conflict. The grief work could proceed only after the pathogenic explanation was uncovered and the conflict was worked through. Unfounded self-blame has some adaptive function by giving a sense of control (albeit unfounded), as mentioned. Such unfounded self-blame, however, usually gives way to a more realistic understanding. Irrational guilt, on the other hand, has the relentless tenacity of a neurotic belief and evokes the profound distress of pathological mourning. The treatment goal is the resolution of the grief; the chronic underlying disturbances or defenses are confronted only when they block mourning. It is not in the patient's interest to address other potential pathogenic factors at this time, because this could add to the narcissistic injury caused by the perinatal loss.

Preexisting interpersonal conflicts tend to become aggravated during mourning and can distract from the resolution of grief. This happens most often in marital relationships when the incongruent grief process accentuates prior unmet needs and revives accumulated resentments. The relationship can become the focus for displaced anger about the loss, arresting further progress toward resolution of the grief. In joint sessions, the treatment goal is to lower the tension of the heightened conflicts by helping the partners to improve the mutual response to their stated needs within the limits of respected personality differences. Once the angry fixation is unblocked, the individual process of mourning can proceed.

What initially appeared as adaptive mourning can turn into pathological grief under the influence of dependent or independent variables. For instance, a subsequent pregnancy soon after the loss may arrest mourning, as can other intervening stressors. When the normal course of mourning derails into one of the several manifestations of pathologic grief, the therapeutic task is to help the patient to affectively revive the loss and "re-grieve."

The second case example may serve as an example of this approach. The patient knew on a rational level that the sacrifices had begun to outweigh the small chances for a positive return. She felt compelled, however, to use all her emotional and financial resources to bolster her defense against grief. Rationally, she was also aware that even a successful outcome would not wipe out the loss of her firstborn, her womb, or the other planned children. She realized that her frantic activity was putting an increasingly heavy burden on the well-being of her family. What had started out as an attempt to avoid "selfish" mourning had become a self-absorbed pursuit.

DSM-III-R (American Psychiatric Association 1987) and the *DSM-IV Options Book* (American Psychiatric Association 1991) include only "uncomplicated bereavement reaction"; unresolved grief is categorized as major depressive disorder. Chronic grief after perinatal loss can present like the latter, but various manifestations of pathologic grief—such as the inhibited mourning process in the case above—would not qualify for that diagnosis (Jacobs and Kim 1990; Rynearson 1990). Unresolved perinatal grief needs to be considered in every psychiatric history. Often women will refrain from mentioning this bereavement when they are asked about losses in general, because it is experienced as a separate part of their lives.

Various psychotherapeutic modalities are suitable for various clinical situations. A joint session with both partners is an essential part of the assessment. For an uncomplicated bereavement, short-term, primarily supportive therapy is appropriate, assisted at times by participation in self-help groups for perinatal loss. Complicated grief, on the other hand, often requires insight-oriented, interpretive, open-ended psychotherapy. When marital tension blocks grief resolution, initial conjoint sessions to achieve a mutually supportive interaction may need to continue at the same time as individual therapy with the woman alone, to help her resolve revived intrapsychic conflicts. The longest and most difficult work is with patients suffering from pathological grief. As mentioned previously, complicated grief reactions are intertwined with other unresolved conflicts and become included in the same tenacious, maladjusted defenses against releasing the affective charge. The unique aspects of perinatal grief relate to mourning of cherished wishes and dreams, which can be more difficult than mourning for memories of a loved one.

CONCLUSIONS

The incidence of perinatal loss will in all probability further decline through medical advances, provided that these are made accessible to all pregnant women. Even under the best of circumstances, however, some losses will be inevitable. Over the course of the last decade, health professionals have become aware of the suffering that such a loss afflicts on the bereaved and its potential to result in long-term psychiatric morbidity. Partners, clinicians, and researchers have alerted health professionals to the crucial role their support has for the bereaved. It is heartening to observe how publications on perinatal grief have spread from psychologically oriented professional journals to the obstetric, pediatric, reproductive, and other medical literature. Further applications of the knowledge gained from perinatally bereaved couples remain to be developed, and much research has yet to be done, but we have begun on the right course.

References

American Psychiatric Association: Diagnostic and Statistical Manual of Mental Disorders, 3rd Edition, Revised. Washington, DC, American Psychiatric Association, 1987

American Psychiatric Association: DSM-IV Options Book: Work in Progress 9/1/91. Washington, DC, American Psychiatric Association, 1991

Benedek T: The psychobiology of pregnancy, in Parenthood: Its Psychology and Psychopathology. Edited by Anthony J, Benedek T. Boston, MA, Little, Brown, 1970

Benfield DG, Leib SA, Vollman JH: Grief response of parents to neonatal death and parents' participation in deciding care. Pediatrics 62:171–177, 1978

Berg B: Nothing to Cry About. New York, Seaview Books, 1981

Borg S, Lasker J: When pregnancy fails. Boston, MA, Beacon Press, 1981

Bourne S: The psychological effects of stillbirths on women and their doctors. J R Coll Gen Pract 16:103–112, 1968

Bourne S: Psychological impact of stillbirth. Practitioner 227:53–60, 1983

Bourne S, Lewis E: Delayed psychological effects of perinatal deaths: the next pregnancy and the next generation. BMJ 289:209–210, 1984

Bowlby J: Attachment and Loss, Vol 1: Attachment. New York, Basic Books, 1969

Bowlby J: Attachment and Loss, Vol 2: Separation. New York, Basic Books, 1973

Bowlby J: Attachment and Loss, Vol 3: Loss. New York, Basic Books, 1980

Condon JT: The parental-fetal relationship—a comparison of male and female expectant parents. Journal of Psychosomatic Obstetrics and Gynaecology 4:271–284, 1985

Condon JT: Prevention of emotional disability following stillbirth—the role of the obstetric team. Aust N Z J Obstet Gynaecol 27:323–329, 1987

Corney RT, Horton FT: Pathological grief following spontaneous abortion. Am J Psychiatry 131:825–827, 1974

Costello A, Gardner SL, Merenstein GB: State of the art perinatal grief and loss. J Perinatol 8:361–370, 1988

Cruikshank DP, Linyear AS: Term stillbirth: causes and potential for prevention in Virginia. Obstet Gynecol 69:841–844, 1987

Cullberg J: Mental reactions of women to perinatal death, in Proceedings of the Third International Congress of Psychosomatic Obstetrics and Gynecology, London 1971. Basel, Switzerland, Karger, 1972, pp 326–329

Davis DL, Stewart M, Harmon RJ: Postponing pregnancy after perinatal death: perspectives on doctor advice. J Am Acad Child Adolesc Psychiatry 28:481–487, 1989

Freeman RK, Dorchester W, Anderson G, et al: The significance of a previous stillbirth. Am J Obstet Gynecol 151:7–13, 1985

Friedman R, Gladstein B: Surviving pregnancy loss. Boston, MA, Little, Brown, 1982

Gardner SL, Merenstein GB: Perinatal grief and loss: an overview. Neonatal Network 5(2):7–15, 1986

Gorer G: Death, Grief, and Mourning. New York, Doubleday, 1965, p 131

Herz EK: Psychological repercussions of pregnancy loss. Psychiatric Annals 14:454–457, 1984

Herz EK: The grief process after pregnancy loss, in The Psychiatric Implications of Menstruation. Edited by Gold JH. Washington, DC, American Psychiatric Press, 1985, pp 63–74

Hutti MH: An examination of perinatal death literature: implications for nursing practice and research. Health Care for Women International 5:387–400, 1984

Hutti MH: A quick reference table of interventions to assist families to cope with pregnancy loss or neonatal death. Birth 15:33–35, 1988a

Hutti MH: Perinatal loss: assisting parents to cope. Journal of Emergency Nursing 14:338–341, 1988b

Jacobs S, Kim K: Psychiatric complications of bereavement. Psychiatric Annals 20:314–317, 1990

Kellner KR, Donnelly WH, Gould SD: Parental behavior after perinatal death: lack of predictive demographic and obstetric variables. Obstet Gynecol 63:809–814, 1984

Kennell JH, Trause MA: Helping parents cope with perinatal death. Contemporary Ob/Gyn 12:53–68, 1978

Klaus M, Kennell J: Interventions in the premature nursery: impact on development. Pediatr Clin North Am 29:1263–1273, 1982

Knapp RJ, Peppers LG: Doctor-patient relationships in fetal/infant death encounters. Journal of Medical Education 54:775–780, 1979

Kubler-Ross E: On Death and Dying. New York, Macmillan, 1969

Lake M, Knuppel RA, Murphy J, et al: The role of a grief support team following stillbirth. Am J Obstet Gynecol 146:877–881, 1983

Lake MF, Johnson TM, Murphy J, et al: Evaluation of a perinatal grief support team. Am J Obstet Gynecol 157:1203–1206, 1987

LaRoche C, Lalinec-Michand M, Engelsmann F, et al: Grief reactions to perinatal death: a follow-up study. Can J Psychiatry 29:14–19, 1984

Leon IG: Psychodynamics of perinatal loss. Psychiatry 49:312–324, 1986

Leon IG: When a Baby Dies. New Haven, CT, Yale University Press, 1990

Leppert PC, Phalka BS: Grieving characteristics after spontaneous abortion: a management approach. Obstet Gynecol 64:119–122, 1984

Lewis E, Page A: Failure to mourn a stillbirth: an overlooked catastrophe. Br J Med Psychol 51:237–241, 1978

Lindemann E: Symptomatology and management of acute grief. Am J Psychiatry 101:141–148, 1944

Lovell A: Some questions of identity: late miscarriage, stillbirth and perinatal loss. Soc Sci Med 17:755–761, 1983a

Lovell A: Women's reactions to late miscarriage, stillbirth and perinatal death. Health Visitor 56:325–327, 1983b

Mandell F, Wolfe LC: Sudden infant death syndrome and subsequent pregnancy. Pediatrics 56:774–776, 1975

Murray J, Callan VJ: Predicting adjustment to perinatal death. Br J Med Psychol 61:237–244, 1988

Naeye RL: Causes of perinatal mortality in the U.S. collaborative perinatal project. JAMA 238:228–229, 1977

Naor S, Assael M, Pecht M, et al: Correlation between emotional reaction to loss of an unborn child and lymphocyte response to mitogenic stimulation in women. Isr J Psychiatry Rela Sci 20:231–239, 1983

Nicholas AM, Lewin TJ: Grief reactions of parental couples: congenital handicap and cot death. Med J Aust 144:292–295, 1986

Nicol MT, Tompkins JR, Campbell NA, et al: Maternal grieving response after perinatal death. Med J Aust 144:287–295, 1986

Parkes CM: Bereavement and mental illness, II: a classification of bereavement reactions. Br J Med Psychol 38:13–26, 1965

Parkes CM: Risk factors in bereavement: implications for the prevention and treatment of pathologic grief. Psychiatric Annals 20:308–313, 1990

Peppers LG, Knapp RJ: Maternal reactions to involuntary fetal/infant death. Psychiatry 43:155–159, 1980a

Peppers LG, Knapp RJ: Husbands and wives: incongruent grieving, in Motherhood and Mourning: Perinatal Loss. New York, Praeger, 1980b, p 66

Poznanski EO: The "replacement child": a saga of unresolved parental grief. Behavioral Pediatrics 81:1190–1193, 1972

Raphael B, Middleton W: What is pathologic grief? Psychiatric Annals 20:308–313, 1990

Rock JA, Zacur HA: The clinical management of repeated early pregnancy wastage. Fertil Steril 39:123–144, 1983

Rynearson EK: Pathologic grief: the queen's croquet ground. Psychiatric Annals 20:295–303, 1990

Seibel M, Graves WL: The psychological implications of spontaneous abortion. J Reprod Med 25:161–165, 1980

Stirtzinger R, Robinson GE: The psychologic effects of spontaneous abortion. Can Med Assoc J 140:799–801, 1989

Stotland NL: Perinatal complications, in Social Change and Women's Reproductive Health Care. Edited by Stotland NL. New York, Praeger, 1988

Stray-Pedersen B, Stray-Pedersen S: Etiologic factors and subsequent reproductive performance in 195 couples with prior history of habitual abortion. Am J Obstet Gynecol 148:140–146, 1984

Theut SK, Pedersen FA, Zaslow MJ, et al: Perinatal loss and parental bereavement. Am J Psychiatry 146:635–639, 1989

Toedter LJ, Lasker JN, Alhadeff JM: The Perinatal Grief Scale: development and initial validation. Am J Orthopsychiatry 58:435–449, 1988

Tudehope DI, Iredell J, Rodgers D, et al: Neonatal death: grieving families. Med J Aust 144:290–292, 1986

Turco R: The treatment of unresolved grief following loss of an infant. Am J Obstet Gynecol 141:503–507, 1981

U.S. Department of Health and Human Services: Health—United States, 1989 and Prevention Profile (DHHS Publ No PHS-90-1232). Hyattsville, MD, Public Health Service, 1990, p 107

Volkan V: Typical findings in pathological grief. Psychiatr Q 44:231–250, 1970

Volkan V: The recognition and prevention of pathological grief. Virginia Medical Monthly 99:535–540, 1972

Wijmak K: Comparison of mother's and father's coping with late fetal death, in Proceedings of the Seventh International Congress on Psychosomatic Obstetrics and Gynaecology, Jerusalem, Israel, 1983

Wilson AL, Fenton LJ, Stevens DC, et al: The death of a newborn twin: an analysis of parental bereavement. Pediatrics 70:587–591, 1982

Wilson AL, Witzke D, Fenton LJ, et al: Parental response to perinatal death: mother-father differences. Am J Dis Child 139:1235–1238, 1985

World Health Organization: World Health Statistics Annual. Geneva, Switzerland, World Health Organization, 1989, pp 13–14

Zeanah CH: Adaptation following perinatal loss: a critical review. J Am Acad Child Adolesc Psychiatry 28:467–480, 1989

SECTION II

GYNECOLOGY

Chapter 9

PSYCHIATRIC ASPECTS OF THE MENSTRUAL CYCLE

Margaret F. Jensvold, M.D.

❖ ❖ ❖ ❖ ❖ ❖ ❖ ❖ ❖ ❖ ❖ ❖ ❖ ❖

Biomedical researchers have commonly viewed the menstrual cycle as a confounding factor in research rather than as a legitimate subject of scientific study, a perspective that has contributed to the exclusion of women of reproductive age from much health research (Kinney et al. 1981). At the same time, a plethora of media articles have conveyed primarily negative images of the menstrual cycle and of premenstrual syndrome (PMS), along with conflicting diagnostic and treatment information and jokes (Chrisler and Levy 1990). If women and their health care providers are confused about the menstrual cycle, there is good reason.

Nevertheless, we do have some knowledge. Research during the past couple of decades has helped to clarify what the questions are and to point to directions for future research. This chapter is not intended to be entirely comprehensive, citing all research findings, but rather to present current research findings and illustrative points to provide a framework for clinicians, researchers, and health care consumers for conceptualizing the role of the menstrual cycle in psychiatry.

Many, if not most, physiologic parameters vary in a circadian manner (e.g., body temperature, cortisol level, thyrotropin-releasing hormone level, sleep-wake cycle), usually without causing symptoms and often with the person not even aware that the changes are occurring. Likewise, many physiologic parameters vary over the course of the normal menstrual cycle, causing no symptoms and often with the woman not aware of the change.

Cultural factors are well documented to have a significant influence on expectations and perceptions related to the menstrual cycle. With both physiologic and cultural factors contributing to changes over the menstrual cycle, how is one to make sense of pathology related to the menstrual cycle? This chapter discusses the physiology of the menstrual cycle, cultural considerations, and related diagnosis and treatment, with attention to methodologic and political concerns.

PHYSIOLOGY

The Normal Menstrual Cycle

The core events of the normal menstrual cycle consist of an integrally interconnected neuroendocrine feedback loop—the hypothalamic-pituitary-ovarian axis.[1] Readers are referred elsewhere for detailed accounts of the endocrine events of the normal menstrual cycle (Severino and Moline 1989; Speroff et al. 1982).

The menstrual cycle can be thought of as consisting of two phases, the follicular phase and the luteal phase, with cyclicity occurring in a number of organs and tissues (Figures 9–1 and 9–2). The suprahypothalamic events that take place over the course of the menstrual cycle are less well understood, but research in animals shows that neurotransmitters cycle catamenially[2] in various parts of the brain (McEwen 1988). The uterus is not a core player in the normal menstrual cycle, but rather is a target organ for hormonal action. Its regular, recurrent menstrual flow is an external indicator that a menstrual cycle has been completed and that another is beginning.

What constitutes the endogenous time clock of the menstrual cycle is relatively unknown at present, although the suprachiasmatic nucleus and associated structures are suspected to play a role (Kawa-

---

[1] A hypothalamic-pituitary-gonadal axis exists in men as well, of course—the hypothalamic-pituitary-testicular axis. The fact that it has no external indicator of its timing does not in itself mean that it does not have an endogenous timing mechanism.

[2] *Catamenial* means of or related to menses or the menstrual cycle.

kami et al. 1980). Circadian cycling is thought to be driven by the suprachiasmatic nucleus, with light input via the retinohypothalamic tract serving as a zeitgeber, or entraining factor that affects the cycle length but does not affect the presence or absence of the circadian cycle alto-

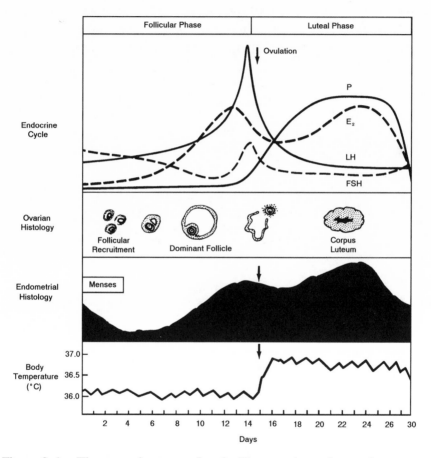

Figure 9–1.   The normal menstrual cycle. Hormonal, ovarian, endometrial, and basal body temperature changes and their relationships throughout the normal menstrual cycle are shown. P = progesterone. E_2 = estradiol. LH = luteinizing hormone. FSH = follicle-stimulating hormone.   *Source.*   Reprinted from Carr BR, Wilson JD: "Disorders of the Ovary and Female Reproductive Tract," in *Harrison's Principles of Internal Medicine,* 11th Edition. Edited by Braunwald E, Isselbacher KJ, Petersdorf RG, et al. New York, McGraw-Hill, 1987, p. 1823. Copyright 1987 McGraw-Hill. Used with permission.

gether. In the absence of light-dark cues, the circadian time clock still cycles in a regular circadian manner, but with a slightly longer average cycle length (27 hours, free running, compared to 24 hours, day-night entrained).

It is not entirely known whether ovarian input to the brain serves as a zeitgeber—simply entraining the timing of a catamenial cycle that would free-run without ovarian input—or whether ovarian input is integral to the continued catamenial cycling of the brain. There is some

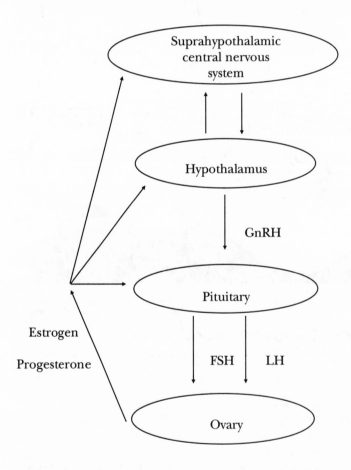

Figure 9–2.   Hypothalamic-pituitary-ovarian axis. The pathways of endogenous and exogenous hormones are shown. GnRH = gonadotropin-releasing hormone. FSH = follicle-stimulating hormone. LH = luteinizing hormone.

evidence in each direction. Evidence from treatment with gonadotropin-releasing hormone agonists indicates that when ovarian input is removed, catamenial cycling of central nervous system symptoms stops (Hammarback and Backstrom 1988). On the other hand, a study of patients with PMS who were using a progesterone antagonist, RU-486, showed that when the normal hormonal milieu of the latter quarter of the menstrual cycle is removed, thus displacing the timing of menstrual flow, menstrually related mood symptoms still occur at the usual time in some patients (Schmidt et al. 1991), indicating either that endocrine events earlier in the cycle ordained the timing of the cyclical mood symptoms or that central nervous system cycling continues independently of the peripheral hormonal milieu, at least for a time.

Variability in the Normal Menstrual Cycle

Although an occasional anovulatory cycle or shortened luteal phase is not uncommon, certain groups of women are more prone to menstrual irregularities, including heavy exercisers, anorexic patients, and women taking neuroleptic medications (Sullivan and Lukoff 1990) or abusing substances. Intercycle variability may be inherent to the self-regulatory mechanisms of normal menstrual cycles (McClintock 1992).

CULTURAL ASPECTS

The evidence for a strong cultural influence on our view of the menstrual cycle comes from a number of fronts. Menstrual taboos have existed across cultures and across time, including today. Deutsch discusses the psychological meaning of menstruation, pointing out the reasons that women deny it and hide it and the tendency to prefer to view it merely as a biological function rather than as having great psychological significance for the woman (Deutsch 1944). The words we use to describe the menstrual cycle convey our tendency to view it negatively, rather than positively (Martin 1987). PMS seems to be to the 20th century what neurasthenia was to the 19th century—a nebulous disorder primarily of women, involving the menstrual cycle, with numerous symptoms, etiologies, and treatments proposed, and conveying a negative view of women (King 1989).

The criteria for a culture-bound syndrome are met by PMS. As such, it constitutes a negotiated reality; its reality is that negotiated between those who treat it and those who suffer it (Morokoff 1991). PMS is unique in the extent to which the societal negotiation process has been overt and public—with research, debates, protests, letters back and forth, and papers supporting various points of view, and with a compromise solution placing late luteal phase dysphoric disorder in the appendix to the DSM-III-R, highlighting its negotiated and controversial status (American Psychiatric Association 1987).

A symbolic analysis of culture-bound syndromes provides an understanding not afforded by the biomedical approach alone (Morokoff 1991). Johnson (1987) argues that PMS addresses the traditional expectations of women and work, reinforcing the cultural double bind of the imperative for women to be both productive and reproductive. Although women with PMS may be unable to work for a limited period (Johnson 1987), they still must interact with others in a manner that is pleasing interpersonally (as is culturally mandated) most of the time. What is new is not the negative view of women as being weak, emotional, and unable to work, which in PMS is captured in the premenstrual phase; but rather the positive view of women as strong, powerful, and capable, which is captured in the nonpremenstrual phases of PMS.

Interpreted literally, PMS allows a woman access to power most of the time, while invalidating her and her experience part of the time. A regularly disabled woman is not seen as a capable woman, and a woman with PMS may be angry or assertive premenstrually and submissive the rest of the time, whether or not this behavior is appropriate to the circumstances (including oppression). Morokoff (1991) argues that PMS captures our cultural ambiguity regarding women and conception, because symptoms occur at the time of greatest ambiguity about whether the woman *has* conceived and, more importantly, whether the woman *should* conceive. PMS appears to constitute a transitional compromise for a culture in which women's roles have changed and men's have not (Morokoff 1991).

Studies show that women report more negative symptoms when they believe they are premenstrual than when they are led to believe that they are not premenstrual. Studies also indicate that women report more premenstrual symptoms when they are aware of the focus of the study than when they are not (Hamilton et al. 1989). These findings substantiate an expectancy component to symptom reporting.

PATHOLOGY AND THE MENSTRUAL CYCLE

Does a unique disorder of primarily psychological symptoms occurring only premenstrually exist? If so, what is its relationship to other psychiatric and medical disorders? Do other psychiatric and medical disorders themselves vary with the menstrual cycle?

A brief history of the term *premenstrual syndrome* is necessary to put into context our modern conceptualization of these questions. When Robert Frank, M.D., coined the term *premenstrual tension* (PMT) in 1931, he distinguished among what he considered to be three different groups of women. The first group had mild symptoms occurring premenstrually, such as fatigue, which he considered to be normal. The second group was characterized by systemic illnesses that varied with the menstrual cycle; he cited two examples, a case of catamenial asthma and a case of catamenial epilepsy. The third group was a small minority who experienced what he called "premenstrual tension," a disorder of severe emotional symptoms occurring premenstrually. These symptoms included, for example, suicidality, a "nervous tension," and "ill considered actions" for which the patients later had remorse, all with relief upon the onset of menses.

Subsequent writers, from the 1930s to the 1950s, added progressively more and more symptoms to the list of possible PMT symptoms. The result was that, by the 1950s, it was recommended that any and all symptoms that vary with the menstrual cycle should be considered as falling under the rubric of PMT, including asthma attacks and seizures. It was also recommended that the name of this clinical entity should be changed to *premenstrual syndrome* to emphasize the wide variety of possible symptoms beyond emotional ones.

With all symptoms related to the menstrual cycle lumped together, however, much confusion has followed. Questions such as the following became necessary: Is there really a single premenstrual syndrome, or many? Is progesterone the drug of choice for *all* cases of PMS, as is widely purported? Lost in the confusion was Frank's original delineation of a severe syndrome that is characterized primarily by psychological symptoms and is distinct from systemic illnesses that vary with the menstrual cycle as well as from normal, mild symptoms. In recent years, research has begun to bring us out of the confusion and, in the process, is pointing us back to Frank's forward-looking original impressions.

Disorders Varying With the Menstrual Cycle

Dysmenorrhea

Dysmenorrhea is defined as recurrent, catamenial pelvic pain. *Primary dysmenorrhea* occurs in the absence of discrete pathophysiology and *secondary dysmenorrhea* in the presence of discrete pathophysiology, including uterine fibromyomas and endometriosis. Now that primary dysmenorrhea is known to be caused by an excess of prostaglandins in the endometrial tissue and is treatable with prostaglandin synthetase inhibitors, it should no longer be considered a manifestation of neurosis or dismissed as "just part of being a woman" or a symptom of PMS.

Medical Disorders

The frequency or intensity of symptoms of a number of medical disorders varies with the phases of the menstrual cycle. These disorders include lupus erythematosus, acute intermittent porphyria, herpes genitalis, pneumothorax, and others (M. Jensvold and G. V. Foster, unpublished data, May 1984). In 10%–70% of women with migraines, the migraines occur regularly during or just before menses (Digre and Damasio 1987). In one study, 35% of women of reproductive age who had asthma reported that their asthma symptoms worsened just before or during menses. Daily spirometry confirmed a significant deterioration in airway resistance during menses only in the group who reported an association of symptoms to the menstrual cycle (Hanley 1981).

Psychiatric Disorders

What is the evidence that psychiatric disorders vary with the menstrual cycle? A few studies have begun to address this question.

Bulimia. In three prospective studies of binge behavior in bulimic women, a modest but statistically significant premenstrual exacerbation of binge eating was found in one study, without an increase in depression (Gladis and Walsh 1987). Another prospective study found a significantly increased frequency of binge episodes in the luteal phase (Price et al. 1987). The third study found no significant changes in eating behavior over the menstrual cycle, although 22% of the women were found to have cyclothymic-type mood changes in association with the menstrual cycle. However, 44% of the women were taking antidepressants or tranquilizers, and 22% had irregular menstrual cycles. In addition, a nonstandard method of data analysis was used, making the results of the latter study difficult to interpret. A report of two patients contrasted one whose bulimic binge increased regularly premenstrually and one whose bulimic binge showed no association with the menstrual cycle (McDaniel 1989).

Panic disorder. In three studies of panic disorder, 40%–90% of the women retrospectively reported worsening of panic or anxiety premenstrually. Using prospective ratings, two of the studies found no evidence of menstrual cycle–related changes in panic (Cook et al. 1990; Stein et al. 1989). The third study found significant worsening in intensity of full-situation panic attacks, the other parameters not showing significant variation. The authors concluded that actual fluctuations in anxiety symptoms across the menstrual cycle were rather small (Cameron et al. 1988).

Affective disorders. Much evidence links affective symptoms and the menstrual cycle. Prevalence rates for premenstrual depression were found to be 65% by several groups examining its prevalence in patients with current or past diagnoses of affective disorder. In patients complaining of premenstrual depression, 39% showed the disorder on daily ratings and 36% showed intermittent depression throughout the cycle (McMillan and Pihl 1987). Lifetime diagnoses of major depressive disorder were found to have prevalence rates of 57%–100% among women in five different samples that met criteria for premenstrual depression. Complaints of premenstrual depression have been found to have predictive value in terms of future depression (Graze et al. 1990).

Data suggest a susceptibility to cycling among women. Most persons with rapid-cycling bipolar disorder are women (Wehr et al. 1988). The same is true of seasonal affective disorder. The mood disorders of only a few of these women, however, cycle in relation to the menstrual cycle (Conrad and Hamilton 1986; Kukopulos et al. 1985; Wehr et al. 1988). The reasons for women's increased susceptibility to cyclicity are not known, and the mechanisms of the interrelationships between mood and cycling are not well understood.

Posttraumatic stress disorders and dissociative disorders.   There is some evidence of a menstrual cycle–related pattern in posttraumatic symptoms and dissociative disorders in some women presenting with complaints of PMS (Jensvold et al. 1989).

PMS and Late Luteal Phase Dysphoric Disorder

Definition

Two definitions of PMS are used most often in the research and clinical literature: 1) a "common" definition of PMS and 2) late luteal phase dysphoric disorder (LLPDD). The common definition of PMS requires a combination of common psychological and physical symptoms that occur premenstrually and are absent during the follicular phase. Commonly cited psychological symptoms include sadness, irritability, and tension or anxiety. Commonly cited physical symptoms include bloating and breast tenderness.

The term *LLPDD*, in contrast, has been used to date only in some of the most recent mental health literature, as would be expected, since LLPDD is a recently available diagnosis. It emphasizes psychological symptoms (physical symptoms being optional), includes a severity criterion, and requires confirmation on daily ratings (Table 9–1) (American Psychiatric Association 1991).

LLPDD as Distinguished From Other Disorders

Women can be identified who report severe symptoms, including occupational or social impairment, only during the premenstrual period; who are confirmed to fulfill the criteria for LLPDD on prospective ratings; and who do not seem to have another current psychiatric illness (Hurt et al. 1992). However, whether the LLPDD, as conceptualized, is reliable and valid as a diagnostic category or is the optimal taxonomic categorization continues to be explored (Halbreich et al. 1983; Hamilton and Gallant 1990; Spitzer et al. 1989). Certainly, rigor is needed in our taxonomic categorizations in order for research and treatment to be most appropriately directed.

Relationship of LLPDD to Other Psychiatric Disorders

One of the diagnostic criteria for LLPDD is that the symptoms are not attributable to another psychiatric disorder. In the presence of another psychiatric disorder, however, it is difficult to determine whether the premenstrual symptoms are attributable to the psychiatric disorder. The nature of the relationship between concurrent LLPDD and other psychiatric disorders remains to be elucidated.

Findings in PMS Research

Prevalence of symptoms.   A number of studies show at least 75% of women reporting at least one symptom occurring premenstrually. The percentage of women who report that symptoms are severe or bothersome enough to warrant treatment, however, is much lower. Psychological symptoms are often reported to be the most distressing. Positive changes also occur premenstrually (Stewart 1989) but often are not looked for. Two studies examined the prevalence of women who fulfill the diagnostic criteria for LLPDD. In one, a community-based survey including prospective ratings, 3.4% of women of reproductive age reported severe symptoms (R. F. Haskett, unpublished

---

Table 9–1. Diagnostic criteria for late luteal phase dysphoric disorder

---

A. In most menstrual cycles during the past year, symptoms in C occurred during the last week of the luteal phase and remitted within a few days after onset of the follicular phase. In menstruating females, these phases correspond to the week before, and a few days after, the onset of menses. (In nonmenstruating females who have had a hysterectomy, the timing of luteal and follicular phases may require measurement of circulating reproductive hormones.)

B. The disturbance markedly interferes with work or with usual social activities or relationships with others.

C. At least five of the following symptoms have been present for most of the time during each symptomatic late luteal phase, at least one of the symptoms being either (1), (2), (3), or (4):

  (1) marked affective lability (e.g., feeling suddenly sad or tearful)

  (2) persistent and marked anger or irritability

  (3) marked anxiety, tension, feelings of being "keyed up," or "on edge"

  (4) markedly depressed mood, feelings of hopelessness, or self-deprecating thoughts

  (5) decreased interest in usual activities (e.g., work, friends, hobbies)

  (6) lethargy, easy fatigability, or marked lack of energy

  (7) subjective sense of difficulty in concentrating

  (8) marked change in appetite, overeating, or specific food cravings

  (9) hypersomnia or insomnia

  (10) other physical symptoms, such as breast tenderness or swelling, headaches, joint or muscle pain, a sensation of "bloating," weight gain

  (11) avoidance of social activities (e.g., staying at home)

  (12) decreased productivity and efficiency at work and at home

  (13) increased sensitivity to rejection

  (14) subjective sense of being overwhelmed ("can't cope")

  (15) subjective sense of feeling "out of control"

  (16) increased interpersonal conflicts

D. The disturbance is not merely an exacerbation of the symptoms of another disorder, such as Major Depressive Disorder, Panic Disorder, Dysthymic Disorder, or a Personality Disorder (although it may be superimposed on any of these disorders).

E. Criteria A, B, C, and D are confirmed by prospective daily self-ratings during at least two symptomatic cycles. (The diagnosis may be made provisionally prior to this confirmation.)

Source. Reprinted from American Psychiatric Association: *DSM-IV Options Book: Work in Progress 9/1/91.* Washington, DC, American Psychiatric Association, 1991, pp. T:3–T:4. Copyright 1991 American Psychiatric Association. Used with permission.

data, May 1987). In the other study, 4.6% of college-age women reported severe symptoms (Rivera-Tovar and Frank 1990). These results suggest that 3%–5% of women of reproductive age may meet the criteria for LLPDD.

Prevalence of Axis I and Axis II disorders.   Only one study has examined the lifetime prevalence of both Axis I and Axis II disorders in women meeting the criteria for LLPDD. Depression was found to be more prevalent in women with LLPDD than in the community-based Epidemiologic Catchment Area (ECA) study, although the prevalence of other psychiatric disorders was similar to ECA figures. Seventy-eight percent of women meeting LLPDD criteria had a lifetime history of Axis I disorders, prior depression being most prevalent. Ten percent met the criteria for Axis II disorders, avoidant personality being most prevalent. Twenty percent were shown to have current psychiatric disorders, despite attempts to exclude women with current psychiatric disorders (Pearlstein et al. 1990).

In a study in which data were pooled from five institutions, 670 women who sought treatment for PMS were examined, of whom 39% were found to have only past psychiatric disorders, 27% had a current psychiatric disorder, and 33% had no psychiatric history. The authors concluded that LLPDD was not simply synonymous with another psychiatric disorder and that a psychiatric history increased the risk of LLPDD, but that having a present psychiatric disorder did not increase the risk of LLPDD. The prevalence of LLPDD varied substantially as a function of the four methods of analyzing daily ratings data (Hurt et al. 1992).

Hormone studies.   Numerous studies have shown no consistent abnormalities in peripheral hormone levels in women with PMS (Rubinow et al. 1988). There is some evidence of a hormone axis instability (Roy-Byrne et al. 1987), and a number of studies have now shown abnormalities in serotonin metabolism (Ashby et al. 1990). Circadian phase shifts may be implicated in some patients (Parry and Wehr 1987). The concept of "multiple cyclic change" occurring as a diversified, dynamic, time-related process (Halbreich et al. 1988, p. 183) is probably more accurate than any hypothesis of unitary abnormalities in accounting for the diversity of symptoms reported with PMS.

Methodologic and Political Issues in PMS Research

Prospective ratings.   The method used in analyzing daily ratings greatly affects the percentage of women meeting the diagnostic criteria for PMS. Currently, daily ratings are seen as the "gold standard" for diagnosis, and negative prospective ratings automatically take precedence over the woman's positive self-report. Cases with discordant retrospective self-report and prospective ratings should be examined more closely for the presence of any of a number of factors contributing to the discordance (Figure 9–3). Reasons to trust prospective ratings over self-report are the evidence of misattributions and negative expectancies. There are a number of reasons, however, for not assuming that prospective ratings are necessarily the ultimate conveyor of truth. These reasons include the possibility of inadvertently creating false-positive or false-negative results by setting cutoffs too low or too high, intercycle variability, and evidence that as many women who do

		Daily ratings (DR)	
		+	−
	+	**Concordant** Positive	**Discordant** False-positive SR or False-negative DR
Self- report (SR)	−	**Discordant** False-negative SR or False-positive DR	**Concordant** Negative

Figure 9–3.   Meeting diagnostic criteria by self-report and daily ratings.

not report having PMS as women who do report having PMS fulfill the diagnostic criteria for PMS on the basis of prospective ratings (Gallant et al. 1992). In addition, when daily ratings were adjusted for range or standard deviation of scale responses (Gallant et al. 1992), no significant differences were found between men's and women's daily ratings. Approaches to discordant cases should be individualized; for example, if there is the presence of a psychiatric disorder in the follicular phase, treatment of that disorder is indicated.

There is some evidence that more severe cases of PMS show greater concordance, with discordance in self-report and daily ratings increasing for less severe cases. In one well-designed study, retrospective reports of PMS were predictive of future major depression, even in women without a personal or family history of depression. Retrospective reports were a better predictor in this study than daily ratings (Graze et al. 1990).

Diagnostic options. Various options exist as to how menstrually related psychiatric symptoms could be denoted in the official psychiatric diagnostic nomenclature. One option is to describe a unique disorder of primarily psychological symptoms that occur premenstrually (LLPDD). Another is the denotation of a psychiatric disorder that has a "menstrual cycle pattern" (similar to the "seasonal pattern" denotation in DSM-III-R). A third alternative is to denote a category of hormone-related disorders, in which male disorders related to hormones could also be included.

Chasm between research and practice. Current research practices automatically exclude from most PMS research women whose self-report and daily ratings are discordant, as well as those who choose not to comply with 2 months of daily ratings. Also, the diagnosis of LLPDD, as currently specified, identifies moderate cases—women who are impaired premenstrually but who can tolerate and are willing to complete 2 months of ratings prior to treatment. The full spectrum of severity of cases, however, presents to clinicians. A chasm, therefore, currently exists between research (which needs rigorously defined homogeneous patient populations) and clinical needs (with the mandate to help all women who present for help).

Political issues. Stotland (1992) points out two main categories of risks to women from an LLPDD diagnosis: 1) the risk that a menstrually related psychiatric disorder poses for all women in terms of potential stigmatization of women and 2) the impact of a narrowly defined LLPDD on the majority of women who now present for treatment of PMS who would be excluded. To say either that all women who have menstrual cycles have a disorder, or that no women who have menstrual cycles have a menstrually related disorder, is to minimize the subject and to not listen to women's experience.

Symptoms is not synonymous with *syndromes* and must be distinguished. The media often portray as mild or moderate PMS what researchers would call normal (Chrisler and Levy 1990). Concern that women with normal menstrual cycles and minimal or no symptoms will be declared to have disorders is not alleviated by the fact that some scales still used in the field classify all women as having varying severities of PMS, with no way of classifying a woman as not having PMS.

No other diagnosis requires prospective ratings to confirm the patient's self-report. The mandatory compliance with daily ratings of sufferers of other disorders has not been studied (Stotland 1992). The assumptions that prospective ratings are always correct, and that discordance between prospective ratings and the woman's retrospective self-report automatically invalidates her self-report, are discriminatory. Hormones contribute to disorders or symptoms in men, such as aggressivity, but do not receive attention as such.

Law. The use of PMS as a legal defense has succeeded in Canada and England, but has been controversial and generally unsuccessful in the United States. A recent case in Virginia received a great deal of publicity, and concern has been expressed that with the use of PMS as a legal defense, all women will be on trial. The barriers to the successful use of PMS as a legal defense seem to be formidable, however (Severino and Moline 1989). Numerous questions remain regarding the implications if PMS is successfully used in this manner. For example, what should be done with the PMS offender who fails or refuses to obtain court-ordered treatment? Is there clear evidence that treatment will succeed (see next section)?

TREATMENT AND THE MENSTRUAL CYCLE

Chronotherapy

Chronobiology has been described as follows (Haen 1988, p. 7):

> ... the broad spectrum of interacting and interdigitating rhythms
> that all together comprise the *time structure* of a living organism. ...
> [By learning the patterns of] biological variations we can compare,
> correlate and finally predict their course. This development makes it
> necessary and possible for physicians to concentrate more closely on
> the individual needs of their patients through *patient-monitoring* and
> *time-specified medications.*

The issue of chronotherapy, or timing therapy, has received much
less attention in psychiatry than it deserves. The following question
arises: If symptoms occur during certain phases of the menstrual cycle
for a particular woman, when should treatment be administered: constantly (throughout the menstrual cycle), periodically (recurrently,
e.g., premenstrually only), or varying (e.g., with increased dosage premenstrually)? The question also arises whether fluctuations in symptoms are caused by physiologic variables (which would occur in any
woman with a normal menstrual cycle), pathologic variables (which
would occur only in persons with the disorder), or as an interactive
process between the two. If the latter, what is the nature of the interaction between fluctuating physiologic and pathologic factors?

Lithium treatment illustrates these concepts well. Individual cases
document that, for some women with bipolar illness, their mood
symptoms and lithium levels vary according to menstrual cycle phases.
In one study, one woman's bipolar illness was in good control except
for premenstrual recurrence of symptoms when she was taking a constant dose of lithium. On a constant lithium dose, her serum lithium
levels dropped premenstrually. When the lithium dose was increased
premenstrually, serum levels remained constant, with good control of
symptoms (Conrad and Hamilton 1986). In another case, a woman
with bipolar illness had regular recurrence of hypomania early in the
cycle, depression late in the cycle, and symptomatic relief with the

onset of menses. Her lithium levels were regularly lowest when she was hypomanic, highest when she was depressed, and intermediate with euthymic mood (Kukopulos et al. 1985).

Do physiologic factors account for these changes in lithium levels? A study of lithium levels in regularly menstruating, normal women found that serum lithium levels following the administration of a single dose of lithium were identical, regardless of the phase of the menstrual cycle and of whether the women were taking oral contraceptives (Chamberlain et al. 1990). This finding indicates that physiologic factors in the normal menstrual cycle do not account for menstrual cycle-related changes in lithium levels, which are probably more related to changes in pathology (e.g., manic or depressive, rather than luteal or follicular). In a study of 54 persons with rapid-cycling bipolar illness, 92% were women, but none were found to switch moods in relation to the menstrual cycle, highlighting the fact that not all women with bipolar illness cycle in relation to the menstrual cycle (Wehr et al. 1988). In addition, Hatotani et al. (1983) found an association between mood and the menstrual cycle in bipolar patients but found that mood was sometimes slightly out of synchronization with the menstrual cycle, raising the issue of what is the actual association between mood and the menstrual cycle.

Why does bipolar illness entrain to the menstrual cycle in some, but not all, regularly menstruating women? What accounts for cycling that moves in and out of synchronization with the menstrual cycle? What is the role of oral contraceptives in entraining pathology to the menstrual cycle, or in freeing it from entrainment? The data discussed here raise as many questions as they answer.

Interaction Between Endogenous Hormones and Psychotropic Medications

Women take more medications, including more psychotropic medications, than do men. Even when the number of medications taken is taken into account, women suffer more adverse effects from medications than do men. Almost certainly one of the contributing factors is lack of attention to the menstrual cycle. The physician who ignores the menstrual cycle runs the twin risks of overtreating or undertreating the patient. If the phase of the menstrual cycle is not considered, cycle-dependent symptoms may be misinterpreted as side effects or as ineffectiveness of the medication.

Clinically significant side effects in relation to sex or hormone levels are known for mood stabilizers (lithium), antidopaminergic and antipsychotic drugs, anticonvulsants (e.g., phenytoin), some benzodiazepines (e.g., diazepam), propranolol, and alcohol (Hamilton 1991). One patient's premenstrual depression was documented to require a varying dose of antidepressant medication throughout the menstrual cycle. A constant low dose of tricyclic antidepressant was well tolerated but only partially effective. A constant higher dose was effective for premenstrual symptoms but was not tolerated in the follicular phase. A varying dose, with a higher dose premenstrually, was effective and well tolerated (Jensvold et al. 1992). Women with catamenial epilepsy had a marked decrease in phenytoin during menses compared with controls and compared with women with noncatamenial epilepsy. Recurrent premenstrual failure of migraine prophylaxis was associated with lower steady-state serum levels of propranolol during menses (Gengo et al. 1984). Some drugs, including salicylates, aminopyrine, nitrazepam, and paracetamol, do not show clearly significant menstrual cycle effects (Hamilton 1991). Without systematically monitoring drug-hormone interactions, the drug differences that have come to our attention can be considered to be the tip of the iceberg. Future studies will show that some drugs do not show any substantial menstrual cycle–related effects, but we do not yet know which drugs those are.

When menstrual cycle–related effects have been found, they often occur in subgroups of women (e.g., those taking lithium or phenytoin), and reported effects generally tend toward increased clearance premenstrually (Hamilton 1991). Sex steroid hormones can have differential effects on partial pathways for various metabolites. Competition between drugs and hormones for the same metabolic sites may account for some differences in metabolic rates in women compared with men or over time (Hamilton 1991). Interindividual differences in the use of alternative metabolic pathways, or in levels of or sensitivity to endogenous sex steroid hormones, may explain why only some women experience menstrual cycle–related effects (Hamilton 1991).

In an additional 37 women whose depressive symptoms varied over the menstrual cycle, 27 were treated adequately with constant antidepressant dosage, whereas 10 required variable dosings over the menstrual cycle to optimize therapeutic benefits or minimize side effects (Jensvold et al. 1992).

Interaction Between Exogenous Hormones and Psychotropic Medications

Oral Contraceptives

In a review of interactions between oral contraceptives and other medications, Teichmann (1990) concluded that medications showing clinically significant interactions with oral contraceptives include antidepressants, antihypertensives, insulin, synthetic glucocorticoids, theophylline, and caffeine. The *Medical Letter Handbook* listed clinically significant interactions of oral contraceptives or estrogens with 29 classes of drugs (Rizack and Hillman 1991).

Oral contraceptives tend to increase the clearance of drugs metabolized by glucuronidation (e.g., some benzodiazepines) and to decrease that of drugs metabolized by oxidative pathways, including the cytochrome P-450 oxidase system (e.g., imipramine, diazepam, caffeine, chlordiazepoxide).

Twenty-seven percent of women of reproductive age in the United States use oral contraceptives, which means that a number of women presenting to psychiatrists are using or will use chemical contraceptive agents. Psychiatric side effects of oral contraceptives were more frequent in the older, higher-dose preparations, but mood effects have been observed with the lower-dose preparations as well. Mood effects from low-dose oral contraceptives have been observed to be responsive to antidepressant medication (J. A. Hamilton, personal communication, June 1991). Oral contraceptives may entrain psychopathology to the menstrual cycle in some cases or may free symptoms from entrainment to the menstrual cycle in others (M. F. Jensvold, unpublished observations, June 1991), although this has been studied very little. In some cases a woman may need to stop hormonal therapy in order to know what role the oral contraceptives are playing in her symptoms:

exacerbating them, ameliorating them, or having no effect.

The oral contraceptive formulations now available to women in the United States include 1) combination medication (in which estrogen and progestogen are taken together for 21 days, followed by a hormone-free week; this is the most commonly used preparation), 2) sequential medication, including triphasic pills (with varying doses of hormones taken sequentially, also commonly used), 3) the "minipill," consisting of low-dose progesterone only (daily oral micronized progesterone, which has fewer side effects but is less commonly used because of its slightly lower effectiveness), and 4) long-acting subcutaneous progesterone (Norplant). Other long-acting progesterone derivatives and chemical contraceptive agents are being tested and used in Europe, Scandinavia, and elsewhere.

Postmenopausal Hormone Replacement Therapy

In a survey study, 32% of postmenopausal women were found to take hormone replacement therapy (HRT) (Harris et al. 1990). HRT differs from oral contraceptives in that it uses natural conjugated estrogens, which do not affect the cytochrome P-450 oxidase system, whereas oral contraceptives use synthetic estrogens (e.g., ethinyl estradiol), which do affect that system. Also, the dosages of hormones are about 1.1–2.5 times higher in oral contraceptives than in HRT.

Nevertheless, HRT can cause mood effects, with progesterone thought to be responsible for recurrent dysphoric moods associated with HRT (Magos et al. 1986). Estrogen, however, has been shown to trigger rapid cycling in vulnerable women (Oppenheim 1984). Consequently, women with histories of affective disorders should be monitored closely for mood effects when HRT is begun.

Postmenopausal HRT is known to cause PMS-like symptoms in some women (Magos et al. 1986), in effect producing iatrogenic PMS. This leads some women to present to psychiatrists for treatment of new-onset or recurrent PMS-like symptoms or mood symptoms. I have found that symptoms can be minimized by decreasing the hormone dose or changing the timing, for example, changing the 10-day interval of progestogen from once monthly to once every 3 months. If these interventions do not provide sufficient relief, consideration should be given to stopping the hormone therapy or adding a psychotropic agent.

Gonadotropin-Releasing Hormone Agonists

Potent gonadotropin-releasing hormone (GnRH) agonists bind powerfully to GnRH receptors at the level of the pituitary, thus blocking the pulsatile action of GnRH. After transiently increasing the release of luteinizing hormone and follicle-stimulating hormone from the pituitary, GnRH agonists paradoxically block the pituitary's normal response to GnRH, thus effecting a "chemical oophorectomy." GnRH agonists are being increasingly used for endometriosis and other conditions. Three forms of GnRH agonists are now available: intramuscular, intranasal, and depot GnRH. The forms vary with respect to ease of administration and in how much control one has over the dose administered. Estrogen deficiency-related symptoms, including hot flushes and osteoporosis, are considerations in the decision regarding whether to use these agents.

Although GnRH agonists have been reported to ameliorate severe premenstrual symptoms, some women experience transient worsening of symptoms in the first month of treatment. One woman had her first hypomanic episode precipitated by GnRH agonists, and in other women mood disorders have remained but become unentrained from the menstrual cycle on these agents.

Gynecologic Versus Psychotropic Medications for Treatment of Premenstrual Symptoms

Because the hypothalamic-pituitary-ovarian axis is an interconnected feedback loop, interventions at different levels of the feedback loop may, at least theoretically, affect a particular targeted, menstrually related symptom.

Gynecologic Treatments

Several methods that have in common the prevention of ovulation have been attempted for the treatment of premenstrual symptoms. Surgical oophorectomy (Casson et al. 1990) and chemical oophorectomy using GnRH agonists (Hammarback and Backstrom 1988) appear to provide lasting relief of severe premenstrual psychological and physical symptoms. Their use is inappropriate for most PMS patients, however, and requires psychiatric screening and long-term follow-up studies. Hysterectomy without oophorectomy provides more variable results, as would be expected, since it removes menses, the external time cue, but the hormonal cycle remains intact. Danazol, an androgenic agent, inhibits ovulation and provides relief for some premenstrual symptoms, particularly mastalgia, but appears to cause or exacerbate depression and irritability in some patients. Oral contraceptives appear to worsen PMS in some women, have no effect in others, and perhaps ameliorate symptoms in still others.

Progesterone as a treatment for PMS is now essentially disproved, as numerous double-blind, controlled studies have failed to show its superiority over placebo (Magos 1990). Additionally, a study using progesterone antagonists appears to disprove the hypothesis that luteal-phase progesterone plays a role in causing catamenial mood symptoms (Schmidt et al. 1991).

Psychotropic Agents

A study of fluoxetine treatment for LLPDD found that premenstrual physical symptoms, as well as psychological symptoms, were ameliorated by fluoxetine (Stone et al. 1991). In Canada, a large, randomized, placebo-controlled, double-blind treatment trial of fluoxetine for LLPDD is nearing completion. A number of smaller trials and reports suggest a role for antidepressant medication in treating LLPDD, and a case report and case series show a role for varying the antidepressant dose in some women to optimize the treatment of menstrual cycle–related depressive symptoms (Jensvold et al. 1992). Studies have shown the efficacy of alprazolam treatment over placebo for LLPDD (Harrison et al. 1990; Smith et al. 1987).

Nonbiologic Treatments of Menstrually Related Symptoms

Dynamic issues regarding the menstrual cycle and what it means to the individual woman are important in some cases. Menstrual cyclicity

188 ❖ *Psychological Aspects of Women's Health Care*

can indirectly affect psychotherapy as well, with some psychother-apeutic work being more possible, more necessary, or more or less effective during certain phases. An example is the woman with state-dependent, recurrent premenstrual flashbacks of earlier trauma (Jensvold et al. 1989). If expectancies or misattributions are thought to play a significant role with a particular patient, then cognitive ther-apy techniques, interpersonal therapy, or feminist therapy, which ex-amines the woman-in-context, including societal influences, rather than narrowly focusing on intrapsychic factors, may be helpful. Sup-port groups may also play a useful role, with group members recogniz-ing dysfunctional behavioral or emotional patterns or expectancies and developing increased insight, confidence, and coping.

CONCLUSIONS

It seems now that Robert Frank was forward-looking in 1931 in distin-guishing among women with a unique psychological disorder occur-ring premenstrually, normal women with mild symptoms, and women whose systemic illnesses varied with the menstrual cycle. Excessive lumping together of disorders over subsequent decades has caused confusion among researchers, clinicians, patients, and the public. State-of-the-art research is now sorting out various threads, addressing questions implied by Frank's clinical observation: Is there validity to a single diagnostic category describing psychological symptoms occur-ring only premenstrually? Do other psychiatric disorders vary with the menstrual cycle? How can one address real problems without stigma-tizing women and without playing into the already excessively nega-tive views of the menstrual cycle and of women? What are the roles of gynecologic and psychotropic agents in treating psychiatric disorders related to the menstrual cycle?

Psychiatric symptoms and the menstrual cycle represent a conflu-ence where mind-body issues can be addressed in interesting and im-portant ways. The potential exists for much to be learned about chronobiology, brain-endocrine interactions, and cultural overlay, as well as the promise of improving the health of our women patients.

REFERENCES

American Psychiatric Association: Diagnostic and Statistical Manual of Mental Disorders, 3rd Edition, Revised. Washington, DC, American Psychiatric Association, 1987

American Psychiatric Association: DSM-IV Options Book: Work in Progress 9/1/91. Washington, DC, American Psychiatric Association, 1991

Ashby C, Carr L, Cook C, et al: Alteration of 5-HT uptake by plasma fractions in the premenstrual syndrome. J Neural Transm Gen Sect 79:41–50, 1990

Cameron O, Kuttesch D, McPhee K, et al: Menstrual fluctuation in the symptoms of panic anxiety. J Affective Disord 15:169–174, 1988

Carr BR, Wilson JD: Disorders of the ovary and female reproductive tract, in Harrison's Principles of Internal Medicine, 11th Edition. Edited by Braunwald E, Isselbacher KJ, Petersdorf RG, et al. New York, McGraw-Hill, 1987

Casson P, Hahn P, Vugt D, et al: Lasting response to ovariectomy in severe intractable premenstrual syndrome. Am J Obstet Gynecol 162:99–105, 1990

Chamberlain S, Hahn P, Casson P, et al: Effect of menstrual cycle phase and oral contraceptive use on serum lithium levels after a loading dose of lithium in normal women. Am J Psychiatry 147:907–909, 1990

Chrisler J, Levy K: The media construct a menstrual monster: a content analysis of PMS articles in the popular press. Women Health 16:89–104, 1990

Conrad C, Hamilton J: Recurrent premenstrual decline in serum lithium concentration: clinical correlates and treatment implications. Journal of the American Academy of Clinical Psychiatry 26:852–853, 1986

Cook B, Noyes R, Garvey M, et al: Anxiety and the menstrual cycle in panic disorder. J Affective Disord 19:221–226, 1990

Deutsch H: The Psychology of Women: A Psychoanalytic Interpretation. New York, Grune & Stratton, 1944

Digre K, Damasio H: Menstrual migraine: differential diagnosis, evaluation, and treatment. Clin Obstet Gynecol 30:417–430, 1987

Frank R: The hormonal causes of premenstrual tension. Arch Neurol Psychiatry 26:1053–1057, 1931

Gallant SJ, Popiel DA, Hoffman DM, et al: Using daily ratings to confirm premenstrual syndrome/late luteal phase dysphoric disorder, Part II: what makes a real difference? Psychosom Med 54:167–181, 1992

Gengo F, Fagan S, Kinkel W, et al: Serum concentrations of propranolol and migraine prophylaxis. Arch Neurol 41:1306–1307, 1984

Gladis M, Walsh B: Premenstrual exacerbation of binge eating in bulimia. Am J Psychiatry 144:1592–1595, 1987

Graze K, Nee J, Endicott J: Premenstrual depression predicts future major depressive disorder. Acta Psychiatr Scand 81:201–205, 1990

Haen E (ed): Chronopharmacology of Reversible Airways Obstruction. Frankfurt, Germany, University of Munich, 1988

Halbreich U, Endicott J, Nee J: Premenstrual depressive changes: value of differentiation. Arch Gen Psychiatry 40:535–542, 1983

Halbreich U, Holtz I, Paul L: Premenstrual changes: impaired hormonal homeostasis. Neurol Clin 6:173–194, 1988

Hamilton J: Clinical pharmacology panel report, in Forging a Women's Health Research Agenda, Conference Proceedings. Edited by Blumenthal SJP, Parry B, Hamilton J, et al. Washington, DC, National Women's Health Resource Center, 1991, pp 1–27

Hamilton JA, Gallant SJ: Debate on late luteal phase dysphoric disorder (letter). Am J Psychiatry 147:1106, 1990

Hamilton J, Gallant S, Lloyd C: Evidence for a menstrual-linked artifact in determining rates of depression. J Nerv Ment Dis 1779:359–365, 1989

Hammarback S, Backstrom T: Induced anovulation as treatment of premenstrual tension syndrome. Acta Obstet Gynecol Scand 67:159–166, 1988

Hanley S: Asthma variation with menstruation. British Journal of Diseases of the Chest 75:306–308, 1981

Harris R, Laws A, Reddy V, et al: Are women using postmenopausal estrogens? a community survey. Am J Public Health 80:1266–1268, 1990

Harrison WM, Endicott J, Nee J: Treatment of premenstrual dysphoria with alprazolam: a controlled study. Arch Gen Psychiatry 47:270–275, 1990

Hatotani N, Kitayama I, Inoue K, et al: Psychoneuroendocrine studies of recurrent psychoses, in Neurobiology of Periodic Psychoses. Edited by Hatotani N, Nomura J. Tokyo, Igaku-Shoin, 1983

Hurt SW, Schnurr PP, Severino SK, et al: Late luteal phase dysphoric disorder in 670 women evaluated for premenstrual complaints. Am J Psychiatry 149:525–530, 1992

Jensvold M, Muller K, Putnam F, et al: Abuse and PTSD in PMS patients and controls. International Society of Psychosomatic Obstetrics and Gynaecology Biannual Meeting, Amsterdam, May 1989

Jensvold MF, Reed K, Jarrett DB, et al: Menstrual cycle–related depressive symptoms treated with variable antidepressant dosage. Journal of Women's Health 1:109–115, 1992

Johnson T: Premenstrual syndrome as a Western culture–specific disorder. Cult Med Psychiatry 11:337–356, 1987

Kawakami M, Arita J, Yoshida E: Loss of estrogen-induced daily surges of prolactin and gonadotropins by suprachiasmatic nucleus lesions in ovariectomized rats. Endocrinology 106:1087–1092, 1980

King C: Parallels between neurasthenia and premenstrual syndrome. Women Health 15:1–23, 1989

Kinney E, Trautmann J, Gold J, et al: Underrepresentation of women in new drug trials. Ann Intern Med 95:495–499, 1981

Kukopulos A, Minnai G, Muller-Oerlinghausen B: The influence of mania and depression on the pharmacokinetics of lithium: a longitudinal single-case study. J Affective Disord 8:159–166, 1985

Magos A: Advances in the treatment of premenstrual syndrome. Br J Obstet Gynaecol 97:7–10, 1990

Magos A, Brincat M, Studd J: Treatment of the premenstrual syndrome by subcutaneous estradiol implants and cyclical oral norethisterone: placebo controlled study. BMJ 292:1629–1633, 1986

Martin E: The Woman in the Body. Boston, MA, Beacon Press, 1987

McClintock MK: Women and their bodies. Presented at the conference on Reframing Women's Health: Multidisciplinary Research and Practice. Chicago, IL, October 1992

McDaniel W: Premenstrual exacerbation of bulimia (letter). Am J Psychiatry 146:807–808, 1989

McEwen B: Basic research perspective: ovarian hormone influence on brain neurochemical functions, in The Premenstrual Syndromes. Edited by Gise L. New York, Churchill Livingston, 1988, pp 21–33

McMillan M, Pihl R: Premenstrual depression: a distinct entity. J Abnorm Psychol 96:149–154, 1987

Morokoff P: Premenstrual Syndrome: Representation of a Cultural Conflict. Washington, DC, Society for Behavioral Medicine, 1991

Oppenheim G: A case of rapid mood cycling with estrogen: implications for therapy. J Clin Psychiatry 45:34–35, 1984

Parry B, Wehr T: Therapeutic effect of sleep deprivation in patients with premenstrual syndrome. Am J Psychiatry 144:808–810, 1987

Pearlstein T, Frank E, Rivera-Tovar A, et al: Prevalence of Axis I and Axis II disorders in women with late luteal phase dysphoric disorder. J Affective Disord 20:129–134, 1990

Price W, Torem M, DiMarzio L: Premenstrual exacerbation of bulimia. Psychosomatics 28:378–380, 1987

Rivera-Tovar A, Frank E: Late luteal phase dysphoric disorder in young women. Am J Psychiatry 147:1634–1636, 1990

Rizack MA, Hillman CDM: The Medical Letter Handbook of Adverse Drug Interactions. New Rochelle, NY, The Medical Letter, 1991

Roy-Byrne P, Rubinow D, Hoban C, et al: TSH and prolactin responses to TRH in patients with premenstrual syndrome. Am J Psychiatry 144:480–484, 1987

Rubinow D, Hoban C, Grover G, et al: Changes in plasma hormones across the menstrual cycle in patients with menstrually related mood disorder and in control subjects. Am J Obstet Gynecol 158:5–11, 1988

Schmidt P, Nieman L, Grover G, et al: Lack of effect of induced menses on symptoms in women with premenstrual syndrome. N Engl J Med 324:1174–1179, 1991

Severino S, Moline M: Premenstrual Syndrome: A Clinician's Guide. New York, Guilford, 1989

Smith S, Rinehart JS, Ruddock VE, et al: Treatment of premenstrual syndrome with alprazolam: results of a double-blind, placebo-controlled, randomized crossover clinical trial. Obstet Gynecol 70:37–43, 1987

Speroff L, Glass R, Kase N: Clinical Gynecologic Endocrinology and Infertility. Baltimore, MD, Williams & Wilkins, 1982

Spitzer RL, Severino SK, Williams JBW, et al: Late luteal phase dysphoric disorder and DSM-III-R. Am J Psychiatry 146:892–897, 1989

Stein M, Schmidt P, Rubinow D, et al: Panic disorder and the menstrual cycle: panic disorder patients, healthy control subjects, and patients with premenstrual syndrome. Am J Psychiatry 146:1299–1303, 1989

Stewart D: Positive changes in the premenstrual period. Acta Psychiatr Scand 79:400–405, 1989

Stone A, Pearlstein T, Brown W: Fluoxetine in the treatment of late luteal phase dysphoric disorder. J Clin Psychiatry 52:290–293, 1991

Stotland N: American Psychiatric Association Component Workshop: Social Implications of a Late Luteal Phase Dysphoric Disorder Diagnosis. Washington, DC, May 1992

Sullivan G, Lukoff D: Sexual side effects of antipsychotic medication: evaluation and interventions. Hosp Community Psychiatry 41:1238–1241, 1990

Teichmann A: Influence of oral contraceptives on drug therapy. Am J Obstet Gynecol 163:2208–2213, 1990

Wehr T, Sack D, Rosenthal N, et al: Rapid cycling affective disorder: contributing factors and treatment responses in 51 patients. Am J Psychiatry 145:179–184, 1988

Chapter 10

INFERTILITY AND THE NEW
REPRODUCTIVE TECHNOLOGIES

Jennifer Downey, M.D.

❖ ❖ ❖ ❖ ❖ ❖ ❖ ❖ ❖ ❖ ❖ ❖ ❖ ❖

Infertility, by the accepted medical definition of a year or more of unprotected coitus without pregnancy, is a common health problem. Medical authorities such as Speroff et al. (1989) estimate that 10%–15% of couples are affected by infertility. The only population-based survey of infertility in women, the National Survey of Family Growth, found in 1982 that, among those who were not surgically sterile, the percentage of infertile couples in the United States was 13.9% of all currently married couples in which the wife was 15–44 years of age (Hirsch and Mosher 1987). In addition, as Hirsch and Mosher noted, there is increasing demand for infertility treatment because of postponement of childbearing, increases in the proportion of infertile couples seeking care, a shrinking supply of adoptable infants, new techniques for treating infertile couples, and increased public awareness of these treatments. In the past, most infertility problems have been attributed to women. In reality, 40%–50% of cases are wholly or in part due to a male factor (Speroff et al. 1989).

PSYCHOLOGICAL EFFECTS OF
INFERTILITY AND ADJUSTMENT TO INFERTILITY

Menning (1980) has proposed that infertility investigation and treatment bring on a life crisis because infertility poses a threat not solvable in the immediate future and it may tax the couple's existing problem-solving resources, threaten their achievement of important life goals, and awaken unresolved key difficulties from the past. She has described a series of feelings experienced by many couples, from surprise through denial, anger, isolation, guilt, and grief, followed by resolution if the feelings are worked through and overcome. Some couples may fail to resolve the problem and continue to seek new treatments, even after every potentially beneficial one has been tried. This model of infertility as a life crisis for many couples is a helpful one that enables the clinician to think about the problem without "pathologizing" it and to organize data by phase in the process of resolution of the problem.

The impact of infertility on marriage appears to vary greatly. It is unknown at present which couples are at risk for marital difficulties when facing involuntary childlessness. Cook et al. (1989) found that 71% of the women in their study reported that infertility had affected their marriage, but among those affected, the proportion of women who felt the impact had been positive was similar to the proportion who felt it had been negative. In some cases, the shared stress of infertility may strengthen a couple's bond. Medical diagnosis and phase of treatment may also affect the likelihood of harmful marital effects. For example, Connolly et al. (1987) found that marital difficulties were more likely if the cause of infertility was a male factor.

When infertility affects a marriage, a key area that often deteriorates is sexual functioning and enjoyment. Negative effects on the sex life of couples have been widely reported; these include impotence, anorgasmia, and lessened sexual desire (Berger 1980; Keye 1984; Lalos et al. 1985). Up to 10% of cases of infertility may be partially or completely explained by sexual dysfunctions in the man (Seibel and Taymor 1982), such as premature ejaculation and impotence. Among both women and men, planned sex for medical tests such as the postcoital examination of cervical mucus has been found to have an adverse impact on sexual functioning (DeVries et al. 1984; Drake and Grunert 1979).

Most investigators have found that women tend to be more distressed by infertility than are their male partners. Keye et al. (1981) reported that 57% of women but only 12% of men thought that infertility was the worst thing they had ever had to face in life. McEwan et al. (1987) found that 40% of women but only 13% of men evinced psychological symptoms of clinical severity and that the women who were most disturbed were younger patients without a clear diagnosis of the infertility problem.

This difference in level of reported distress between men and women is found throughout the phases of infertility evaluation and treatment. Wright et al. (1991) found that at the time of a couple's first visit to an infertility clinic, women had significantly more overall psychiatric symptomatology, depression, anxiety, and hostility and reported more stress and less self-esteem than did men. Assessing men and women after the failure of a first episode of in vitro fertilization treatment—the other end of the spectrum usually reached after years of unsuccessful treatment—Newton et al. (1990) reported that 25.4% of women were experiencing mild or more serious depressions, defined by scores on the Beck Depression Inventory (Beck 1978) of 10–18 for "mild" and scores of greater than 18 for "serious." Only 10% of male participants were depressed, and most were only mildly so.

Effects on the infertile couple's family and social relationships can be profound. The parents of the couple are often eager for grandchildren and exert spoken or unspoken pressure on their grown offspring to reproduce. Cultural and religious affiliations that place a high value on bearing children may increase the infertile couple's sense of failure and public embarrassment. Siblings and friends who have already conceived and borne children may be avoided because exposure to them exacerbates the infertile couple's sadness or because they are objects of envy. Since fertility is inevitably linked to sexual function, affected couples may feel embarrassed to reveal their problem or to have others allude to it. A frequent result is social isolation as the couple begins to avoid family gatherings, where their childless state may be remarked upon, and other social events where pregnant women and small children may be present.

The financial burden of infertility can be considerable. Because of the ambiguous status of infertility as a medical problem, government-sponsored medical insurance programs such as Medicaid usually do not cover infertility treatment, and private insurance may reimburse only part of it. Treatments with in vitro fertilization, for instance—which currently cost between $4,000 and $6,000 per cycle in the United States—are usually not covered. Adoption is also expensive:

legal and other fees often average above $10,000. The result is that infertility treatment is usually available only to couples of at least middle-class financial status, and that couples undergoing treatment may make significant financial sacrifices such as foregoing vacations and using the money they had saved for a down payment on a house.

Months and sometimes years of infertility treatment affect patients' views of reality in sometimes subtle ways. Commonly, couples may become so focused on pregnancy as the concrete solution to their dilemma that they develop the attitude that all their life problems will be resolved if pregnancy occurs. Such patients can be particularly resistant to psychiatric interventions when needed, because their belief is that pregnancy is the only necessary treatment for whatever is bothering them.

Studies on the psychological sequelae of successful fertility treatment are limited, but clearly the consequences can be deleterious. Pregnancy in reality may be unexpectedly uncomfortable and fraught with excessive anxiety (Shapiro 1986). Parenthood may not have been anticipated in a realistic way. Use of the new reproductive technologies is associated with an increased incidence of multiple births, which carry their own risks of physical and psychological morbidity (Attia and Downey 1992). These pregnancies are often complicated with treatment requiring months of bed rest. Once the babies are born, the parents find that having more than one infant to care for can be physically, emotionally, and financially overwhelming. Further, it is not clear that the offspring of infertility treatment grow up without harm. Secrecy about use of techniques such as artificial insemination by donor and uncertainty about parentage which affects all involved parties when gamete donation has been used constitute risks to a happy childhood and family life (Sokoloff 1987). Studies of the psychological well-being of offspring of the new reproductive technologies are critically needed.

SPECIFIC INFERTILITY INTERVENTIONS AND THEIR PSYCHOLOGICAL EFFECTS

The infertility evaluation usually begins with a history taken from the couple, a physical examination of the female partner, and a few basic studies. These include a basal body temperature chart kept by the woman for 1–2 months. The temperature is taken each morning before the woman rises and is charted on a graph; days when intercourse occurs are also noted. The rationale for the chart is that a rise in temperature signals the time of the surge of luteinizing hormone and ovulation and thus indicates the beginning of the woman's fertile period. Other early studies almost invariably include a postcoital examination or a sperm count. For the postcoital examination, a sample of cervical mucus, usually collected within 8 hours of the last intercourse, is assessed for its receptivity and for the number of sperm per high-power field that are present and moving. Semen specimens may also be examined to assess the number of motile sperm and the percentage with normal morphology.

These early studies may be repeated numerous times in the course of infertility evaluation and treatment, and although simple both in concept and execution, they are associated with psychological morbidity. The need to take and chart one's temperature daily is a constantly repeated reminder of the couple's failure to conceive and leads in many cases to a loss of spontaneity and enjoyment in sexual intercourse, the timing of which is determined by "fertile days" by the chart. The postcoital examination also requires scheduled sexual activity and has the additional drawback of symbolically "inviting" a third person (the physician and/or laboratory technician) as an observer to the sexual act. Under these conditions, the incidence of both female anorgasmia and male impotence increases. Semen specimens usually must be studied within hours after collection, and production of semen by masturbation in a bathroom at the medical facility near the laboratory is often suggested. Under these conditions of intense performance anxiety, a significant number of men have difficulty obtaining the specimen, and the infertility evaluation becomes acutely embarrassing.

The female partner's failure to ovulate regularly is a relatively common cause of infertility, occurring in 40% of the cases in which the infertility is attributable to the woman. Treatment consists of one of several hormonal regimens. If the woman does not have ovarian failure (that is, if she has not already undergone menopause, in which case no hormonal therapy will work), clomiphene, a nonsteroidal drug that blocks estrogen receptors, is usually the first drug used. The psychiatric side effects of this drug include nervousness, insomnia, and depression. Human menopausal gonadotropins (Pergonal) by daily injection is often used if clomiphene is not effective. The treatment is expensive, costing $1,000 or more per cycle for the drug alone. Multiple ovulation is associated with human menopausal gonadotropins: 30% or more of pregnancies achieved with the drug are multiple, and three or more fetuses are present in 5% of these cases. Ovarian hyperstimulation syndrome is a potentially life-threatening complication of treatment with human menopausal gonadotropins, and close monitoring by a knowledgeable physician is essential. As with clomiphene, ovulation and conception may not occur during the first cycle, in which case repeated cycles become necessary. In some cases, bromocriptine (Parlodel) or gonadotropin-releasing hormone administered intravenously with a pump may be used for ovulation induction. (The reader is referred to the latest edition of Speroff et al.'s [1989] *Clinical Gynecologic Endocrinology and Infertility* or Gilman et al.'s [1990] *Pharmacological Basis of Therapeutics* for additional information.)

To date, there are virtually no published reports describing the psychiatric side effects of ovulation-inducing agents. The astute clinician will recognize, however, that hormonal treatments that affect the pituitary axis have potential for effects on mood and thinking. Further, the associated stresses are significant—taking such regimens of medication month after month with their multiple physical side effects, the close medical monitoring required, the high cost, the necessity for scheduled intercourse, the risks to health, and the possibility of multiple pregnancy if conception occurs. Thus, the usual clinical situation is that the couple indeed shows signs of psychiatric distress, but it is not immediately evident which of the many potential contributing factors are affecting this particular couple.

If the female partner has normal mucus and appears to ovulate and the male partner has normal sperm count and morphology, a hysterosalpingogram (X-ray examination of the female reproductive tract using radiopaque dye) and/or laparoscopy (direct visualization of the female reproductive organs performed with anesthesia and a small incision through which a laparoscope is inserted) may be performed to establish whether any anatomical abnormalities exist that might hinder the successful movement of an ovum through the fallopian tubes to the uterus. Such abnormalities include adhesions from previous pelvic surgery or infections, endometriosis from implants of the uterine lining that have seeded elsewhere in the reproductive tract, and congenital anomalies such as a bicornuate uterus. Obstruction of the fallopian tubes is a common factor in female infertility (30%–50% of cases). Thin adhesions and implants from endometriosis may be treated through the laparoscope. In other cases, hormonal therapy to shrink endometrial implants or surgery to restore the patency of the tubes (tuboplasty) may be attempted. Hormones used to suppress endometriosis include estrogen-progestin combinations (birth control pills) given continuously, medroxyprogesterone acetate (Provera), and danazol, an androgenic compound that is a derivative of the steroid 17α-ethinyltestosterone. All these compounds may cause symptoms of depression or emotional lability. The success of tuboplasty, which may require microsurgical techniques, is variable depending largely on the preoperative condition of the tubes, and it cannot be relied on to produce a successful pregnancy.

About 10% of cases of infertility are attributed to "cervical factors" after a series of poor postcoital tests. Sometimes this is due to excessively thick cervical mucus, which may be modified by treatment with low-dose estrogen or circumvented by the intrauterine insemination of sperm. In other cases, "sperm allergy," on the part of either the male or the female partner, may be suspected. Interventions have included corticosteroid therapy, use of condoms for periods of time to reduce exposure to semen, and intrauterine inseminations of washed sperm. All have been of equivocal benefit so far. A major contributing factor when postcoital tests are poor is often poor coital technique. A careful sexual history may reveal that there is an impotence problem and that vaginal intercourse may not occur, or the couple may be using vaginal lubricants, which have a spermicidal effect.

Among the new reproductive technologies are in vitro fertilization (IVF) and gamete intrafallopian transfer (GIFT), both interventions that are usually reached after years of unsuccessful infertility treatment. With IVF, the female partner is usually treated with ovulation-enhancing drugs and undergoes laparoscopy for the retrieval of eggs.

These are then cultured, fertilized in vitro with the male's sperm, and implanted in the uterus. The technique of GIFT is similar except that fertilization takes place in the fallopian tube, where follicles and sperm are placed. Such treatment is intense and expensive and success is uncertain. For years, pregnancy rates from a single cycle of IVF have hovered around 15%, but technical advances are beginning to improve these odds.

A couple who does conceive is at high risk of having a multifetal gestation, with its attendant increases in medical risks, rate of pregnancy loss, expense, and difficulties of simultaneously raising more than one child. Couples who do not conceive have spent years and large amounts of financial resources in a "go-for-broke" situation that has proven unsuccessful. This failure has significant psychological sequelae for some couples. For instance, Newton et al. (1990) reported that both men and women experienced increased depressive and anxiety symptoms and depressive disorders after unsuccessful IVF treatment and that childless women were at particular risk.

The new reproductive technologies acquire an increased degree of psychological risk when gametes (sperm or eggs) are donated or a surrogate is involved to carry the pregnancy. Artificial insemination by donor (AID) is actually not new and is medically very simple to perform. It is also highly successful in producing pregnancy when the female partner's fertility is intact but the male partner has a low sperm count (oligospermia) or no viable sperm (azoospermia). Egg donation is a much newer and more elaborate procedure and involves locating an anonymous donor or a cooperative friend or relative. The donor and the infertile woman are then treated with medications to synchronize their cycles. At the appropriate time, the eggs are harvested from the donor, and an IVF or GIFT procedure is used to fertilize the egg with the male partner's sperm. The infertile woman then carries the pregnancy. In cases where the infertile woman has sufficient eggs but for some reason cannot carry a pregnancy, a reverse of this procedure may be employed and a gestational surrogate may be found to "lend" her uterus for the duration of the pregnancy. Another variation is for AID to be used to impregnate the woman who is a surrogate; she then both contributes the egg and carries the pregnancy to delivery.

Berger (1980) has reported on the severe stress couples experience when a male is diagnosed as azoospermic or severely oligospermic. Sixty percent of the men studied developed transient impotence, and their wives reported a high frequency of rageful dreams and fantasies of leaving the infertile partner. AID is so medically simple to perform that couples may proceed with it before fully exploring their feelings regarding incorporating a (usually) unknown man's genetic heritage into their relationship. In addition to the couple's shame at their deficiency, legal and religious ambiguity about the status of the procedure is conducive to the couple's trying to keep it a secret. Total secrecy is a burden to maintain, however, and in the heat of some family crisis, the fact of the insemination is likely to be blurted out in a harmful way (Sokoloff 1987). Knowledge of one's genetic parentage is increasingly being seen in the United States as the birthright of every adult individual, a situation that complicates the task of maintaining secrecy.

On the other hand, when the donor of the gametes is known (which is much more likely if the donor is female), other complicating factors arise: the infertile couple's ongoing relationship with the donor, the donor's feeling of emotional proprietorship, and the possibility that the offspring may have "multiple parents" to deal with. Additionally, when the woman who carries the pregnancy is not to keep the baby, she may encounter unforeseen difficulties in relinquishing it to the parents. This is understandable, since women who volunteer to be surrogates are often motivated not only by financial need, the desire to be pregnant, and the wish to give a baby to an infertile couple, but also by the desire to master unresolved feelings about a previous pregnancy loss (Parker 1983).

PSYCHOLOGICAL TREATMENT ISSUES FOR INFERTILITY PATIENTS

Numerous studies have suggested that one response to infertility treatment, especially if unsuccessful, is depressive symptoms. An episode of depression by DSM-III-R criteria (American Psychiatric Association 1987) needs, of course, to be distinguished from feelings of distress and discouragement, which commonly occur and do not constitute an episode of depressive disorder. Mood swings may occur (with or without the presence of exogenous hormones and with or without a history of premenstrual mood symptoms) over the course of the month as women grow hopeful or anxious during the days before and after ovulation, only to become frustrated and disappointed with the onset of menstruation. I have seen women who appeared to have moderately severe agitated depressions around the time of menses who were asymptomatic 2 weeks later and repeated this cycle every month.

Any depression needs careful evaluation, especially with regard to severity, since among a small number of both female and male infertility patients psychiatric illness may develop or be exacerbated by the stress of the infertility workup. Some episodes will be manageable with the physician's support and variations in the pace of infertility treatment. Others will require psychotherapy; a few, the addition of psychotropic medications. At this point, great tact on the part of the mental health practitioner is necessary (as well as the support of the gynecologist or urologist), since infertility treatment is often deferred when patients are taking other medications and patients bent on achieving fertility may refuse any medication that would delay their efforts to conceive.

Although few women or men undergoing infertility treatment will develop a psychiatric disorder, many are so focused on achieving their goal of pregnancy that they will lose the ability to keep the problem in perspective with the rest of their lives. An infertile couple may feel that time is so pressing that even a respite of a few weeks during which they do not pursue treatment is unacceptable. The psychiatrist may be able to help such exhausted or symptomatic couples to take a holiday from treatment. This is often the first intervention when distress seems to be building toward dysfunction, and in some cases it may be the only one needed.

It is important for the treating clinician not to have preconceptions about how the infertility problem will affect the couple's relationship. Some women are more anxious about being childless than are their partners and feel isolated as a result. Other women find that facing this life crisis with their partners has strengthened their relationship. The emotional benefits of approaching infertility as a shared problem suggest that when one member of an infertile couple seeks psychological help, it is valuable for the clinician to see both partners, at least as part of the initial assessment, so that the less symptomatic partner can be brought into the treatment as needed.

Couples undergoing infertility treatment may be under such pressure to perform sexually in order to comply with the many requirements of the evaluation and treatment that they begin to develop sexual dysfunctions, such as impotence, anorgasmia, or lack of sexual desire. Frequently, the sexual symptoms will lessen with relatively simple interventions, such as limiting the taking of basal body temperature or taking 1–2 months' break from treatment. Persistent, severe sexual dysfunction needs more extensive exploration.

One of the most common problems infertility patients face has to do with the "relaxed attitude" often advised by their friends and family as an aid to enhancing fertility. It is innately stressful and not at all relaxing to be struggling to reach a difficult goal such as conception. Although it may be beneficial to learn relaxation techniques to enhance coping strategies, there is as yet no good evidence that relaxation enhances fertility. Adoption, while it may relieve the pressure to conceive, has also not been shown to enhance fertility beyond the effects of additional time during which unprotected intercourse may lead to conception (Collins et al. 1983; Lamb and Leurgans 1979).

Couples seeking conception are prone to accept responsibility for the infertility problem when it does not have to do with their behavior, for instance, by assuming that conflicts about pregnancy may be causing their infertility. Clinicians can be most beneficial to such patients by clarifying that stress and conflicts do not ordinarily affect fertility, and that difficulties conceiving are not the patients' fault.

A perceived loss of control is perhaps the most common stress of infertility. For women accustomed to planning their careers and other aspects of their lives, infertility may be experienced as their first major disappointment and as an unjust shock. Envy of friends and family members who conceive easily is common: "Why them and not us?" couples ask. Anger toward the treating physician is also common, and one of the tasks of the mental health professional is helping the infertility patient determine when his or her expectations of the physician are unrealistic.

A central task in the clinical management of infertility patients is helping them to achieve a sense of mastery in managing their treatment. As more and more new reproductive technologies are becoming available, it becomes increasingly difficult for patients to decide when "enough is enough" (Taylor 1990). The internal pressure to persist no matter what the emotional and financial cost is intense. The patient may need help from the mental health professional as he or she seeks a clear statement from the physician of the chances of achieving pregnancy so that together they can make an informed decision. Once the couple has this information, they may need help in weighing the benefits and costs for themselves in relation to the other alternatives open to them, such as adoption or living without children.

The appropriate mode of psychiatric treatment, if indicated, will depend on the couple's or patient's presenting symptoms, their psychiatric history, and their characterological strengths and deficits. Conjoint marital or sexual therapy may be indicated, as may individual psychotherapy or briefer periods of counseling. Support group–oriented therapies available in an infertility clinic setting or given under the aegis of RESOLVE (the national self-help organization for infertile couples) are appropriate when couples are willing to seek help in a group setting and are not too anxious and suggestible.

Speroff et al. (1989) have stated the goals of infertility treatment in their text for gynecologists (p. 540):

> to accomplish a thorough investigation, to treat any abnormalities that are uncovered, to educate the couple to the workings of the reproductive system, to give the couple some estimate of their fertility potential, to counsel for adoption when appropriate, and to provide emotional support.

Inherent in this advice is the idea that for all of us who treat patients with infertility problems, the goal is not to achieve pregnancy at any cost, but rather to assist couples in resolving their infertility crisis and becoming able to move on in life. This may mean having a birth child, adopting or fostering a child or children, or adopting a child-free way of life in which a couple's creativity and urge to contribute to the benefit of the next generation can find expression.

REFERENCES

American Psychiatric Association: Diagnostic and Statistical Manual of Mental Disorders, 3rd Edition, Revised. Washington, DC, American Psychiatric Association, 1987

Attia E, Downey J: Psychological consequences of successful treatment: a case report of a pregnancy assisted by in vitro fertilization–embryo transfer. Psychosomatics 33:218–221, 1992

Beck AT: Depression Inventory. Philadelphia, PA, Center for Cognitive Therapy, 1978

Berger DM: Couples' reactions to male infertility and donor insemination. Am J Psychiatry 137:1047–1049, 1980

Collins JA, Wrixon W, Janes LB, et al: Treatment-independent pregnancy among infertile couples. N Engl J Med 309:1201–1206, 1983

Cook R, Parsons J, Mason B, et al: Emotional, marital and sexual functioning in patients embarking upon IVF and AID treatment for infertility. Journal of Reproductive and Infant Psychology 7:87–93, 1989

Connolly KJ, Edelmann RJ, Cooke ID: Distress and marital problems associated with infertility. Journal of Reproductive and Infant Psychology 5:49–57, 1987

DeVries K, Degani S, Eibschitz I, et al: The influence of the post-coital test on the sexual function of infertile women. Journal of Psychosomatic Obstetrics and Gynaecology 3:101–106, 1984

Drake TS, Grunert GM: A cyclic pattern of sexual dysfunction in the infertility investigation. Fertil Steril 32:542–547, 1979

Gilman AG, Rall TW, Nies AS, et al: The Pharmacological Basis of Therapeutics, 8th Edition. New York, Pergamon, 1990

Hirsch MB, Mosher WD: Characteristics of infertile women in the United States and their use of infertility services. Fertil Steril 47:618–625, 1987

Keye WR: Psychosexual responses to infertility. Clin Obstet Gynecol 27:760–766, 1984

Keye WR, Deneris A, Wilson T, et al: Psychosexual responses to infertility: differences between infertile men and women (abstract). Fertil Steril 36:426, 1981

Lalos A, Lalos O, Jacobsson L, et al: Psychological reactions to the medical investigation and surgical treatment of infertility. Gynecol Obstet Invest 20:209–217, 1985

Lamb EJ, Leurgans S: Does adoption affect subsequent fertility? Am J Obstet Gynecol 134:138–144, 1979

McEwan KL, Costello CG, Taylor PG: Adjustment to infertility. J Abnorm Psychol 96:108–116, 1987

Menning BE: The emotional needs of infertile couples. Fertil Steril 34:313–319, 1980

Newton CR, Hearn MT, Yuzpe AA: Psychological assessment and follow-up after in vitro fertilization: assessing the impact of failure. Fertil Steril 54:879–886, 1990

Parker PJ: Motivations of surrogate mothers: initial findings. Am J Psychiatry 140:117–118, 1983

Seibel MM, Taymor ML: Emotional aspects of infertility. Fertil Steril 37:137–145, 1982

Shapiro CH: Is pregnancy after infertility a dubious joy? Social Casework 67:306–313, 1986

Sokoloff BZ: Alternative methods of reproduction: effects on the child. Clin Pediatr 26:11–17, 1987

Speroff L, Glass RH, Kase NG: Clinical Gynecologic Endocrinology and Infertility. Baltimore, MD, Williams & Wilkins, 1989

Taylor PJ: When is enough enough? Fertil Steril 54:772–774, 1990

Wright J, Duchesne C, Sabourin S, et al: Psychosocial distress and infertility: men and women respond differently. Fertil Steril 55:100–108, 1991

Chapter 11

INDUCED ABORTION

Nada L. Stotland, M.D.

❖ ❖ ❖ ❖ ❖ ❖ ❖ ❖ ❖ ❖ ❖ ❖ ❖ ❖

T he elective termination of a pregnancy is a weighty decision and a powerful act. It is imbued with significant psychological meanings and implications. These meanings and implications arise from origins encompassing religion, interpersonal relationships, and biology. Induced abortion is an act enmeshed in its social surroundings in every respect: its genesis, its performance, and its sequelae. It is a medical intervention that has evoked so much feeling in the United States that elections for public office are won and lost on the basis of the avowed attitudes of candidates toward abortion funding, access, availability, acceptable grounds, and the right of potentially concerned parties other than the pregnant woman herself to be informed of or to consent to the procedure (Tribe 1990).

Organized psychiatry, as represented by the American Psychiatric Association, has taken an official position on abortion. This position, adopted in 1978, is as follows (American Psychiatric Association 1978):

> The emotional consequences of unwanted pregnancy on parents and their offspring may lead to long-standing life distress and disability, and the children of unwanted pregnancies are at high risk for abuse, neglect, mental illness, and deprivation of the quality of life. Pregnancy that results from undue coercion, rape, or incest creates even greater potential distress or disability in the child and the parents. The adolescent most vulnerable to early pregnancy is the product of adverse sociocultural conditions involving poverty, discrimination, and family disorganization, and statistics indicate that the resulting pregnancy is

laden with medical complications which threaten the well-being of mother and fetus. The delivery that ensues from teenage pregnancy is prone to prematurity and major threats to the health of mother and child, and the resulting newborns have a higher percentage of birth defects, developmental difficulties, and a poorer life and health expectancy than the average for our society. Such children are often not released for adoption and thus get caught in the web of foster care and welfare systems, possibly entering lifetimes of dependency and costly social interventions. The tendency of this pattern to pass from generation to generation is very marked and thus serves to perpetuate a cycle of social and educational failure, mental and physical illness, and serious delinquency.

Because of these considerations, and in the interest of public welfare, the American Psychiatric Association 1) opposes all constitutional amendments, legislation, and regulations curtailing family planning and abortion services to any segment of the population; 2) reaffirms its position that abortion is a medical procedure in which physicians should respect the patient's right to freedom of choice—psychiatrists may be called on as consultants to the patient or physician in those cases in which the patient or physician requests such consultation to expand mutual appreciation of motivation and consequences; and 3) affirms that the freedom to act to interrupt pregnancy must be considered a mental health imperative with major social and mental health implications.

Several other professional medical organizations have taken a similar stance, although the American Medical Association has decided to leave it to the individual practitioner. Although this official position probably represents the stance of a sizable majority of psychiatrists, there are those whose cherished values and beliefs are violated by it. They question the appropriateness of such a stance within a profession dedicated to the preservation of life, the relevance of abortion policy to psychiatry in particular, and the effectiveness of access to abortion in eliminating or reducing the problems to which the American Psychiatric Association's statement addresses itself: child abuse, neglect, and deprivation. On the other hand, some psychiatrists regard abortion as such a fundamental human right that they threatened to boycott a psychiatric convention scheduled in a state in which the legislature had passed statutes limiting abortion access. Of particular importance to the practice of psychiatry are the issues of physician-patient confidentiality, the right and obligation of physicians to see that patients have access to and knowledge about all therapeutic options without barriers, and the autonomy of the pregnant woman, regardless of her age, to make decisions about her care in consultation with the health professionals who provide that care.

The issue of abortion is so contentious that fundamental realities are often overlooked in the debate. The consideration of these realities is essential not only for policy-making, but also for clinical practice and scientific study. For example, there is the fact that abortion is performed only on women who are pregnant. If an abortion is not performed (and barring complications such as spontaneous abortion), these women will go on to deliver. This fact is overlooked in attempts to study the outcome of abortion whenever the outcome is not compared with the sequelae of labor, delivery, and motherhood. The only truly appropriate control group may be women who found their pregnancies similarly problematic, who sought abortion, and who were unable to obtain it. The findings from the few such studies that have been performed are summarized here. Women considering abortion are not only pregnant, but pregnant under circumstances they experience as untenable. The circumstances also make a substantive contribution to whatever outcome obtains; the abortion procedure does not have an impact in isolation. Last, the effects of social and medical context on the experience and outcome of abortion are often overlooked. These considerations will be expanded in the section on psychiatric issues.

GYNECOLOGIC AND PUBLIC HEALTH ISSUES

The data in this section are taken from *Public Health Policy Implications of Abortion*, a handbook for health professionals that was developed collaboratively by a group of medical organizations, including the American College of Obstetricians and Gynecologists, the American Medical Association, and the American Psychiatric Association, and which was published in January 1990. It can be obtained through those organizations. Statistics were derived from the Centers for Disease Control and the National Center for Health Statistics.

Procedures to terminate a pregnancy vary somewhat by trimester. Until recently, second-trimester abortions were generally induced by the intrauterine instillation of chemical agents, such as urea or saline, which precipitated the onset of uterine contractions and the expulsion of the fetus. Currently, second-trimester pregnancies are also terminated by methods similar to those used in the first trimester: cervical dilation and uterine evacuation. Since 1981, 90% of all abortions have been performed by using suction curettage. Under local anesthesia, the cervix is dilated and the uterine contents suctioned. The procedure takes 10–12 minutes.

At least half of all induced abortions in the United States are performed within the first 8 weeks, and 90% within the first trimester, of pregnancy. During this time, the risk of medical complications is less than 0.5%. Abortions performed after 20 weeks of gestation constitute fewer than 1% of all such procedures; most of these occur at 21–23 weeks. Most abortions are performed in freestanding (nonhospital) clinics, where the cost is about one-third (average, $213) of that in a hospital and the safety equivalent (for early and uncomplicated abortions), access, and psychological experience are easier. The maternal mortality from abortion performed under safe conditions is 0.5 per 100,000 procedures; the rate from childbirth is 25 times greater. During the 1960s, before abortion was legalized in the United States, illegal abortion led to approximately 20% of pregnancy-related admissions to hospitals in major population centers and 20% of all deaths from pregnancy and childbirth.

Access to abortion is geographically uneven; the vast majority of abortion providers are in urban areas. Eighty-two percent of all counties in the United States lack a facility performing abortions; the 30% of women who live in a county without a provider obtain, on average, substantially fewer abortions than women in areas with a provider. The large majority of general hospitals perform no abortions, and many of the hospitals that do perform very few. Other barriers to service include the federal ruling that Medicaid funds cannot be used for abortion services except to save the mother's life, and requirements for notification or consent of the patient's parents or spouse. Evidence indicates that such barriers deter timely and safe care and lead to adverse public health consequences (Berger 1978).

The antiprogestin mifepristone (RU-486) is 95% effective in inducing abortion when taken orally and followed by a dose of prostaglandin. It is associated with minimal side effects and with no known complications or long-term health implications. It is available and in use in China and in France; clinical trials are under way in other countries all over the world. The U.S. Food and Drug Administration has not approved the use of mifepristone. Anti-abortion groups have reportedly threatened to initiate major actions, including boycotts, against any pharmaceutical company that seeks to market the drug in this country. There is also a federal ban on the study of abortifacients.

EPIDEMIOLOGY

Rates of induced abortion in the United States have been compiled according to race, age, and marital and reproductive status. The figures quoted here were published by the American College of Obstetricians and Gynecologists in 1990 (American College of Obstetricians and Gynecologists 1990). Approximately 70% of women who undergo abortions are white. Fifty-seven percent are nulliparous, and 35% have one or two children. Sixty-one percent have not undergone an induced abortion previously. Eighty-one percent of all women, and 96% of teenage women, who have induced abortions are unmarried. Marriage occasioned by pregnancy places teenagers at higher risk for abuse, school failure, and dependence on public support (Zuravin 1991).

The ages of women who have abortions are as follows: over 60% are younger than 25 years, and 42% of pregnancies in teenagers are terminated by induced abortion. Though women over 40 years become pregnant more rarely and account for relatively few induced abortions, 51% of their pregnancies are terminated by induced abortion. The numbers and rates of induced abortion have remained fairly constant throughout the 1980s and approximate those before abortion was legalized. In 1986, approximately 33 million legal and 27 million illegal abortions were performed throughout the world (Tietze and Henshaw 1986).

HISTORY AND ANTHROPOLOGY

Induced abortions have been performed throughout recorded history, in every part of the world, and in virtually every sort of culture (Devereux 1976). Mention of abortion practices and beliefs in selected cultures serves to put the practice in some perspective (Newman 1991).

Induced abortion is mentioned—and proscribed—in the Hippocratic oath. Therefore, it must have been practiced and discussed in ancient Greece (Edelstein 1989). In the former Soviet Union, an officially atheist state that sought to increase its population, abortions were provided by the state health system (though supplementary, sub-rosa fees are required for anesthesia), and women underwent an average of nine abortions each (Page 1989).

In China, it is reported that the number of induced abortions is at least equal to the number of live births. Population control is a major national priority, and considerable pressure may be exerted on a woman or a couple when conception has occurred without prior approval by the work group to which the individual(s) belong (Engelhardt 1989). Abortions are also widely performed in officially Roman Catholic countries, where they are completely illegal, available only illicitly, and lead to thousands of maternal deaths.

Induced abortions are legal, common, safe, and accepted in Japan. This accepting social context is not associated with a lack of meaning and feeling, however. Japanese religious and cultural belief holds that the soul of the embryo may cause health and other problems for the mother if not laid to rest in a religious observance. There is a goddess who takes a special interest in embryos and young children. Shrines dedicated to her are hung with offerings of baby toys and bibs (Ohnuki-Tierney 1984).

In the United States, approximately 1.5 million induced abortions are performed each year. The number was not much lower before the *Roe v. Wade* decision by the Supreme Court legalized abortion in 1973. Although the absolute numbers have remained about the same, the percentage of pregnancies terminated by induced abortion has fallen somewhat in the last few years (Cates 1982). The *Roe v. Wade* decision declared a right to privacy between a woman and her physician concerning the decision of whether to have an abortion, a right to abortion during the first 12 weeks of pregnancy. During the second trimester, the state was permitted to regulate abortion only to protect maternal well-being. The U.S. Congress, however, has enacted legislation enjoining the use of federal funds to support abortion services. The Supreme Court has recently upheld state laws limiting abortion and is expected to overturn *Roe,* overtly or in effect.

As mentioned above, access to abortion services has become the subject of heated controversy. Seemingly irreconcilable factions argue that it is murder or that it is an imperative for women's autonomy and equity in society. Induced abortion has come to signify major social concerns and fears: the continuity of the nuclear family structure and traditional sex roles, the erosion of sexual morality, the liberation of women from oppression and abuse, the opportunity for children to enter the world as wanted members of loving families with the resources to provide for them. Cultural icons have crystallized around these positions: the fetus for groups self-identified as "pro-life," the bloody coat hanger of the back-alley abortionist for those "pro-choice."

ETHICAL ISSUES

These cultural symbols are also reflections of the varying foci and levels of discourse about the ethics of induced abortion. The levels of discourse reflect the medical, psychological, and social complexities of the procedure (B. Brody 1982; Warren 1982). Abortion is the termination of a pregnancy. Society has an interest in the successful propagation of the species. A particular pregnancy may advance or deter that goal. Pregnancy almost always occurs as the result of sexual intercourse between a man and a woman. The intercourse may be more or less consensual or coercive, and the sexual partners may have congruent, divergent, or contradictory investments in procreation and intentions with regard to the parenting of a potential child.

Fertilization may also take place deliberately, without intercourse, by recourse to more (in vitro fertilization) or less (artificial insemination by turkey baster) sophisticated technological means. It always involves the genetic material of a male and a female human individual, although the genetic, gestational, and social parent(s) may all be different persons. Since procreative maturity precedes psychological and legal maturity (the age of majority), pregnancy can and does occur in minor women, whose capacity to weigh alternatives and whose moral rights to make decisions about their own care and futures is a complicating subject of debate.

Induced abortion may be performed by a lay attendant, attempted by the pregnant woman herself, or carried out by a physician or other medically trained and licensed professional health care provider. This array of possibilities raises analogous ethical problems for the gynecologist and psychiatrist alike. Abortion may be viewed as a service that doctors are obligated to provide on request, a procedure for which physicians are the appropriate gatekeepers (many court decisions and official organizational positions stipulate that the decision is to be made "by a woman and her doctor"), or a prima facie violation of medical ethics. The possibility or probability of substantial dangers of abortion performed outside the medical system is weighed in the ethical decisions made by doctors about the procedure as well (Jacobson 1988).

Another question of responsibility often raised in discussions of the ethics of induced abortion concerns the woman's responsibility for conception and the embryo thus engendered. There is the more or less explicit image of the sexually wanton female who seeks to rid herself of the predictable outcome of her sexual pleasure at the expense of the life of her potential child. In point of fact, many realities constrain women's control over sexual activity and contraception. These include not only rape and incest, but lack of access to information about reproduction and contraception, lack of access to contraceptive devices and medical services, and sexual activity in which financial, social, and psychological coercion falls short of narrowly defined sexual assault (DaVanzo et al. 1991). Contraceptives also fail.

Alternatively posed is the image of the virtuous woman who accepts the responsibility to maintain the pregnancy once conceived and makes the personal sacrifice involved in the experience of pregnancy, labor, delivery, and either child care or child relinquishment to adoption in the interests of her child (Vaux 1989). This stance imbues the woman in the earliest stages of pregnancy with the role and moral obligations of the parent of a child already born. It also raises the issue that pregnancy, delivery, parenthood, and the potential child become the instruments by which the woman is faced with, in fact punished for, sexual intercourse. The argument that most sentimentalizes the attachment to the potential child sometimes conceptualizes that child as a retribution rather than a blessing.

Other issues must be raised and discussed before the ethical issues surrounding induced abortion can be joined. There is the question of when in relation to fertilization and/or conception human life begins, which overlaps with the question of the definition of "human life." A fertilized ovum is living matter with the genetic composition of a human being, and the potential to develop into a human being, though only within a woman's body. Embryologic research indicates that the differentiation of cells that results in the formation of a normal organism can occur only in a given sequence and in the matrix and structure of embryonic development as a whole. The cells that are to differentiate into, for example, liver cells can do so only if the rest of development is proceeding normally around them at each of the requisite stages. Put another way—a way relevant to the ethics of abortion—the cells and tissues of the preembryo and embryo are not inevitably destined to become a human being.

Even given the circumstances of normal development, there is no clear or consensual definition of human life. It may be defined by genetic composition, human form, the appearance of brain waves, the ability to experience sensation, or the awareness of the self and other people as human. What distinguishes human life from other forms of life, and what privileges, if any, does our humanity confer upon us? Both humans and animals experience pleasure and pain, and both exert strenuous effort to stay alive. Although cells biopsied from human tissue are alive, capable of reproduction, and endowed with a full complement of human chromosomes, it would be difficult to argue that such a collection of cells constitutes human life, or a human being. The assertion that any particular stage of human development constitutes the beginning of "human life" is fraught with variously problematic implications.

Fetal viability has been raised as an issue both by ethicists and lawmakers. Publicity about the survival of some infants born extremely prematurely has led the public to believe that the medical community is steadily moving back the point in pregnancy at which the fetus can live outside the mother. Scientific evidence does not support this belief, however, and perinatologists think it likely that we have already approached the limits of our abilities to support extrauterine life in prematurely born infants.

All of these problems complicate attempts to apply the usual standards of beneficence, autonomy, and justice to the consideration of the ethics of abortion. The American Psychiatric Association's position statement seems to imply that it can be beneficent to a potential child not to allow it to come into being. Abortion ends a potential or an actual life, as well as the hopes and interests of those who wanted to see it realized, although it may further the good of the woman whose pregnancy and potential motherhood she experiences as intolerable. The availability of abortion may hurt society insofar as it undermines respect for potential life and for support during pregnancy and childrearing. It may benefit society insofar as it diminishes the social burden of unwanted and poorly cared-for children and the loss or injury of women who resort to unsafe attempts to terminate their pregnancies.

PSYCHIATRIC SEQUELAE OF INDUCED ABORTION

Psychiatrists help patients make decisions about problem pregnancies and deal with their short- and long-term reactions to induced abortion. In 1988, C. Everett Koop, M.D., the Surgeon General of the United States, was charged by the president of the United States to determine the medical and psychological effects of abortion on American women and to publish a review of the findings. Dr. Koop, whose published personal stance was that of opposition to abortion, solicited opinion and scientific information from a wide variety of medical and interest groups, including the American Psychiatric Association, and concluded that there was insufficient information to assert that abortion had negative sequelae (Koop 1991).

The public is nevertheless quite concerned about the psychiatric sequelae of abortion. The popular press and antiabortion groups have published allegations that abortion causes serious, disabling, permanent psychological damage: an "abortion trauma syndrome" (DeVeber et al. 1991). This term, which is absent from the peer-reviewed literature, seems to have been coined to resemble posttraumatic stress disorder. There have also been allegations that the medical community is deliberately withholding or overlooking data supportive of this position (Pro-Life Action Ministries, undated). Psychiatrists are the appropriate source for accurate scientific findings concerning the psychological sequelae of induced abortion.

Public confusion often arises for two reasons: because of the failure to differentiate passing negative feelings from psychiatric syndromes, and the failure to accurately identify the source of the distress some women feel upon having an induced abortion. Semantic ambiguity compounds the problem. In the English language, *depression* is used both as a description of a mood and as a technical term to denote the diagnosis of a major psychiatric illness. Women's reactions to induced abortion arise not only from the brief procedure itself, but from psychological, social, and political circumstances and the communicated attitudes and behaviors of the personnel who perform the procedure. Abortion is only considered for and performed on women who are pregnant—and pregnant in problematic circumstances. The psychosocial impact of finding oneself to have conceived an unanticipated and undesired pregnancy is, in and of itself, considerable.

The process of arriving at the conclusion that the pregnancy cannot be maintained is an additional stress, often involving confrontation with such realities as poverty; the implications of interrupting one's work or education; the end or threatened end of the relationship with one's partner, who may be the father of one's other children; genetic defects; or overwhelming burdens of caring for other young children. A woman's religion or significant others may disapprove of abortion, even to the point of excluding a woman who has undergone an abortion from membership in the religious community or protection and regard of the family. Abortion may be accessible only illicitly, or only through a complex process such as obtaining parental approval, judicial bypass, or medical justification. Of particular importance for psychiatric study is the fact that women may choose abortion because they have psychiatric illnesses that make pregnancy and motherhood problematic. Given these realities, it is difficult or even impossible to assess the impact of the abortion in isolation.

Published results of psychological reactions to induced abortion have, at least to some degree, paralleled prevailing social attitudes and expectations. A large (479 women) Swedish study concluded in 1955 that three-quarters of the subjects had experienced no regrets or self-reproach, and all of the 1% with psychiatric problems had had prior psychiatric illness (Ekblad 1955). Despite these findings, authors tended to assume negative effects until the early 1960s. Since that time, a succession of studies have been published, and methodology has been consistently improved. All studies agree that negative emotional effects are nearly always transient, that most women who choose abortion tend to feel increasingly relieved and comfortable with their decisions, and that in many cases their overall life satisfaction and success are improved (Addelson 1973; H. Brody et al. 1971; Ford et al. 1971; Lask 1975; Marder 1970; Niswander and Patterson 1967; Osofsky and Osofsky 1972; Peck and Marcus 1966; Schusterman 1976; Simon et al. 1967). Women who were denied abortion tended to have poorer outcomes, especially if the burdens of motherhood were compounded by great multiparity or lack of social support (Pare and Raven 1970).

The reactions of men to their partners' induced abortions have not been well studied. Male partners are often overlooked and their psychological needs not attended to. In one study of men accompanying women to an urban hospital abortion service, abortion was found to be a developmental challenge. Some men retreated to dependence on their parents, leaving their wives or girlfriends to obtain the necessary information and make the decision largely without their support. Most mastered the challenge, however, and emerged from the experience with an enhanced feeling of fatherliness and responsibility (Rothstein 1991). Like women who undergo abortion, they had decided that parenthood should be the result of a considered decision that one could provide for a child, and not undertaken by chance.

The incidence of major psychiatric illness following induced abortion has been studied and, in the best studies, compared with the occurrence of major psychiatric illness after delivery and in patients denied abortion. A large study in Great Britain reported that the incidence of psychosis was 0.3/1,000 after abortion and 1.7/1,000 postpartum (Brewer 1977). All other studies report similar findings. A 1989 study performed by a researcher at Johns Hopkins University followed adolescents who presented to a school health clinic seeking pregnancy tests (Zabin et al. 1989). Some were not pregnant; of those who were, some chose to abort and some to carry to term. Those who terminated their pregnancies experienced the most favorable outcomes in terms of psychological adjustment and completion of education, excelling even over those young women who had not been pregnant.

No specific illness or pattern of pathologic response to induced abortion has been described in the scientific literature. Patients who are at risk for psychiatric illness following induced abortion include those with prior psychiatric illness, those pressured or coerced into undergoing the abortion, those markedly ambivalent about the decision, and those with a paucity of social supports (Blumenthal 1991). Negative attitudes of those who provide care during and after the procedure also increase the risk of psychiatric sequelae. Psychiatrists treating patients who are considering abortion can best help them by providing the above information and by helping them, in collaboration with significant others of their own choosing, to arrive at autonomous decisions that reflect their own circumstances, religious beliefs, and values.

PSYCHIATRIC IMPLICATIONS OF LEGAL CONSTRAINTS ON ABORTION

In a global sense, restrictions on abortion services threaten all women with unintended motherhood or illegal abortion, outcomes likely to be psychologically stressful. Insofar as restrictions limit access for some women, but not others, they raise ethical and public health questions for all physicians. The Hyde Amendment passed by the U.S. Congress proscribes the use of federal funds for abortion services. Therefore, Medicaid funds other obstetric and gynecologic services, but not abortion. Women with social support, means, and sophistication have always been able to obtain safe abortions. This differentiation imposes two standards of care on all medical practice.

Psychiatrists are particularly concerned with induced abortion for several reasons. The procedure is usually conceived as a medical one, and psychiatrists are physicians. In times and places where abortion services are not available to women on demand, psychiatric grounds may be among those that allow access to these services. Where abortion is available only to save the mother's life, the clinical conclusion that a pregnant woman is suicidal has been used to justify the procedure. This justification was sometimes perceived to have been overused or incorrectly used, and some states and the military specifically disallowed abortion to be performed on psychiatric grounds. Other laws have been more liberal, allowing psychiatric factors to be considered on a par with other medical factors that had a significant likelihood of impairing the mother's health were the pregnancy to be allowed to continue (Shepler 1991).

Either of these legal circumstances raises problems for psychiatry. Excluding suicide or mental health indications isolates psychiatric illness from the rest of medicine and reinforces the stigma surrounding psychiatric patients and practitioners. Allowing psychiatric indications for abortions that are otherwise restricted places psychiatrists in an untenable position in several respects. Suicidality and other adverse psychiatric outcomes are not predictable with scientific accuracy, especially when the patient who is providing the data for the decision is in the midst of a crisis and has a vested interest in obtaining a particular procedure. Studies indicate that patients who are denied abortions that are requested on psychiatric or psychosocial grounds, as well as their children, suffer adverse outcomes as compared with control families, but that they seldom complete the act of suicide during the pregnancy (Dagg 1991).

The psychiatrist may be in a bind because the clinical evidence in a case may not warrant the conclusion that the patient is suicidal, although the patient or the psychiatrist (or both) may feel strongly that an abortion would be in the patient's best interest. The psychiatrist must then either lie about the findings or see the patient denied care. If the designation of serious psychiatric illness or suicidality is applied, that label may well follow the patient, who is likely to be a young woman, through her life, to hamper her career development and to impair her eligibility for health insurance.

Psychiatrists have a particular interest and expertise in the psychosocial circumstances associated with the conception of unplanned pregnancies. These range from ignorance, poverty, and lack of contraceptives to abuse, immaturity and impulsivity, various degrees of interference with reality testing, and more subtle psychodynamics. Many psychiatrists treat patients with histories of severe psychiatric complications and sequelae of pregnancy and delivery. They treat patients who appear or have been shown to be unable to master the responsibilities of motherhood, including patients who have suffered further exacerbations of psychiatric illness after losing custody of children in the past. They treat patients who have taken psychotropic medications in the early days and weeks of pregnancy, with unknown effects on the embryo and fetus (see Chapter 5), and patients who require psychotropic drugs to forestall decompensations.

Limitations on access to abortion restrict patient autonomy and therapeutic options for both the patient and the psychiatrist and may even put the psychiatrist in a legal bind. For example, the 1989 Supreme Court decision affirming the Missouri law in the case of *Webster v. Reproductive Health Services* lets stand language stating that public funds may not be used to advise or counsel a woman to have an abortion. A psychiatrist might be bound to advise a woman with a history of severe postpartum psychiatric illness, loss of custody, severe psychiatric vulnerability, or treatment with psychotropic drugs in early pregnancy of the full range of therapeutic options, including abortion. At the same time, if the patient's care is publicly funded, or takes place in a publicly funded facility, such a law may proscribe the discussion of abortion. (Similar wording has been enacted in states other than Missouri.) Antiabortion activists have threatened to visit doctors' offices with simulated psychiatric histories in order to expose physicians who violate the law. Even if access to abortion is not restricted by law, a patient may encounter difficulty in attempting to explore a full range of therapeutic options if her psychiatrist is morally opposed to induced abortion under any circumstances. However, if there were no legal repercussions, such a psychiatrist might be more likely to refer patients who want to consider pregnancy termination to colleagues.

Recent U.S. Supreme Court decisions have precipitated the passage of a rash of restrictive state laws. Some legislative and judicial restrictions on abortion are couched in terms of notification and consent of third parties. The Pennsylvania legislature passed a bill requiring the signature of a woman's husband. It was vetoed by the governor. Several states have enacted laws requiring the notification and/or consent of the parents of a minor woman seeking abortion. These laws have been found to be constitutional so long as they include a provision for "judicial bypass," a procedure whereby the young woman can apply to a court for permission to terminate her pregnancy when her parents have denied permission, when they cannot be located, or when she believes that informing them of the pregnancy would pose a psychological or physical risk to her well-being (Shepler 1991).

These laws have a clear emotional appeal to the public's sentiments about parental protection of minor children and the sanctity of the family. They ignore, however, realities about adolescent development, troubled families, and the judicial process. All major medical organizations support the physician's role in advising and helping most pregnant young women to inform and enlist the support of their families. Unfortunately, adolescents from abusive and neglectful families are at increased risk of unintended pregnancy; forcing them to tell their parents further exposes them to the risk of abuse, expulsion from the home, and self-destructive behavior, including suicide. Mandating this intervention is also a contratherapeutic intrusion in the physician-patient relationship.

The "judicial bypass" requires that an adolescent without adequate family support, and in the middle of the crisis precipitated by an unwanted pregnancy, must manage to find out that she must contact a court. She must locate the court, make excuses to absent herself from home and school, and present herself at the court. In rural areas, she may have to travel a considerable distance. Once at the court, she must make her intentions known to staff so that she can be directed to the appropriate room. In rural areas, both the court staff and the judge may well know her and her family. In Minnesota, where such a law was passed, it was studied and found to produce no positive outcome. The judges who heard the cases almost invariably allowed the abortion to take place. For all these reasons, all major medical societies, including the American Academy of Pediatrics, have take official positions against parental notification laws.

While recognizing the deeply felt religious and moral aversion of some psychiatrists to induced abortion, and the profound decision most feel it to be, the American Psychiatric Association, in concert with other medical and public interest organizations, has taken a strong stance in opposition to legislation that places dangerous and inequitable restrictions on women's access to safe abortion services, as well as limitations on all physicians' ability to discuss, recommend, and provide services for their patients. There is a real tragedy in the psychosocial inadequacies that lead to the occurrence of so many problem pregnancies in a world that has the scientific knowledge to prevent them.

REFERENCES

Addelson F: Induced abortion: source of guilt or growth? Am J Orthopsychiatry 43:815–823, 1973

American College of Obstetricians and Gynecologists: Public Health Policy Implications of Abortion: A Government Relations Handbook for Health Professionals. Washington, DC, American College of Obstetricians and Gynecologists, 1990

American Psychiatric Association: Position Statement on Abortion. Washington, DC, American Psychiatric Association, 1978

Berger LR: Abortions in America: the effects of restrictive funding. N Engl J Med 298:1474–1477, 1978

Blumenthal SJ: Psychiatric consequences of abortion: overview of research findings, in Psychiatric Aspects of Abortion. Edited by Stotland NL. Washington, DC, American Psychiatric Press, 1991, pp 17–37

Brewer C: Incidence of post-abortion psychosis: a prospective study. BMJ 1:476–477, 1977

Brody B: The morality of abortion, in Contemporary Issues in Bioethics, 2nd Edition. Edited by Beauchamp TL, Walters L. Belmont, CA, Wadsworth Publishing, 1982, pp 201–211

Brody H, Meikle S, Gerritse R: Therapeutic abortion: a prospective study. Am J Obstet Gynecol 109:347–352, 1971

Cates W: Legal abortion: the public health record. Science 215:1586–1590, 1982

Dagg P: The psychological sequelae of therapeutic abortion—denied and completed. Am J Psychiatry 148:578–585, 1991

DaVanzo J, Parnell AM, Foege WH: Health consequences of contraceptive use and reproductive patterns: summary of a report from the U.S. National Research Council. JAMA 265:2692–2696, 1991

DeVeber LL, Ajzenstat J, Chisholm D: Post abortion grief: psychological sequelae of induced abortion. Humane Medicine 7:203–208, 1991

Devereux G: A Study of Abortion in Primitive Societies, Revised Edition. New York, International Universities Press, 1976

Edelstein L: The Hippocratic oath: text, translation, and interpretation, in Cross-Cultural Perspectives in Medical Ethics: Readings. Edited by Veatch R. Boston, MA, Jones & Bartlett, 1989, pp 6–24

Ekblad M: Induced abortion on psychiatric grounds—a followup study of 479 women. Acta Psychiatr Scand Suppl 99:1–238, 1955

Engelhardt HT: Bioethics in the People's Republic of China, in Cross-Cultural Perspectives in Medical Ethics: Readings. Edited by Veatch R. Boston, MA, Jones & Bartlett, 1989, pp 112–119

Ford CV, Castelnuovo-Tedesco P, Long KD: Abortion: is it a therapeutic procedure in psychiatry? JAMA 218:173–178, 1971

Jacobson JL: Choice at any cost. World-Watch, March–April 1988, pp 30–38

Koop CE: Former Surgeon General Koop speaks out on health care reform and policy. Hospitals 65(20):57–58, 1991

Lask B: Short-term psychiatric sequelae to therapeutic termination of pregnancy. Br J Psychiatry 126:173–177, 1975

Marder L: Psychiatric experience with a liberalized therapeutic abortion law. Am J Psychiatry 126:1230–1236, 1970

Newman LF: Historical and cross-cultural perspectives on abortion, in Psychiatric Aspects of Abortion. Edited by Stotland NL. Washington, DC, American Psychiatric Press, 1991, pp 39–49

Niswander K, Patterson R: Psychologic reaction to therapeutic abortion. Obstet Gynecol 29:702–706, 1967

Ohnuki-Tierney E: Illness and Culture in Contemporary Japan: An Anthropological View. Cambridge, England, Cambridge University Press, 1984

Osofsky JD, Osofsky HJ: The psychological reaction of patients to legalized abortion. Am J Orthopsychiatry 42:48–60, 1972

Page B: Eastern Europe in the twentieth century, in Cross-cultural Perspectives in Medical Ethics: Readings. Edited by Veatch R. Boston, MA, Jones & Bartlett, 1989, pp 98–105

Pare C, Raven H: Follow-up of patients referred for termination of pregnancy. Lancet 1:635–658, 1970

Peck A, Marcus H: Psychiatric sequelae of therapeutic interruption of pregnancy. J Nerv Ment Dis 143:417–425, 1966

Pro-Life Action Ministries: What They Won't Tell You at the Abortion Clinic. St. Paul, MN, Pro-Life Action Ministries (undated)

Roe v Wade, 410 U.S. 113 (1973)

Rothstein A: Male experience of elective abortion: psychoanalytic perspectives, in Psychiatric Aspects of Abortion. Edited by Stotland NL. Washington, DC, American Psychiatric Press, 1991, pp 145–158

Schusterman LR: The psychosocial factors of the abortion experience: a critical review. Psychology of Women Quarterly 1:79–106, 1976

Shepler LT: The law of abortion and contraception—past and present, in Psychiatric Aspects of Abortion. Edited by Stotland NL. Washington, DC, American Psychiatric Press, 1991, pp 51–73

Simon N, Senturia A, Rothman D: Psychiatric illness following therapeutic abortion. Am J Psychiatry 126:1224–1229, 1967

Tietze C, Henshaw SK: Induced Abortion: A World Review, 6th Edition. New York, Alan Guttmacher Institute, 1986

Tribe LH: Abortion: The Clash of Absolutes. New York, Norton, 1990

Vaux K: Birth Ethics: Religious and Cultural Values in the Genesis of Life. New York, Crossroad, 1989

Warren DG: The law of human reproduction: an overview. J Leg Med 3(1):1–57, 1982

Webster v Reproductive Health Services, 109 S.Ct. 3040 (1989)

Zabin LS, Hirsch MB, Emerson MR: When urban adolescents choose abortion: effects on education, psychological status, and subsequent pregnancy. Fam Plann Perspect 21:248–255, 1989

Zuravin SJ: Unplanned childbearing and family size: their relationship to child neglect and abuse. Fam Plann Perspect 23:155–161, 1991

Chapter 12

MENOPAUSE: MYTHS AND REALITIES

Barbara B. Sherwin, Ph.D.

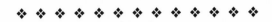

Menopause is both a natural and a universal event in the human female life cycle. A set of defining characteristics for this biological event was formulated at the first International Congress on Menopause (Utian and Serr 1976, pp. 2–3). Three criteria were established:

1. The climacteric is that phase of life in the aging process of women marking the transition from the reproductive to the nonreproductive stage of life.
2. Menopause indicates the final menstrual period and occurs during the climacteric. Present estimates date this at a mean of 51 years, on average.
3. The climacteric is sometimes, but not necessarily always, associated with symptomatology.

The formulation then went on to describe three major etiologies (and their possible interaction) that give rise to menopausal symptoms and complaints:

1. Decreased ovarian activity with subsequent hormonal deficiency resulting in early symptoms (hot flushes, perspiration, and atro-

The preparation of this manuscript was supported by a grant from the Medical Research Council of Canada (#MT-11623) awarded to B.B.S.

phic vaginitis), and late symptoms related to the metabolic change in the affected organ.
2. Sociocultural factors determined by the woman's environment.
3. Psychologic factors, dependent on the nature of the woman's character.

Considering the fact that menopause is a universal phenomenon, it is curious that it was only in 1976 that an international definition of this event was first formulated and published. One explanation may be related to changes in statistics regarding female life expectancy. As recently as 1900, the average life span of a woman living in the United States was approximately 50 years. In 1988, the life expectancy for North American women was 80 years, and the projected female life expectancy for the year 2000 is 84 years (Cope 1976). Therefore, women now live one-third of their lives beyond cessation of their reproductive capacity, and the quality of life during the latter one-third of the life span has, understandably, become a major issue of concern to both health professionals and women themselves.

During the past century, the age of menopause has remained remarkably stable at 50–51 years (Treolar 1981). Because of the increase in life expectancy, however, there is an increasing number of postmenopausal women in the United States population; this number is now estimated to be approximately 40 million.

Surgical menopause occurs when both ovaries are removed before the natural menopause has occurred. Before the 1970s, bilateral oophorectomy was performed fairly commonly in association with hysterectomy undertaken for benign gynecologic conditions. The rationale underlying this practice was 1) the prevention of ovarian cancer and 2) the view that ovarian function was expendable if pregnancy was no longer possible. Epidemiologic evidence suggesting that, in the absence of a family history, women have a low risk of ovarian cancer served to curtail the practice of indiscriminately removing normal-appearing ovaries at the time of hysterectomy undertaken for benign disease. An even more compelling reason for retaining the ovaries in premenopausal women emerged when it became clear that acceleration of cardiovascular disease (Parrish et al. 1967) and osteoporosis (Lindsay et al. 1980) were associated with early oophorectomy. For these reasons, the conservation of normal ovaries at the time of hysterectomy has become the more common practice in North America.

Consistent with the 1976 definition of the climacteric syndrome (Utian and Serr 1976), the etiology and frequency of symptomatology that may occur at this time are discussed in this chapter from neurohormonal, sociocultural, and psychological perspectives and an attempt is made to synthesize this material.

NEUROHORMONAL PROCESSES

Changes in Sex Hormone Secretion in Menopausal Women

In premenopausal women, the ovary secretes 95% of the estradiol that enters the circulation (Lipsett 1986). After menopause, the ovary virtually stops producing estradiol, and estrone, a much weaker estrogen, becomes the predominant estrogen that arises from peripheral conversion of androstenedione (Longcope 1981). Although it was once thought that the drastic decrease in ovarian estradiol secretion at the time of menopause was due solely to follicle depletion and ovarian senescence, it is now clear that age-related alterations in hypothalamic function also occur (Wise et al. 1989). Thus, the transition to menopause is a multifactorial process involving both neural and ovarian factors.

In women, both the adrenal and the ovary contain the biosynthetic pathways necessary for androgen synthesis and secretion. The ovary produces approximately 25% of plasma testosterone, 60% of androstenedione, and 20% of dehydroepiandrosterone (DHEA), whereas the adrenal produces 25% of circulating testosterone, 40% of androstenedione, 50% of DHEA, and 90% of DHEA sulfate. The remainder of circulating androgens in the female are thought to arise through peripheral conversion, which probably accounts for the production rate of 50% of testosterone and 25% of DHEA (Longcope 1986). Although ovarian production of estrogens decreases drastically, about 50% of women produce even greater amounts of androgens after menopause due to ovarian stromal hyperplasia that occurs under the influence of high levels of luteinizing hormone (Judd et al. 1974). When it occurs, however, this increase in ovarian testosterone production is time limited, so that eventually, testosterone levels decrease in all women.

Neurobiological Effects of Estrogen and Androgen

Estrogen has both inductive and direct effects on neurons. This hormone induces ribonucleic acid (RNA) and protein synthesis via genomic mechanisms that, in turn, cause changes in levels of specific gene products, such as neurotransmitter synthesizing enzymes (Luine et al. 1975). Other prolonged neuronal regulatory effects include the expression of gonadal hormone receptors in specific brain areas. On the other hand, direct effects of estrogen on the brain appear to take place more rapidly. For example, estrogens can alter electrical activity of neurons in the hypothalamus (Kelly et al. 1977).

Autoradiographic studies have demonstrated that neurons containing specific cytosolic receptors for estrogen are found in specific areas of the brain, predominantly in the pituitary, hypothalamus, limbic forebrain (including the amygdala and lateral septum), and the cerebral cortex (McEwen 1980). Moreover, a number of neurotransmitter systems, including serotonergic, adrenergic, γ-aminobutyric acid (GABA), and opioid systems, have been suggested to be responsive to estrogen, although not all of these effects have been demonstrated in vivo or at physiological conditions (McEwen et al. 1979).

It has also been demonstrated by means of autoradiographic studies that specific cytosolic receptors for testosterone are predominantly found in the preoptic area of the hypothalamus, with smaller concentrations in the limbic system (amygdala and hippocampus) and in the cerebral cortex (Chamness et al. 1979). Moreover, the brain contains aromatizing enzymes necessary to convert androgens to estrogens. The anterior hypothalamus is the most active aromatizing central tissue, although limbic system structures also convert androgens to estrogens (Naftolin and Ryan 1975). Thus, it is clear that sex steroids may exert direct actions on portions of the brain thought to subserve emotion and sexuality.

Peripheral Effects of Estrogen

Because the integrity of the tissues of the female reproductive tract is dependent on estrogen, degenerative changes in these structures ensue when levels of estrogen decrease after menopause. The vaginal mucosa of postmenopausal women who do not receive estrogen therapy becomes attenuated and pale due to a decrease in vascularity. Marked atrophic changes may result in atrophic vaginitis. In this condition, the vaginal epithelium is very thin and may become inflamed or even ulcerated (Bergman and Brenner 1987). These changes, in turn, may lead to a severe diminution in vaginal lubrication and/or dyspareunia. The urethral epithelium is also estrogen dependent (Ostergard 1980), and urge incontinence is not an infrequent complaint in untreated postmenopausal women (Brenner 1988).

Consequences of Hormonal Changes at Menopause

Physical symptoms.   In view of the fact that estrogen affects a multitude of organ systems, it is evident that the drastic changes in the hormonal milieu that occur around the time of menopause may have consequences for both physical and psychological functions. Hot flushes, the cardinal menopausal symptom, occur in 60%–90% of menopausal women, albeit with a high degree of variability in their frequency and intensity. For 65% of postmenopausal women, the vasomotor phenomena of hot flushes and cold sweats persist for at least 1 year, and for 20%, these symptoms continue for more than 5 years (Brenner 1988). Because hot flushes occur more frequently at night, sleep is often disrupted. Hot flushes are reliably relieved by estrogen replacement therapy (Coope et al. 1975), and although some researchers have noted a simultaneous beneficial effect of exogenous estrogen on hot flushes and sleep quality (Schiff et al. 1980), others have found these two things to be dissociable (Sherwin and Gelfand 1984). What does seem to be clear is that if sleep disturbance is associated with frequent awakenings during the night due to hot flushes, estrogen administration will probably eliminate both symptoms. The efficacy of exogenous estrogen is less well established, however, for sleep disturbances not associated with nocturnal flushes.

Psychological symptoms.   Historically, myriad psychological symptoms have been associated with menopause, the most prominent of which are depression, irritability, and mood lability. It is now generally thought that affective disorders that occur during menopause do not constitute a distinct subtype of depression. Winokur (1973) found that women were not at greater risk for a first episode of depression at the time of menopause than they were other times during the life span. In that study, however, more stringent severity criteria for the diagnosis of depression during menopause were used because of the high frequency with which symptoms of depression and nervousness occurred in his sample of menopausal patients. The circularity of this reasoning makes the results difficult to interpret. In a sample of female outpatient admissions with diagnosis of major nonbipolar depression, it was concluded that there was insufficient evidence to consider onset of depression at menopause as a distinct entity (Weissman 1979), despite the fact that 47% of the depressed menopausal and 65% of the depressed postmenopausal women had no history of depression. Moreover, Brown et al. (1984) reported that involutional-onset depression was associated with a lower family history of depression than that observed in women with early-onset depression. Taken together, these observations suggest that it may be timely to reexamine both the biological and the psychosocial aspects of mood disorders occurring during the menopausal years.

   Although some epidemiologic studies of normal women have failed to find an increased incidence of depression and minor psychological symptoms in peri- and postmenopausal women (Kaufert and Syrotuik 1981; S. M. McKinlay and Jeffreys 1974; Thompson et al. 1973), others have documented an increase in the prevalence of depressive symptomatology at this time (Bungay et al. 1980; Greene and Cooke 1980; Hunter and Whitehead 1989). Perhaps even more important is the fact that, of women who seek medical consultation for menopausal symptoms, 79% have physical symptoms and 65% have varying degrees of depression (Anderson et al. 1987). The suggestion that symptomatic women who seek health care are "atypical," although having some merit (J. B. McKinlay and McKinlay 1986), does not negate the considerable incidence of physical and psychological disturbances associated with menopause that come to the attention of health professionals.

The most commonly used experimental technique to investigate the effects of the sex steroids on affect has been to measure changes in mood in perimenopausal women before and after a trial of hormone replacement therapy. Many earlier studies were uncontrolled with respect to blindness (George et al. 1973), the presence of malignant disease (Chakravarti et al. 1977), and concurrent psychiatric illness (Dennerstein et al. 1979), thus rendering their findings difficult to interpret. In studies in which the investigators controlled for these factors, reported discrepancies may be related to both the psychiatric status of the populations investigated in individual studies and the doses of estrogen administered.

Several studies of nonpsychiatric populations of postmenopausal women have reported on changes in affect as a function of circulating levels of sex hormones. In two prospective studies of women who had undergone oophorectomy, depression scores covaried inversely with circulating levels of both estradiol and testosterone (Sherwin 1988; Sherwin and Gelfand 1985). Moreover, depression scores increased when a placebo was substituted for estrogen in these surgically menopausal women. These results therefore confirmed the positive association between mood and plasma sex hormone levels in healthy, nondepressed women.

It is also important to note that, in both studies, the positive correlations between mood and sex hormone levels occurred when both variables fluctuated within the normal range; that is, these women never became clinically depressed, and the doses of hormones administered induced circulating levels that were within the physiologic range for women of reproductive age.

In another study, affective responses to exogenous estrogen were investigated in postmenopausal women who differed at pretreatment with regard to the intensity of their depression (Schneider et al. 1977). Of 10 women whose pretreatment depression scores were in the "mildly depressed" range, 9 women improved after treatment with 1.25 mg of conjugated equine estrogen daily, whereas 6 of the 10 women who were clinically depressed before treatment actually became more depressed with the same dose of exogenous estrogen. When women with severe, refractory depression were given very large pharmacologic doses of conjugated equine estrogen (15–25 mg/

day), depression scores decreased in most of the women after 3 months (Klaiber et al. 1979). On the basis of these findings and those of our own studies of nondepressed women (Sherwin 1988; Sherwin and Gelfand 1985), it now seems reasonable to suggest that the administration of estrogen in doses conventionally used to treat menopausal symptoms enhances mood in nondepressed women but is therapeutically ineffective with respect to mood disturbances of a clinical magnitude.

Several mechanisms of estrogenic action on indoleamine metabolism could account for its mood-enhancing effect. First, it has been demonstrated that exogenous estrogen decreases monoamine oxidase (MAO) activity in the amygdala and hypothalamus of rats (Luine et al. 1975). Since MAO is the enzyme that catabolizes serotonin, the net effect of estrogen administration would be to maintain higher serotonin levels in the brain. Indeed, it has been found that regularly cycling depressed women have higher levels of plasma MAO activity than do nondepressed women (Klaiber et al. 1972).

A second mechanism of action that may explain the putative beneficial effect of estrogen on mood is related to its impact on tryptophan in plasma. Tryptophan, the precursor of serotonin, is displaced from its binding sites to plasma albumin by estrogens both in vitro and in vivo (Aylward 1973), thereby allowing more free tryptophan to be available to the brain, where it is metabolized to serotonin. A significant negative correlation between depression scores and free plasma tryptophan was reported in women who had undergone oophorectomy and whose mood and free tryptophan levels were enhanced after treatment with exogenous estrogen (Aylward 1976). The results of this clinical study provide some, albeit indirect, support for an estrogenic effect on neurotransmitter concentrations.

Finally, a recent prospective study of surgically menopausal women found an increase in the density of tritiated imipramine binding sites on platelets coincident with higher estradiol levels and lower depression scores (Sherwin and Suranyi-Cadotte 1990). To the extent that estrogen increases serotonin concentrations or the amount of time this neurotransmitter remains in the synapse, it will, in accordance with the biogenic amine hypothesis of depression (Schildkraut 1965), enhance mood.

GYNECOLOGIC ASPECTS

Gynecologic Assessment

The premenopausal period is characterized by changes in the regularity of the menstrual cycle and in the duration and volume of menstrual bleeding. Menopause is said to have occurred when 12 successive menstrual cycles have been missed. Gonadotropin levels increase because of the lack of positive feedback resulting from the vastly diminished ovarian production of estradiol. Follicle-stimulating hormone levels of greater than 50 IU/ml and luteinizing hormone levels of greater than 35 IU/ml are considered, in the absence of organic disease, to be diagnostic of menopause (Jaffe 1989). The vaginal epithelium becomes atrophic, and decreased lubrication may be apparent. When the endometrium is biopsied with a curette after menopause, atrophy of this tissue is noted (Benirschke 1986). In time, a decrease in the size of the uterus and breasts occurs. Probably because of the persistence of testosterone production by the postmenopausal ovary in some women that is unopposed by the premenopausal levels of estrogen, there may be an increase in hair on the upper lip and the chin (Jaffe 1989). Because menopausal women are in a high-risk age group for cancer of the breast, most gynecologists recommend breast self-examination and yearly mammography for menopausal and postmenopausal women.

Hormone Replacement Therapy

The ideological dispute as to whether menopause is a normal reproductive event or whether it is an endocrine deficiency disease or an endocrinopathy requiring medical intervention continues to rage. Indeed, it is unlikely that it will ever be resolved, simply because this is a conceptual and not an empirical issue. The differing conceptualizations of this female reproductive event have a major impact on whether medical intervention ought to play a role. That is, does menopause need to be "managed," or is it a reproductive event, like menarche, to be simply experienced? Perhaps a more dispassionate and more useful approach is one that weighs the short- and long-term consequences of estrogen deprivation for each individual woman.

The variability among women with respect to the intensity and frequency of the early symptoms of hot flushes and cold sweats means that some are greatly disturbed by these vasomotor phenomena, whereas others experience them so mildly that they do not pose any negative influence on daily functioning. Highly symptomatic women may be treated with hormone replacement therapy (HRT) for a limited period until its gradual withdrawal does not provoke a resurgence of vasomotor disturbances. Another consideration is that, irrespective of the severity of vasomotor symptoms, all untreated women will, in time, develop atrophy of the estrogen-dependent urogenital tissues, which may give rise to symptoms such as atrophic vaginitis and urge incontinence. Whether a woman wishes to begin HRT to effectively alleviate these symptoms usually depends on her own assessment of the degree of discomfort she is experiencing. On the other hand, there is now incontrovertible evidence that HRT can protect against degenerative diseases that seriously compromise the quality of life beyond the sixth decade. The two most compelling reasons for long-term HRT derive from the reliable finding that estrogen helps to maintain bone density, thereby protecting against osteoporosis (Lindsay et al. 1980). Second, estrogen administration reduces mortality from cardiovascular disease by two-thirds (Bush et al. 1987) and ultimately reduces mortality from all causes by 10%–60% (Henderson et al. 1991). The accumulated research findings from the 1980s therefore strongly suggest that postmenopausal women who receive HRT experience both increased longevity and an enhanced quality of life during the latter decades of their life span.

Risks of HRT

It became clear in 1975 that the use of unopposed estrogen was associated with a marked increase in the incidence of endometrial cancer (Weiss et al. 1976). Adding a progestin to the therapy for 10–12 days a month effectively protects the endometrium from the stimulatory effects of estrogen (Gelfand and Ferenczy 1989), and combined estrogen-progestin regimens are now recommended as HRT for women in whom the uterus is intact.

Orally administered estrogen induces changes in hepatic metabolism that could have adverse influences. Among these potential changes are increased production of renin substrate and decreased production of antithrombin III (DeLignieres et al. 1986). No increased incidence of hypertension or thrombosis has been noted, however, in postmenopausal women receiving oral estrogen replacement (Ettinger 1988).

Considerable controversy has existed regarding the association between HRT and the incidence of breast cancer in postmenopausal women. A recent review of 31 studies that investigated the relationship between HRT and breast cancer found consistent evidence that a daily dosage of 0.625 mg of conjugated estrogens for several years does not appreciably increase the risk of breast cancer. Neither was there convincing evidence of a positive relationship between duration of treatment and the risk of breast cancer with this dosage (Dupont and Page 1991).

Despite the knowledge gained during the past 10 years with respect to the beneficial effects of HRT for postmenopausal women, it is not mandated for all such women. For example, not every woman is at risk for the development of osteoporosis. Indeed, it has been established that Caucasian, tall, slim, small-boned women who smoke are at greatest risk. The decision as to whether an individual woman is a suitable candidate for HRT, therefore, should be predicated on assessing her risks and providing her with information so that she can be a partner in the decision-making process.

PSYCHOSOCIAL ISSUES FOR WOMEN IN MIDLIFE

Psychological Theories

Historically, psychological theorizing with respect to the etiology of menopausal symptoms first occurred within the psychoanalytic framework. The psychological loss theory of menopause is based on the contention that the ability to bear children is central to the meaning of a woman's life. Logically, then, to lose this ability is to lose life's meaning (Deutsch 1945). Other Freudians have expressed the view that menopause is "symbolic castration" (Benedek 1950) and deprives the woman of any means of compensating for the anger, hopelessness, and frustration she has always felt at not being born a male (Prados 1967). With regard to treatment of symptoms that arise at this time, psychoanalytic theory is geared to helping women accept the "mortification of menopause" (Deutsch 1944).

Sociocultural Theories

The sociocultural model posits that the major determinants of psychological disturbance at the time of menopause are role changes and cultural attitudes toward aging. The culture of a given society may be regarded as that which attributes meaning to reality and which thereby transforms a natural or biological event into a cultural event. It follows that the psychological impact of menopause will be strongly influenced by the importance attached by a particular culture to procreation, fertility, aging, and female roles (vanKeep and Prill 1975). Cross-cultural studies have shown that menopause is indeed experienced differently in different cultures. In general, in those cultures where women receive rights at the time of menopause that were denied them during their fertile period, menopausal symptoms are minimal (Flint 1975; Maoz et al. 1977). The facts that North American society is youth oriented and that stereotypes of aging women are largely negative do not serve to provide a supportive environment for menopausal women in our culture.

Level of education and socioeconomic factors also seem to influence the experience of menopause. Several authors from different countries have reported that menopausal women with less education and from lower socioeconomic classes have a higher degree of symptomatology at menopause than do more advantaged women (vanKeep and Kellerhals 1974; Jaszmann et al. 1969; Maoz et al. 1977).

The Postparental Phase and
Other Transitional Phenomena

Menopause, of course, occurs during midlife, a time that is commonly regarded as a period of psychosocial transition and readjustment.

Women who heretofore had heavily invested their emotion and energy in childrearing are forced to redefine their role at menopause as children are growing up and leaving the home and reproductive capacity ceases. From the perspective of role theory, it would be important at this time to develop new, alternate roles in order to maintain self-esteem when old roles lose importance (Havighurst 1966). The departure of grown children from the parental home that tends to occur coincident with menopause has come to be known as the postparental stage of life. Some authors hold that this change inevitably constitutes a psychological loss because the mother loses one of her major roles and thus the rewards that accompanied it (Blood and Wolfe 1960). This formulation, therefore, points to the conclusion that depression occurring during menopause may be due to the "empty-nest syndrome."

In fact, a careful reading of the literature suggests that this conclusion is a function of the population studied. For example, menopausal women who are hospitalized with a major depressive disorder after their last child has left home have been characterized as having had overprotective or overinvolved relationships with their offspring (Bart 1971; Bart and Grossman 1978). Results of general population surveys tell another story. In nonclinical populations, middle-age women whose children had left home reported somewhat greater happiness, enjoyment of life in general, and greater marital harmony than did women of similar age with at least one child still living at home (Glenn 1975). The findings of this cross-sectional study are consistent with those of retrospective (Deutscher 1964) and longitudinal (Clausen 1972) investigations of the postparental stage in nonclinical populations. This evidence indicates that, for previously well-functioning middle-age women, the so-called "crisis of the empty nest" is mythical.

Certain life stresses may be temporally linked with menopause. Some of the negative events that may occur in a woman's life at this time are onset of a major illness or disability in her spouse, death of her spouse, employment uncertainty for either partner, the need to care for one's own elderly parent(s), and loss of support from important friends or family through illness, death, or geographic relocation. It is clear that stressful life events, in particular losses or bereavements, may lead to somatic or psychological symptoms for women during the climacteric (Greene and Cook 1980), just as they do during other life phases.

Studies of the impact of marital status on the experience of menopause are equivocal, probably because it is the quality and not the fact of the relationship that determines whether it serves as a buffer against other life stresses (Gove et al. 1983). Studies in the United States (J. B. McKinlay et al. 1987) and in England (Hunter 1990) found that single women were least likely to be depressed, followed by married women and those who were widowed, divorced, or separated. Moreover, it was the less well-educated women who were widowed, divorced, or separated who were the most likely to be depressed (Hunter 1990).

Sexuality

Survey data generally show a considerable incidence of problems in various aspects of sexual functioning in postmenopausal women. Various studies have reported a 10%–85% decrease in sexual interest (Cutler et al. 1987; McCoy and Davidson 1985) and a 16%–48% decrease in the frequency of orgasm (Hallström 1977; Kinsey et al. 1953) in menopausal women. Although numerous studies have found that exogenous estrogen alleviates atrophic vaginitis and associated dyspareunia and increases vaginal lubrication (Morrell et al. 1984; Myers and Morokoff 1986), exogenous estrogen failed to increase sexual desire or libido. Several prospective studies of surgically menopausal women, however, have demonstrated that the addition of testosterone, which is normally produced by the ovaries, to an estrogen replacement regimen increased sexual desire, sexual arousal, and the frequency of sexual fantasies compared with women treated with estrogen alone (Sherwin et al. 1985; Sherwin and Gelfand 1987). The consistency between these findings and those of investigators in England (Cardozo et al. 1984) and Australia (Burger et al. 1984) who used subcutaneously implanted pellets containing both estradiol and testosterone strongly suggests that in women, as in men, testosterone is the sex steroid that is critical for the maintenance of sexual desire.

Numerous nonhormonal factors may also influence sexual functioning in postmenopausal women. Clearly, one such factor is the desire and capacity of the partner for sexual activity (Davidson et al. 1983). There is also a positive relationship between previous sexual interest or importance of sex with frequency of sexual activity in later middle life (Pfeiffer and Davis 1972). Finally, cultural and societal notions of sexual attractiveness and attitudes concerning the expression of sexuality beyond the reproductive years also have a significant influence on the maintenance of sexual activity in middle-age and elderly women.

"Life Begins at 50"

With so much emphasis on the negative impact of the changing hormonal milieu and the losses and life stresses that often occur coincident with menopause, the fact that this reproductive event is welcomed as a positive event by many women is frequently ignored. For example, the departure of children from the home also means that women are able to redirect their time and energy to tasks and activities that bring other important sources of gratification. Reentering the work force and devoting more time to an already established career, travel, and other leisure activities are all potential benefits of the postparental years. Solid marital relationships may become closer and more intimate at a time when a couple has more opportunity to spend time alone together. Moreover, the absence of menstrual cycles and the accompanying freedom from the need to be concerned about birth control methods may serve to enhance the sexual relationship. Although the climacteric can be characterized as potentially offering the opportunity for freedom to explore new roles, it should be noted that this freedom presumes both the time and the personal and economic resources for such explorations, which a middle-class bias often ignores.

MENOPAUSE AND THE MENTAL HEALTH PROFESSIONAL

The most common reason for referral of a menopausal woman to a mental health professional is for the diagnosis and treatment of a depressive disorder that is associated with the endocrine changes occurring during this reproductive event. Recent studies have failed to confirm the existence of involutional melancholia as a distinct sub-type of depressive illness, leading to its removal from current psychiatric nomenclature. There is a great deal of evidence, however, that depressive symptoms, if not a distinctive syndrome, are experienced by many women at the time of menopause. Clinical observations suggest that women who experienced premenstrual syndrome during their reproductive years and those with a history of depressive illness may be at a greater risk for the development of a depressive episode at the time of menopause than are women without such a history. Unfortunately, little empirical evidence exists to support these observations, because the critical studies have not yet been attempted.

The initial approach to the management of mood and behavioral disturbances in menopausal women requires the determination of the woman's symptoms and the hormonal context in which they occur, a personal history of depression, a family history of affective disorder, feelings about aging and mortality, and concurrent life stresses. If a woman is experiencing distressing signs of estrogen deficiency, such as hot flushes and vaginal dryness, and has no contraindications to HRT (such as a history of breast cancer), then a trial of HRT may be indicated as a first approach. Women who have undergone surgical menopause usually experience more severe symptoms of estrogen deficiency, owing to the abruptness of the change in their hormonal milieu. In the absence of contraindications, HRT would be particularly important for these women. In these cases, it is also critical to explore the psychological impact of the hysterectomy and bilateral oophorectomy and the reasons that necessitated the surgery.

Because of the demonstrated ability of estrogen to alter the concentrations or availability of neurotransmitters in the synapse, it is possible that menopausal women with affective symptoms in the presence of mild or minimal hypoestrogenic somatic symptoms may also respond to a trial of HRT. It is important to note, however, that at present there is no evidence to suggest that a major depressive illness will be significantly alleviated by the doses of estrogen conventionally used to treat postmenopausal women. The decision to institute adjunctive psychopharmacotherapy will depend on the severity and duration of the depressive symptoms and on the premorbid and family history of affective illness.

REFERENCES

Anderson E, Hamburger S, Liu JH, et al: Characteristics of menopausal women seeking assistance. Am J Obstet Gynecol 156:428–433, 1987

Aylward M: Plasma tryptophan levels and mental depression in post-menopausal subjects: effects of oral piperazine-oestrone sulphate. IRCS Journal of Medical Science 1:30–34, 1973

Aylward M: Estrogens, plasma tryptophan levels in perimenopausal patients, in The Management of the Menopause and Post-Menopausal Tears. Edited by Campbell S. Baltimore, MD, University Park Press, 1976, pp 135–147

Bart PB: Depression in middle-aged women, in Women in Sexist Society. Edited by Gornick V, Morgan BK. New York, Basic Books, 1971, pp 163–186

Bart PB, Grossman M: Menopause, in The Woman as Patient. Edited by Notman M, Nadelson C. New York, Plenum, 1978

Benedek T: Climacterium: a developmental phase. Psychoanal Q 11:19–26, 1950

Benirschke K: The endometrium, in Reproductive Endocrinology, 2nd Edition. Edited by Yen SSC, Jaffe RB. Philadelphia, PA, WB Saunders, 1986, pp 385–405

Bergman A, Brenner PF: Alterations in the urogenital system, in Menopause: Physiology and Pharmacology. Edited by Mishell DR. Chicago, IL, Year Book Medical, 1987, pp 67–75

Blood RO, Wolfe DM: Husbands and Wives: The Dynamics of Married Living. New York, Free Press, 1960

Brenner PF: The menopausal syndrome. Obstet Gynecol 72 (suppl):6–11, 1988

Brown RP, Sweeney J, Loutsch E, et al: Involutional melancholia revisited. Am J Psychiatry 141:24–28, 1984

Bungay GT, Vessey MP, McPherson CK: Study of symptoms in middle-life with special reference to the menopause. BMJ 2:181–183, 1980

Burger HG, Hailes J, Menelaus M, et al: The management of persistent menopausal symptoms with oestradiol-testosterone implants: clinical, lipid and hormonal results. Maturitas 6:351–358, 1984

Bush TL, Barrett-Connor E, Cowan LD, et al: Cardiovascular mortality and noncontraceptive use of estrogen in women: results from the Lipid Research Clinics Program Follow-Up Study. Circulation 6:1102–1109, 1987

Cardozo L, Gibb DMF, Tuck SM, et al: The effects of subcutaneous hormone implants during the climacteric. Maturitas 5:177–184, 1984

Chakravarti S, Collins WP, Newton JR: Endocrine changes and symptomatology after oophorectomy in premenopausal women. Br J Obstet Gynecol 84:769–776, 1977

Chamness GC, King TW, Sheridan PJ: Androgen receptors in the rat brain—assays and properties. Brain Res 161:267–273, 1979

Clausen JA: The life course of individuals, in Aging and Society, Vol 3. Edited by Riley MW, Johnson M, Foner A. New York, Russel Sage Foundation, 1972

Coope J, Thompson J, Poller L: Estrogen administration and hot flushes in menopausal women. BMJ 4:139–143, 1975

Cope E: Physical changes associated with the postmenopausal years, in The Management of the Menopausal and Post-Menopausal Years. Edited by Campbell S. Lancaster, UK, MTP Press, 1976, pp 29–42

Cutler WB, Garcia CR, McCoy NL: Perimenopausal sexuality. Arch Sex Behav 16:225–235, 1987

Davidson JM, Chen JJ, Crapo L, et al: Hormonal changes and sexual function in aging men. J Clin Endocrinol Metab 51:19–28, 1983

DeLignieres B, Basdevant A, Thomas G, et al: Biological effects of estradiol-17 beta in postmenopausal women: oral versus percutaneous administration. J Clin Endocrinol Metab 62:536–541, 1986

Dennerstein L, Burrows GD, Hyman GJ: Hormone therapy and affect. Maturitas 1:247–259, 1979

Deutsch H: The Psychology of Women. New York, Grune & Stratton, 1944

Deutsch H: The Psychology of Women, Vol 2. New York, Grune & Stratton, 1945

Deutscher J: The quality of postparental life. Journal of Marriage and the Family 26:52–59, 1964

Dupont WD, Page DL: Menopausal estrogen replacement therapy and breast cancer. Arch Intern Med 151:67–72, 1991

Ettinger B: Optimal use of postmenopausal hormone replacement therapy. Obstet Gynecol 82 (suppl):31–36, 1988

Flint M: The menopause: reward or punishment? Psychosomatics 16:161–173, 1975

Gelfand MM, Ferenczy A: A prospective one-year study of estrogen and progestin in postmenopausal women: effects on the endometrium. Obstet Gynecol 74:398–402, 1989

George GCW, Beaumont PJV, Beardwood CJ: Effects of exogenous estrogens on minor psychiatric symptoms in postmenopausal women. S Afr Med J 47:2337–2248, 1973

Glenn ND: Psychological well-being in the postparental stage: some evidence from national surveys. Journal of Marriage and the Family 32:105–110, 1975

Gove WR, Hughes M, Style CB: Does marriage have positive effects on the psychological well-being of the individual? J Health Soc Behav 24:122–131, 1983

Greene JG, Cooke DJ: Life stress and symptoms at the climacterium. Br J Psychiatry 136:486–491, 1980

Hallström T: Sexuality in the climacteric. Clin Obstet Gynecol 4:227–239, 1977

Havighurst RJ: Changing roles of women in the middle years, in Potentialities of Women in the Middle Years. Edited by Gross J. Lansing, Michigan State University Press, 1966

Henderson BE, Paganini-Hill A, Ross RK: Decreased mortality in users of estrogen replacement therapy. Arch Intern Med 151:75–78, 1991

Hunter MS: Psychological and somatic experience of the menopause: a prospective study. Psychosom Med 52:357–367, 1990

Hunter MS, Whitehead MJ: Psychological experience of the climacteric and postmenopause, in Menopause: Evaluation, Treatment and Health Concerns. Edited by Hammond CB, Haseltine FP. New York, Alan R Liss, 1989, pp 211–224

Jaffe RB: The menopause and postmenopausal period, in Menopause: Evaluation, Treatment and Health Concerns. Edited by Hammond CB, Haseltine FP. New York, Alan R Liss, 1989, pp 406–423

Jaszmann L, Van Lith WD, Zoat JL: The perimenopausal syndrome: the statistical analysis of a survey. Medical Gynecology 4:268–272, 1969

Judd HL, Judd GE, Lucas WE, et al: Endocrine function of the postmenopausal ovary: concentrations of androgens and estrogens in ovarian and peripheral vein blood. J Clin Endocrinol Metab 139:1020–1026, 1974

Kaufert P, Syrotuik J: Symptom reporting at the menopause. Soc Sci Med 15:173–184, 1981

Kelly MJ, Mass RL, Dudley CA: The effect of microelectrophoretically applied estrogen, cortisol and acetylcholine on medial preoptic-septal unit activity through the estrous cycle of the female rat. Exp Brain Res 30:53–64, 1977

Kinsey AC, Pomeroy WB, Martin CE, et al: Sexual behavior in the human female. Philadelphia, PA, WB Saunders, 1953

Klaiber EL, Broverman DM, Vogel W, et al: Effects of estrogen therapy on plasma MAO activity and EEG driving responses of depressed women. Am J Psychiatry 128:1492–1498, 1972

Klaiber EL, Broverman DM, Vogel W, et al: Estrogen therapy for severe persistent depression in women. Arch Gen Psychiatry 36:550–554, 1979

Lindsay R, Hart DM, Forrest C, et al: Prevention of spinal osteoporosis in oophorectomized women. Lancet 2:1151–1154, 1980

Lipsett MB: Steroid hormones, in Reproductive Endocrinology, Physiology, Pathophysiology and Clinical Management. Edited by Yen SSC, Jaffe RB. Philadelphia, PA, WB Saunders, 1986

Longcope C: Metabolic clearance and blood production rates in post-menopausal women. Am J Obstet Gynecol 111:779–785, 1981

Longcope C: Adrenal and gonadal steroid secretion in normal females. J Clin Endocrinol Metab 15:213–220, 1986

Luine VN, Khylchevskaya RJ, McEwen B: Effect of gonadal steroids on activities of monoamine oxidase and choline acetylase in rat brain. Brain Res 86:293–306, 1975

Maoz B, Antonovsky A, Apter A, et al: The perception of menopause in five ethnic groups in Israel. Acta Obstet Gynaecol Scand 65:69–76, 1977

McCoy NL, Davidson JM: A longitudinal study of the effects of menopause on sexuality. Maturitas 7:203–209, 1985

McEwen BS: The brain as a target organ of endocrine hormones, in Neuro-endocrinology. Edited by Kreiger DT, Hughes JS. Sunderland, MA, Sinauer Associates, 1980, pp 33–42

McEwen BS, Davis PG, Parsons B, et al: The brain as a target for steroid hormone action. Ann Rev Neurosci 2:65–112, 1979

McKinlay JB, McKinlay SM: Health status and utilization behavior associated with the menopause. Am J Epidemiol 125:110–121, 1986

McKinlay JB, McKinlay SM, Brambilla D: The relative contribution of endocrine changes and social circumstances to depression in mid-aged women. J Health Soc Behav 28:345–363, 1987

McKinlay SM, Jeffreys M: The menopausal syndrome. British Journal of Preventive and Social Medicine 28:108–115, 1974

Morrell MJ, Dixon JM, Carter S, et al: The influence of age and cycling status on sexual arousability in women. Am J Obstet Gynecol 148:166–174, 1984

Myers LS, Morokoff PJ: Physiological and subjective sexual arousal in pre- and postmenopausal women taking replacement therapy. Psychophysiology 23:283–290, 1986

Naftolin F, Ryan KJ: The metabolism of androgens in central neuroendocrine tissues. J Steroid Biochem 6:993–997, 1975

Ostergard DR: Embryology and anatomy of the female bladder and urethra, in Gynecologic Urology: Therapy and Practice. Edited by Ostergard DR. Baltimore, MD, Williams & Wilkins, 1980, pp 3–10

Parrish HM, Carr CA, Hall DG, et al: Time interval from castration in premenopausal women to development of excessive coronary atherosclerosis. Am J Obstet Gynecol 99:155–162, 1967

Pfeiffer E, Davis GC: Determinants of sexual behavior in middle and old age. J Am Geriatr Soc 4:151–160, 1972

Prados M: Emotional factors in the climacterium of women. Psychother Psychosom 15:231–244, 1967

Schiff I, Regenstein Q, Schinfeld J, et al: Interactions of oestrogens and the hours of sleep on cortisol, FSH, LH, and prolactin in hypogonadal women. Maturitas 2:179–183, 1980

Schildkraut JJ: The catecholamine hypothesis of affective disorders: a review of supporting evidence. Am J Psychiatry 122:509–522, 1965

Schneider MA, Brotherton PL, Hailes J: The effect of exogenous oestrogens on depression in menopausal women. Med J Aust 2:162–163, 1977

Sherwin BB: Affective changes with estrogen and androgen replacement therapy in surgically menopausal women. J Affective Disord 14:177–187, 1988

Sherwin BB, Gelfand MM: Effects of parenteral administration of estrogen and androgen on plasma hormone levels and hot flushes in the surgical menopause. Am J Obstet Gynecol 148:552–557, 1984

Sherwin BB, Gelfand MM: Sex steroids and affect in the surgical menopause: a double-blind cross-over study. Psychoneuroendocrinology 10:325–335, 1985

Sherwin BB, Gelfand MM: The role of androgen in the maintenance of sexual functioning in oophorectomized women. Psychosom Med 49:397–409, 1987

Sherwin BB, Suranyi-Cadotte BE: Up-regulatory effect of estrogen on platelet 3H-imipramine binding sites in surgically menopausal women. Biol Psychiatry 28:339–348, 1990

Sherwin BB, Gelfand MM, Brender W: Androgen enhances sexual motivation in females: a prospective, cross-over study of sex steroid administration in the surgical menopause. Psychosom Med 47:339–351, 1985

Thompson B, Hart SA, Durno D: Menopausal age and symptomatology in a general practice. Journal of Biology and Social Science 5:71–82, 1973

Treolar AE: Menstrual cyclicity and the pre-menopause. Maturitas 3:249–264, 1981

Utian W, Serr D: The climacteric syndrome, in Consensus on Menopause Research. Edited by vanKeep PA, Greenblatt R, Fernet A. Lancaster, UK, MTP Press, 1976, pp 1–14

vanKeep PA, Kellerhals JM: The impact of socio-cultural factors on symptom formation. Psychother Psychosom 23:251–263, 1974

vanKeep PA, Prill HJ: Psycho-sociology of menopause and post-menopause, in Estrogens in the Postmenopause. Edited by Lauritzen C, vanKeep PA. Basel, Switzerland, Karger, 1975

Weiss NS, Szekely R, Austin DF: Increasing evidence of endometrial cancer in the United States. N Engl J Med 294:1259–1262, 1976

Weissman MM: The myth of involutional melancholia. JAMA 242:742–744, 1979

Winokur G: Depression in the menopause. Am J Psychiatry 130:92–93, 1973
Wise PM, Weiland NG, Scarbrough K, et al: Changing hypothalamopituitary function: its role in aging of the female reproductive system. Horm Res 31:39–44, 1989

Chapter 13

CHRONIC GYNECOLOGIC PAIN

John F. Steege, M.D.
Anna L. Stout, Ph.D.

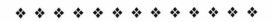

This chapter will review vulvovaginitis and chronic pelvic pain, two of the most vexing problems in clinical gynecology. Both problems are marked by their often chronic and intractable nature, as well as by the frequent contribution of psychological factors to their severity. They represent opportunities for effective collaboration between the gynecologic and mental health specialties.

TYPES OF CHRONIC GYNECOLOGIC PAIN

Vulvovaginitis

Vaginal yeast infections, trichomoniasis, and the mixed infection of bacterial vaginosis are extremely common. Monilial (yeast) vaginitis typically is marked by a white, cheesy discharge; trichomoniasis (*Trichomonas vaginalis* infection), by a frothy, mildly malodorous discharge; and bacterial vaginosis, by a chronic, intermittent, irritating, and malodorous discharge. Women with such clearly identifiable acute symptoms and signs will seldom require mental health consultation. Many women with these disorders, however, may later develop chronic, continuing vaginal and vulvar symptoms, even though the bacteriological precipitants may have been brought under control. The possible role of psychological factors in perpetuating symptoms may lead to referral for psychological evaluation.

More troubling than these entities is the patient who undergoes careful, frequent examinations with no pathogenic organisms visualized. Gynecologists often recognize that such individuals may be unduly focused on any perceived irregularities of vaginal sensation or secretion. Intense symptoms of vaginal discomfort may be a "calling card" or presenting symptom for affective disorders, anxiety disorders, marital discord, somatization tendencies, or sexual dysfunction. For example, continued dyspareunia may be due to vaginismus triggered by repeated uncomfortable vaginal events associated with vaginitis. When pain persists, the patient may return to her physician, claiming that her "vaginitis is back," assuming that any pain in this area must be due to recurrent infection. This situation may benefit from collaboration between the gynecologist and the mental health clinician.

In the postmenopausal patient, specific vaginal infections are far less common, except for atrophic vaginitis in women who are not taking estrogen replacement therapy. Postmenopausal women, however, are prone to the development of vulvar dystrophies, which can present with intense vulvar burning and itching in the absence of any significant vaginal infection. These distressing symptoms can become such an impediment to normal functioning that they may precipitate depressive episodes. Conversely, vulvar symptoms may represent a depressive equivalent.

Chronic Pelvic Pain

Pelvic pain is usually defined as chronic when it has lasted for 6 months or more on a continuous or a cyclic basis. It may be useful to distinguish between patients who have pain that is chronic and those who have a true chronic pain syndrome. In chronic pain syndrome, the pain is accompanied by impaired function in recreational activities and household responsibilities, possible vegetative signs of depression (especially sleep disturbance), and significant alterations of the patient's roles within her family (Steege et al. 1991). Psychological evaluation and treatment are often helpful in such patients.

Dyspareunia.   Dyspareunia, or painful intercourse, is usually described as being either introital (in the area around the opening of the vagina) or deep (Steege 1984). Patients often describe introital dyspareunia as pain "at the opening" or as "trouble getting in" during intercourse. The pain is usually continuous but can be exacerbated perimenstrually in the presence of contributing factors, such as recurrent monilial vaginitis or inflammation of the vestibule. Deeper pelvic pain is often described as "pain inside" or by noting that the partner's penis feels as though it "hits something." Traditionally, deep dyspareunia has been felt by gynecologists to be more likely due to organic factors, whereas introital dyspareunia is more often psychologically based. Although these generalizations are still partly valid, enough exceptions occur to impel careful inquiry into all aspects of the problem. A careful history should delineate the location of the pain, the relationship of the pain to the sexual response cycle, and any alterations of the sexual response cycle. Tactful inquiry should be made regarding any variation of symptoms with different sexual partners.

General pelvic pain.   Pain that is present over the entire lower pelvic area, sometimes greater in intensity on one side than on the other, may occur on either a cyclic or a continuous basis. Cyclic discomforts are more typically associated with endometriosis, although pain associated with pelvic adhesive disease can also be somewhat cyclic, being worse before and during menstruation. Similarly, pain that is possibly attributable to pelvic congestion (overdistention of the pelvic venous system) will often be worse premenstrually (Beard et al. 1989). Worsening endometriosis often starts out as cyclic dysmenorrhea, with the pain gradually subsuming more and more of the menstrual month as time goes on. Continuous pain is more often due to adhesive disease that is either postinfectious or postsurgical in nature. Dyspareunia may be present along with chronic daily pain. It is more common when the pelvic pathology is central in location rather than in the adnexal areas.

The role of organic pathology in the pathophysiology of chronic pelvic pain is poorly understood (Steege et al. 1991), despite research efforts. Most series in the literature report that no abnormal laparoscopic findings are present in approximately 10%–60% of women undergoing this procedure for evaluation of chronic pelvic pain. These numbers, however, may be an overestimation of the percentage of "negative" pelvic findings, since most of the studies were published before it was recognized that endometriosis can present in atypical or unpigmented forms. A woman with negative findings on laparoscopy may nevertheless have some physical contributions to her pain, such as trigonitis, urethritis, functional pelvic musculoskeletal problems, postural changes, or irritable bowel syndrome. Some of the studies describing psychological profiles in women with negative laparoscopies fail to describe evaluations for such problems.

Sizable fractions of women with organic pathology also demonstrate substantial psychological changes on psychometric testing and clinical or structured interview (Castelnuovo-Tedesco and Krout 1970). This confusing picture makes it clinically difficult to decide in a given individual case whether the primary difficulty is physiologic or psychologic. For example, several studies document that women with organic pathology, most often endometriosis or adhesions, will more often have pelvic pain than those without any organic pathology. Although the location of the pain often correlates with the location of the pathology, however, the intensity of the pain demonstrates no quantitative relationship to the amount of tissue change present (Fedele et al. 1990; Stout et al. 1991). It therefore remains a matter of difficult clinical judgment to decide on the appropriate medical or surgical treatments of the organic pathology.

DIAGNOSIS AND TREATMENT

Vulvovaginal Symptoms

Vulvovaginitis. A complete evaluation of vulvovaginitis includes a careful history of sexually transmitted diseases, use of intrauterine devices, the medical and medication risk factors described previously in this chapter, and a sexual history. The examination should include a complete routine pelvic examination, along with a microscopic examination of the vaginal secretions for the detection of trichomonads, a search for the clue cells indicative of bacterial vaginosis, and a rough quantitation of yeast forms. Specific cultures for yeast are seldom of benefit, since often they are positive in asymptomatic women and do not provide a quantitative measure. *T. vaginalis* cultures may be useful in the rare instance when symptoms appear to be typical of that disease, but the microscopic test is not diagnostic. Cultures for bacterial vaginosis are useful only on a research basis.

In the postmenopausal woman with intense vulvar symptoms, careful visual inspection of the vulva is essential, and a biopsy should be performed to evaluate any suspected abnormalities. Vulvar carcinoma is notoriously difficult to recognize visually, and the vulvar dystrophies are so varied in appearance that biopsy is often necessary for proper diagnosis.

In many situations, these diagnostic tests are indeterminate, yet the symptoms persist. Often the gynecologist in this situation may prescribe topical steroids and other vaginal medications as therapeutic trials. When the mental health professional sees such a patient, it is often useful to initiate a candid dialogue with the gynecologist to better understand the degree to which bacteriological or fungal diagnoses are truly well established.

Vulvodynia.   The problem of vulvar pain without any evidence of visual or intraepithelial change is a most perplexing problem for both the gynecologist and the mental health professional. Investigation by routine histologic and culture techniques is often unrevealing. Present studies are focused on the potential role of human papillomavirus in this disorder, but results are far from conclusive. While allowing the possibility of as-yet undiscovered organic etiologies, health professionals must be prepared to deal with the often simultaneous problems of significant depression and despair for such patients in the face of continuing symptoms. These symptoms may also be somatic symptoms of a primary psychiatric condition.

Chronic Pelvic Pain

Adequate assessment of chronic pelvic pain includes a careful chronologic history of development of the pain as it affects the woman's daily life. Disability often develops gradually, and particular inflection points in the curve of disability may be punctuated by external life events or events within the family. A careful history should also include the chronology of the development of any particular sexual dysfunctions. Although such dysfunctions may be initially triggered by organic events, they may become chronic. Sexual dysfunctions may be more apt to occur in women with previous difficulties in sexual adjustment.

In a careful physical examination for chronic pelvic pain, the examiner should systematically look for vulvar epithelial changes and sensitivity, vaginal introital muscle tone and control, levator plate tension, cervical motion tenderness, and general pelvic tenderness during the bimanual and rectovaginal examinations. The two conditions most often associated with chronic pelvic pain—endometriosis and adhesions—are often difficult to detect by physical examination and imaging techniques. Laparoscopy should be freely used for diagnosis and probably for the treatment of these conditions. In one encouraging report of laparoscopic adhesiolysis, long-term relief was noted in 75% of women without a chronic pain syndrome as defined previously in this chapter and in 40% of those with chronic pain syndrome (Steege and Stout 1991). Other reports have noted improvement rates of 50%–85% following such procedures (Sutton and MacDonald 1990; Daniell 1989), depending to some extent on the degree of adhesive disease treated.

PSYCHOLOGICAL ASPECTS OF CHRONIC GYNECOLOGIC PAIN

Early reports in the medical literature implied that women who reported chronic pelvic pain had a high degree of feminine identity problems arising from conflicts regarding adult sexuality (Gidro-Frank et al. 1960), psychiatric disturbance characterized by mixed character disorders with predominant schizoid features (Castelnuovo-Tedesco and Krout 1970), and high neuroticism and unsatisfactory relationships (Beard et al. 1977). Studies by Duncan and Taylor (1952) and Benson et al. (1959) reported an association between the onset of symptoms of pelvic pain and emotional stress.

Although these initial studies served to identify the importance of psychological factors in patients with chronic pelvic pain, some of the generalizations about psychopathology have been questioned from several perspectives. Because some physical abnormalities that cannot be identified on pelvic examination can often be observed on laparoscopic surgery, women who were considered to have normal pelvic examinations in early studies may have been diagnosed with some type of organic pathology if they had been evaluated by currently accepted diagnostic procedures. In a study of 1,200 women undergoing diagnostic laparoscopy for pelvic pain, Cunanan et al. (1983) found that 63% of the women with normal pelvic examinations before diagnostic laparoscopy had abnormal findings on diagnostic laparoscopy. On the other hand, questions have been raised about the assumption of a cause-and-effect relationship between physical findings and pain symptoms. Kresch et al. (1984) identified some possible pathologic conditions in 29% of asymptomatic women who underwent laparoscopic surgery for tubal ligation.

Other methodologic issues that have raised questions about the conclusions from previous studies suggesting the high prevalence of psychopathology include 1) a selection bias in the sample of patients who were studied psychologically because of high refusal rates for psychological assessment that are reported in some studies, 2) a potential bias of psychological evaluators who were not blinded to the presence or absence of organic disease, and 3) lack of appropriate control groups to establish population base rate data for psychosocial factors, such as marital and sexual adjustment difficulties. In all studies of which we are aware, limited information is available on the psychological status of the pelvic pain samples before the onset of pain.

Some of the confusion about the relative contribution of psychological factors in chronic gynecologic conditions has also arisen probably because of varying definitions of chronic pelvic pain and other gynecologic conditions. At least three different types of operational definitions of chronic pelvic pain appear in the literature with some frequency. These definitions focus on the following aspects of the chronic condition:

1. *Duration*—Any type of chronic pelvic or gynecologic pain that has lasted 6 months or longer, a time marker used in other chronic pain conditions
2. *Anatomic*—Chronic pelvic or gynecologic pain that lacks an apparent physical cause sufficient to explain the pain

3. *Affective-behavioral*—Pain accompanied by significant disturbance of mood and altered physical activities (i.e., work, recreational, or sexual activity)

Studies in which psychological inquiry has been focused on patients for whom no apparent physical findings can be identified may reflect more psychological contributions to the pain. Obviously, chronic pelvic pain samples that are selected on the basis of an accompanying affective disturbance may be expected to reflect a strong association with depressive symptoms. Other studies that have selected patients with chronic pelvic pain on the basis of duration of pain may include women with documented organic pathology, most commonly endometriosis and pelvic adhesive disease; however, these women may report varying levels of pain severity and impairment. Stout et al. (1991) reported that the extent of physical disease evaluated by diagnostic laparoscopy did not correlate significantly with ratings of pain levels or a number of other indices of impairment. These findings confirmed the need for exploration of other factors, such as psychological variables, which have been shown to account for a significant portion of individual differences in functional impairment in other pain conditions.

In the literature on chronic pain, investigators have examined a number of personality variables, including anxiety; depression; and certain patterns on personality inventories that have been described as neurotic, particularly those characterized by hypochondriasis and somatization tendencies (Sternbach 1974). In several studies (Chaturvedi 1988; Papciak et al. 1987; Postone 1986), alexithymia (lack of words for feelings) has been investigated as a personality characteristic that may serve to promote and maintain pain symptoms. Bradley et al. (1981) point out that an important shortcoming of many personality studies is that most such studies of patients with chronic pain present composite responses, therefore fostering an inaccurate picture of homogeneity in these patients. Keefe et al. (1986) found that depression was a significant predictor of pain behavior in patients with low-back pain independent of demographic or medical status variables; however, psychological variables (depression, anxiety, helplessness) were not found to be independent predictors of pain behaviors in patients with rheumatoid arthritis (Anderson et al. 1988), pointing out the danger of generalizing from one chronic population to another.

In reviewing studies of chronic pelvic pain (specifically focusing on those in which a diagnostic laparoscopy was used to investigate the organic component) and other chronic gynecologic conditions, an association has been noted between these conditions and certain psychological variables. Rosenthal et al. (1984) administered the Minnesota Multiphasic Personality Inventory (MMPI) (Hathaway and McKinley 1970) to 163 consecutive patients referred for chronic pelvic pain, 60 of whom had diagnostic laparoscopy. The most frequent finding was a "somatizing" pattern (elevations on scales 1 and 3). Abnormal physical findings were present in 75% of the women who underwent diagnostic laparoscopy; however, three-quarters of those patients thought to have an organic cause for their pain also had evidence of psychopathology on the MMPI. The MMPI was therefore a poor predictor of organic pathology.

Magni et al. (1986) examined the psychological characteristics of 30 women who had diagnostic laparoscopies for chronic pelvic pain and 30 matched controls using the Middlesex Hospital Questionnaire (Crown and Crisp 1966) and the Zung Self-Rating Depression Scale (Zung 1965). No differences in somatization scores were observed in patients with chronic pelvic pain with or without organic pathology, although both groups had higher scores than did controls. Those patients with pelvic pain and without observed physical pathology were, however, more depressed than were the patients with organic pelvic pain and controls.

In a study in which a structured psychiatric interview (the National Institute of Mental Health Diagnostic Interview Schedule; Robbins et al. 1981) was conducted with 25 women with chronic pelvic pain and 30 women with other gynecologic concerns, Harrop-Griffiths et al. (1988) found that patients with chronic pelvic pain had a significantly higher prevalence of lifetime major depression, current major depression, lifetime substance abuse, adult sexual dysfunction, and somatization. Stout and Steege (1991) found that 50% of 294 women seeking evaluation at a pelvic pain clinic scored in the depressed range (≤ 16) on the Center for Epidemiologic Studies–Depression Scale (Radloff 1977) at the time of their initial visit. Slocumb et al. (1989) found that patients with abdominal pelvic pain syndrome scored higher as a group on Hopkins Symptom Checklist (Derogatis et al. 1974) scales of anxiety, depression, anger-hostility, and somatization; they also pointed out, however, that 56% of the patients with pain rated themselves within the normal range on all scales. Stewart et al. (1990) found that women with clinically unconfirmed vulvovaginitis were significantly more emotionally distressed than women with confirmed vulvovaginitis and healthy controls.

Sexual history has been explored in several inquiries indicating that women seeking treatment have a high incidence of sexual trauma, including molestation, incest, and rape (Beard et al. 1977; Duncan and Taylor 1952; Gross et al. 1980; Haber and Roos 1985; Raskin 1984; Reiter and Gambone 1990; Schei 1991; Walker et al. 1988). In the study by Harrop-Griffiths et al. (1988) cited previously in this chapter, the two groups undergoing diagnostic laparoscopies were also administered a structured interview on sexual abuse. The patients with chronic pelvic pain with or without positive laparoscopy findings were more likely than control subjects to have experienced childhood and adult sexual abuse. In the study by Reiter and Gambone (1990) 48% of 106 women with chronic pelvic pain had a history of major psychosexual trauma (molestation, incest, and rape), as compared to 6.5% in a control group of 92 pain-free control subjects presenting for annual routine gynecologic examinations ($P < .001$). Rapkin et al. (1990) did not find a higher prevalence of childhood or adult sexual abuse in a group of women with chronic pelvic pain than in women with chronic pain in other locations or in control subjects, although women with chronic pelvic pain reported a higher prevalence of childhood physical abuse. These researchers concluded that their findings failed to support the hypothesis that pelvic pain is specifically and psychodynamically related to sexual abuse and suggest that abusive experiences, whether physical or sexual, may promote the chronicity of many different painful conditions.

As might be expected, many of these same studies also report a high incidence of marital distress. Stout and Steege (1991) found that 56% of 220 married women presenting for evaluation of chronic pelvic pain scored in the maritally distressed range (<100) on the Locke-Wallace Marital Adjustment Scale (Locke and Wallace 1959).

Women presenting with chronic gynecologic conditions often also present with concomitant sexual dysfunction, particularly dyspareunia. Although establishing accurate baseline functioning is difficult, some women report satisfactory sexual functioning before the onset of pain symptoms, whereas others appear to have long-standing sexual difficulties. In any case, sexual dysfunction is highly associated with chronic gynecologic pain, either as an antecedent or as a consequence. Decreased sexual desire and conditioned vaginismus are correlates of this problem that often need specific intervention in addition to any indicated medical treatment.

Since studies to date have been cross-sectional in design, it is not possible to determine whether the negative psychological states reported are a predisposing factor or a reaction to the pain condition. It is important to note that no significant differences in personality or psychosocial variables have been found in most studies of women with chronic pelvic pain with or without identified organic pathology, perhaps suggesting that chronic pelvic pain in some women may be more closely associated with psychosocial factors than with organic factors. In reviewing the literature regarding the relationship between chronic pain and depression, Romano and Turner (1985) concluded that there may be at least two distinct groups of chronic pain patients: one subgroup in whom pain and depression are a final common presentation reached by a number of pathways, and another group who develop depression in reaction to pain, as in some other acute and chronic medical diseases. Patients with chronic gynecologic conditions also appear to be a heterogeneous group; however, the high prevalence of sexual trauma, marital and sexual dysfunction, and emotional distress in previously studied samples of these patients warrants specific attention to these areas in any clinical evaluation. Further research is needed to explore whether these psychosocial factors have a specific relationship to the development and persistence of chronic gynecologic conditions.

MANAGEMENT OF CHRONIC GYNECOLOGIC PAIN

In current gynecologic practice, the woman usually referred for psychiatric care has had a negative laparoscopy—that is, the referring physician believes that the gynecologic causes have been "ruled out." Unfortunately, it is far more common for the patient to have some organic pathology and to have been repeatedly subjected to medical and surgical measures in pursuit of pain relief. Many of these women have developed a chronic pain condition, characterized by significant changes in mood and activities, that needs behavioral and psychological approaches as well as psychopharmacologic treatment, in some cases. This group of patients with chronic pain presents an opportunity for fruitful collaboration between the gynecologic and mental health specialties. In most of these cases, it is clinically difficult to diagnose any particular underlying psychopathology as the precise cause for the pain. More often, clinical judgment will determine that attention to both physical and psychological factors may be important, that both should proceed simultaneously, and that the hope of assigning a particular degree of responsibility to either element must be surrendered. In some cases, the treatment of intrapelvic pathology by laparoscopic approaches, such as lysis of adhesions or vaporization of endometriosis, may be useful. When the parameters of a chronic pain syndrome described here are also present, however, behavioral and psychological assistance is also required.

Reports of controlled trials of psychological interventions specifically for chronic pelvic pain are quite limited; however, increasing evidence substantiates that combined medical and psychological approaches are likely to result in greater improvement than are gynecologic treatments alone in many women with chronic pelvic pain. Pearce et al. (1987) reported the results of a prospective, randomized, controlled trial of two different psychological interventions in the treatment of chronic pelvic pain. Seventy-eight women with chronic pelvic pain of at least 6 months' duration and with no obvious pathology observed on laparoscopy were allocated to a pain analysis, a stress analysis, or a minimal-intervention control group. All groups received an explanation of the pain as being due to abnormalities in pelvic blood flow. In addition, the stress analysis group received training in identifying and implementing alternative cognitive and behavioral responses to concerns other than pain and in applying Jacobsonian relaxation strategies in stressful situations. The pain analysis group focused on monitoring and modifying events antecedent and consequent to pain, graded exercise, and reinforcement of "well behaviors." Both the stress analysis and the pain analysis group reported significantly lower pain intensity ratings at 6-month follow-up visits than did the control group.

In two recent studies by Kames et al. (1990) and Peters et al. (1991), significant improvement in pain ratings and functioning have been reported following multidisciplinary pain management approaches. Peters et al. (1991) randomly assigned 106 patients with chronic pelvic pain to either a standard-approach group or an integrated-approach group. The standard approach consisted of excluding organic pathology by diagnostic laparoscopy and then referring the patient for psychological treatment if no somatic cause could be found. The integrated approach included attention to somatic, psychological, dietary, environmental, and physiotherapeutic factors from the beginning of the evaluation. After a 1-year interval, women in the integrated-approach group showed significantly greater improvement in general pain experience, disturbance of daily activities, and associated pain symptoms. Since the particular types of treatments applied to any individual patient were not standardized in either of these studies, it is unfortunately not possible to identify the effective therapeutic components in these combined approaches.

In general, the psychological treatment component of chronic gynecologic conditions appears to be most effective when psychosocial factors are evaluated simultaneously with organic factors. Although patients with chronic pelvic pain are often unwilling to view their pain symptoms as other than organically based, many individuals are aware of some factors that worsen their pain, such as worry, muscle tension, or depression. A crucial aspect of successful psychotherapeutic intervention is making a connection with the patient at her own level of conceptualization of the pain problem.

Therapeutic interventions for the patient with chronic pelvic pain usually focus initially on exploring behavioral and cognitive patterns that exacerbate the pain symptoms and developing coping strategies to interrupt these patterns. New information is often obtained by having the patient record pain ratings across the day. Depending on the relative influence of particular factors on pain ratings, psychological treatment interventions have often included relaxation training di-

rected at reducing muscle tension components, stress analysis to identify difficult life areas, assertiveness training to teach skills for dealing
more directly with people or circumstances that may be controlled or
avoided by the patients' complaints of pain, and cognitive interventions directed at specific emotional responses to pain that may feed
back to increase anxiety, depression, and perceived pain.

Psychological approaches may also involve spouses or families to
assist in defining a valued role in the family despite some possible limitations in previous activities. Changes in sexual activity often accompany pelvic pain, and specific education and counseling may be
required to allow the patient to return to a level of comfort. Sexual
counseling suggestions often include information about adequate
physiological arousal, changes in sexual positions, and instruction in
vaginal relaxation exercises to treat a conditioned vaginismus response. As a trusting therapeutic relationship is established and coping skills are developed, some women may be receptive to pursuing
psychotherapeutic approaches that are inclusive of broader issues related to unresolved emotional issues from past experiences.

The medical management of chronic pelvic pain may include the
use of antidepressants, although therapeutic trials of these agents in
the treatment of chronic pelvic pain are lacking. Tricyclic antidepressants and the newer serotonergic agents are used by many clinics providing care for patients with chronic pelvic pain. Although analgesic
prescriptions should be limited to nonnarcotic agents, chronic pain is
better treated by the continuous use of such medications, thereby
eliminating the tendency for medication to act as a reinforcer of pain
behaviors or complaints. Other medications aimed at the symptomatic relief of bladder and bowel dysfunction are often additive. We
have found that it is often better to treat various contributing factors
simultaneously.

Nonpharmacologic methods are also useful in selected individuals.
Alterations of gait or stance that might be traced to a musculoskeletal
problem can be best evaluated by a physical therapist. Appropriate
muscle strengthening, stretching, and relaxation exercises can also
help. Transcutaneous nerve stimulators have been used sparingly in
patients with pelvic pain but are sometimes useful.

When pain and related disability are severe, many clinicians feel that intensive inpatient treatment is warranted (Fogel and Stoudemire 1986; Maruta et al. 1989; Stoudemire and Fogel 1986). In such a case, a multispecialty team, particularly on a combined medical-psychiatric unit, is the most productive approach, as it may best maintain a balanced approach to the often complicated and integrated psychological and physical components to chronic pelvic pain.

CONCLUSIONS

Chronic pelvic pain is a common complaint. Although a minority of women will present with this problem in the absence of any organic pathology, in most, chronic pain will have developed in the presence of disease processes, such as adhesions and endometriosis. It is often clinically impossible to assign specific degrees of responsibility to physical and psychological contributions to pain. Clinical care is therefore facilitated when needs in both areas are addressed as clinically appropriate and efforts to assign degrees of responsibility are suspended. This approach requires close collaboration between the gynecologist and the mental health professional.

The patient experiencing chronic pain in the total absence of organic pathology presents a more difficult problem and often represents more long-standing and complicated psychopathologic processes. Again, collaborative management will be useful in order to evaluate and minimize unnecessary treatment while continually offering psychological assistance aimed at helping the patient and her family cope with her difficulties.

REFERENCES

Anderson KO, Keefe FJ, Bradley LA, et al: Prediction of pain behavior and functional status of rheumatoid arthritis patients using medical status and psychological variables. Pain 33:25–32, 1988

Beard RW, Belsey EM, Lieberman BA, et al: Pelvic pain in women. Am J Obstet Gynecol 128:566–570, 1977

Beard W, Reginald PW, Wadsworth J: Clinical features of women with chronic lower abdominal pain and pelvic congestion. Br J Obstet Gynecol 95:153–161, 1989

Benson RC, Hanson KH, Matarazzo JD: Atypical pelvic pain in women: gynecologic and psychiatric considerations. Am J Obstet Gynecol 77:806–825, 1959

Bradley LA, Prokop CK, Gentry WD, et al: Assessment of chronic pain, in Medical Psychology: Contributions to Behavioral Medicine. Edited by Prokup CK, Bradley LA. New York, Academic Press, 1981, pp 35–52

Castelnuovo-Tedesco P, Krout BM: Psychosomatic aspects of chronic pelvic pain. Int J Psychiatry Med 1:109–126, 1970

Chaturvedi SK: Chronic pain patients with and without alexithymia. Can J Psychiatry 33:830–833, 1988

Crown S, Crisp AH: A short clinical diagnostic self-rating scale for psychoneurotic patients: The Middlesex Hospital Questionnaire. Br J Psychiatry 112:917–923, 1966

Cunanan RG, Courey NG, Lipes J: Laparoscopic findings in patients with pelvic pain. Am J Obstet Gynecol 146:589–591, 1983

Daniell JF: Laparoscopic enterolysis for chronic abdominal pain. Journal of Gynecologic Surgery 5:61–66, 1989

Derogatis LR, Lipman RS, Rickels K, et al: The Hopkins Symptom Checklist (HSCL): a self-report symptom inventory. Behav Sci 19:1–15, 1974

Duncan CH, Taylor HC: A psychosomatic study of pelvic congestion. Am J Obstet Gynecol 64:1–12, 1952

Fedele L, Parazzini F, Bianchi S, et al: Stage and localization of pelvic endometriosis and pain. Fertil Steril 53:155–158, 1990

Fogel BS, Stoudemire A: Organization and development of combined medical-psychiatric units, II. Psychosomatics 27:417–428, 1986

Gidro-Frank L, Gordon T, Taylor HC Jr: Pelvic pain and female identity: a survey of emotional factors in 40 patients. Am J Obstet Gynecol 79:1184–1202, 1960

Gross R, Doerr J, Caldirola D, et al: Borderline syndrome and incest in chronic pelvic pain patients. Int J Psychiatry Med 10:79–96, 1980

Haber J, Roos C: Effects of spouse abuse and/or sexual abuse in the development and maintenance of chronic pain in women, in Advances in Pain Research and Therapy, Vol 9. Edited by Fields HL, et al. New York, Raven, 1985, pp 889–895

Harrop-Griffiths J, Katon W, Walker E, et al: The association between chronic pelvic pain, psychiatric diagnoses, and childhood sexual abuse. Obstet Gynecol 71:589–594, 1988

Hathaway SR, McKinley JC: Minnesota Multiphasic Personality Inventory, Revised. Minneapolis, University of Minnesota, 1970

Kames LD, Rapkin AJ, Naliboff BD, et al: Effectiveness of an interdisciplinary pain management program for the treatment of chronic pelvic pain. Pain 41:41–46, 1990

Keefe FJ, Wilkins RH, Cook WA, et al: Depression, pain and pain behavior. J Consult Clin Psychol 54:665–669, 1986

Kresch AJ, Seifer DB, Sachs LB, et al: Laparoscopy in 100 women with chronic pelvic pain. Obstet Gynecol 64:672–674, 1984

Locke MJ, Wallace KM: Short marital adjustment and predictions tests: their reliability and validity. Marriage and Family Living 21:251–255, 1959

Magni G, Anderoli C, de Leo D, et al: Psychological profile of women with chronic pelvic pain. Arch Gynecol Obstet 237:165–168, 1986

Maruta T, Vatterott MK, McHardy MJ: Pain management as an anti-depressant: long-term resolution of pain-associated depression. Pain 36:335–337, 1989

Papciak AS, Feuerstein M, Belar CD, et al: Alexithymia and pain in an outpatient behavioral medicine clinic. Int J Psychiatry Med 16:347–357, 1987

Pearce S, Matthews AM, Beard RW: A controlled trial of psychological approaches to the management of pelvic pain in women. Paper presented at the 8th annual scientific sessions of the Society of Behavioral Medicine, Washington, DC, March 1987

Peters AAW, van Horst E, Jellis B, et al: A randomized clinical trial to compare two different approaches in women with chronic pelvic pain. Obstet Gynecol 77:740–744, 1991

Postone N: Alexithymia in chronic pain patients. Gen Hosp Psychiatry 8:163–167, 1986

Radloff LS: The CES-D Scale: a self-report depression scale for research in the general population. Applied Psychological Management 1:385–410, 1977

Rapkin AJ, Kames LD, Darke LL, et al: History of physical and sexual abuse in women with chronic pain. Obstet Gynecol 76:92–96, 1990

Raskin DE: Diagnosis in patients with chronic pelvic pain (letter). Am J Psychiatry 141:824, 1984

Reiter RC, Gambone JC: Demographic and historic variables in women with idiopathic chronic pelvic pain. Obstet Gynecol 75:428–432, 1990

Robbins LN, Helzer JD, Croughan J, et al: National Institute of Mental Health Diagnostic Interview Schedule: its history, characteristics and validity. Arch Gen Psychiatry 38:381, 1981

Romano JM, Turner JA: Chronic pain and depression: does the evidence support a relationship? Psychol Bull 97:18–34, 1985

Rosenthal RH, Ling FW, Rosenthal TL, et al: Chronic pelvic pain and laparoscopic findings. Psychosomatics 25:833–841, 1984

Schei B: Sexual factors in pelvic pain. Journal of Psychosomatic Obstetrics and Gynaecology 12 (suppl):99–108, 1991

Slocumb JC, Kellner R, Rosenfeld RC, et al: Anxiety and depression in patients with the abdominal pelvic pain syndrome. Gen Hosp Psychiatry 11:48–53, 1989

Steege JF: Dyspareunia and vaginismus. Clin Obstet Gynecol 23:750–759, 1984

Steege JF, Stout AL: Resolution of chronic pelvic pain following laparoscopic adhesiolysis. Am J Obstet Gynecol 165:278–283, 1991

Steege JF, Stout AL, Somkuti SG: Chronic pelvic pain in women: toward an integrative model. Journal of Psychosomatic Obstetrics and Gynaecology 12 (suppl):3–30, 1991

Sternbach RA: Pain Patients: Traits and Treatment. New York, Academic Press, 1974

Stewart DE, Whelan CI, Fong IW, et al: Psychosocial aspects of chronic, clinically unconfirmed vulvovaginitis. Obstet Gynecol 76:852–856, 1990

Stoudemire A, Fogel BS: Organization and development of combined medical-psychiatric units, I. Psychosomatics 27:341–345, 1986

Stout AL, Steege JF: Psychosocial and behavioral self-reports of chronic pelvic pain patients. Paper presented at the meeting of the American Society of Psychosomatic Obstetrics and Gynecology, Houston, TX, March 1991

Stout AL, Steege JF, Dodson WC, et al: Relationship of laparoscopic findings to self-report of pelvic pain. Am J Obstet Gynecol 164:73–79, 1991

Sutton C, MacDonald R: Laser laparoscopic adhesiolysis. Journal of Gynecologic Surgery 6:155–159, 1990

Walker EW, Katon W, Harrop-Griffiths J, et al: Relationship of chronic pelvic pain to psychiatric diagnoses and childhood sexual abuse. Am J Psychiatry 145:75–80, 1988

Zung WWK: A self-rating depression scale. Arch Gen Psychiatry 12:63–70, 1965

Chapter 14

GYNECOLOGIC DISORDERS AND SURGERY

Paula J. A. Hillard, M.D.

❖ ❖ ❖ ❖ ❖ ❖ ❖ ❖ ❖ ❖ ❖ ❖ ❖ ❖

Gynecologic disorders and gyne-
cologic surgery have the potential to evoke significant emotional responses. A sexually transmitted disease, contracted from a partner
with whom a woman has been intimate, suggests betrayal and violation of trust. The fact that some sexually transmitted diseases are
incurable, with the potential for carcinogenesis or death as a consequence, is understandably terrifying.

From the time of menarche, women learn to identify monthly cycles and rhythms of menstrual function, and disturbances of normal
functioning are often distressing. Surgeries on the genital organs may
be threatening to a woman's childbearing potential, her sense of feminine identity, and her sexual functioning.

This chapter provides information on a number of common gynecologic concerns and discusses their impact. Issues covered in this
chapter include sexually transmitted diseases, in utero exposure to diethylstilbestrol, common gynecologic procedures, and liaison between
the psychiatrist and gynecologist. Although the potential for adverse
psychological consequences for the individual woman is significant
and the number of women with these common gynecologic problems
is large and increasing, little attention has been directed to the study of
the psychological consequences of many of these problems.

SEXUALLY TRANSMITTED DISEASES

The current complement of sexually transmitted diseases (STDs) is an
alphabet soup of abbreviations, including infections caused by the fol-

lowing organisms: *Neisseria gonorrhoeae* (referred to by the abbreviation GC, for gonococcus), herpes simplex virus (HSV), human papillomavirus (HPV), human immunodeficiency virus (HIV), *Chlamydia trachomatis* (as yet without a common abbreviation), and *Treponema pallidum* (which causes syphilis).

An increasing number of individuals have experienced disease related to one of these organisms, with some types of infections reaching epidemic proportions, primarily among young adults and adolescents. Whereas some of the bacterial infections are easily treated and cured with antibiotics, the viral infections are usually incurable. There may be potential sequelae for future health and fertility, as with chlamydial infection–associated pelvic inflammatory disease. The potential for HPV-associated cervical, vulvar, and vaginal intraepithelial neoplasia may be significant, and the potential lethality of HIV infection is well known, even among the lay public. Individuals who initiate sexual activity at an early age and those who have had multiple sexual partners are at greater risk for contracting an STD. Sexually active adolescents and young people are a particularly high-risk group (Bell and Hein 1984).

Public health reporting of STDs is required in all states for gonorrhea, syphilis, and acquired immunodeficiency syndrome (AIDS) (but not HIV seropositivity). The incidences of HSV, HPV, and chlamydia are estimates only. The Centers for Disease Control surveillance reported a decline in the incidence of gonorrhea in 1989 from previous years, with approximately 733,000 cases reported (Centers for Disease Control 1990). The greatest number of cases occurred in the age group of 20–24 years. *Chlamydia trachomatis* causes an estimated 3–5 million infections annually in the United States (Judson 1985), particularly among sexually active adolescents and young adults (Bell 1990). Syphilis is making a comeback, primarily among drug users who trade drugs for sex. Approximately 111,000 cases of syphilis in all stages were reported in 1989 (Centers for Disease Control 1990). There has been a concomitant increase in the incidence of congenital syphilis. It has been estimated that more than 2 million cases of genital herpes occur annually in the United States (Droegemueller et al. 1987). The rate of consultations with private physicians for this disease and for genital warts (HPV infections) has increased markedly (Becker et al.

1987). Nearly 1.2 million office visits for genital warts were reported in 1988 (Biro and Hillard 1990).

Cervical HPV infection is associated with cervical dysplasia and abnormal Pap smears. The reported rates of cervical dysplasia and abnormal Pap smears appear to be increasing, especially among adolescents (P. J. A. Hillard et al. 1989a). The degree of abnormality reported on the Pap smear may range from mild squamous atypia to frankly invasive carcinoma, although this spectrum of abnormalities is often not appreciated by the lay public, who may view the Pap (or "cancer") smear as having only one of two possible results: normal and indicative of cancer. Significant anxiety often accompanies the diagnosis of an abnormal Pap smear. The provision of accurate information about the spectrum of abnormalities, the procedures needed to evaluate abnormal results (colposcopy and biopsy), and any planned treatment and expected outcome can help to alleviate this concern (P. J. A. Hillard et al. 1989b).

In selected patients with mild cervical abnormalities on biopsy, observation without specific therapy may be recommended, as regression may occur in up to 40% of patients (Krebs 1982). Compliance with recommendations for subsequent Pap smears is essential, as progression may also occur. Fear about possible progression may sometimes paradoxically result in failure to keep subsequent appointments or in other behaviors that may be maladaptive (Biro et al. 1991).

Higher-grade abnormalities (moderate dysplasia, severe dysplasia, carcinoma in situ) generally require ablative therapy, which may range from office laser vaporization, cervical cryotherapy, or excision with electrical current to hysterectomy. Cervical cryotherapy and laser vaporization have been shown to have essentially similar rates (85%–90%) of eradication of the lesion (Townsend and Richart 1983) and thus have largely replaced hysterectomy as therapy for cervical dysplasia in the absence of other gynecologic problems that would warrant a hysterectomy. Reassurances of this fact should be given to the patient at the onset of a diagnostic workup, as the fear of hysterectomy with its real and perceived losses may be an unstated concern. Loop electrical excision is a much newer technique whose efficacy appears good, but most clinicians in the United States have had little experience with its use. The type of treatment recommended depends primarily upon the training and preferences of the treating physician and the available treatment modalities.

In patients who do not fulfill the criteria for outpatient ablative therapy, cervical conization is necessary. This procedure preserves childbearing potential, with little detrimental effect on future fertility or childbearing. Criteria for conization include the inability to completely visualize the lesion with disease of the endocervical canal, or a significant discrepancy between Pap smear and biopsy results. Cervical conization involves the removal of a cone-shaped biopsy specimen by using a laser or conventional scalpel. This procedure is usually performed in an operating room with a general or regional anesthetic, and in the absence of complications, the patient can be admitted and discharged on the same day.

The potential for resolution of cervical dysplasia, also called cervical intraepithelial neoplasia, is good with therapy, but follow-up and surveillance are critical, as recurrences are possible. One of the most psychologically distressing aspects of HPV-associated genital lesions is the evidence suggesting that the virus itself is not eradicated by treatment. The prospect of an "incurable" disease is associated with anxiety. In addition, with HPV-related disease, much is unknown about how the virus is transmitted (although it is generally considered to be an STD, the possibility of nonsexual transmission has been raised), how infectious it is, and the degree of risk of progressive disease. The fact that these questions with very practical implications are as yet unanswered by scientific evidence is often distressing. Medical professionals who acknowledge the current degree of uncertainty related to HPV are sometimes viewed as incompetent or insensitive to the patient's true concerns.

The psychological effects of STDs have been addressed in only a limited manner. STDs have been characterized as "among the most stigmatizing diseases that most Americans . . . acquire" (Darrow and Pauli 1984, p. 66). The psychologic effects have been most extensively studied among participants of genital herpes self-help groups, but to some extent, the psychological reactions that have been described with herpes may occur with any STD. With herpes, as with other serious diseases, the initial diagnosis of the infection may lead to shock. After the diagnosis is made, there is a search for a cure. Subsequently, there is a sense of isolation and loneliness and, with herpes, a realization of its incurability (Luby and Gillespie 1981).

Other, curable STDs, such as gonorrhea and chlamydia, may not result in such feelings, but HPV infections share the characteristic incurability of herpes. As these concerns increase, anger becomes important. Initially, the anger is directed toward the partner who transmitted the infection, but the anger can also be directed toward the physician who is unable to cure the viral disease. Subsequently, anxiety and fears about the infectious nature of the disease, its impact on future childbearing and fertility, and the potential risks of cancer may generalize to other areas of the individual's life. Fears about the impact of the disease on sexual activity, sexuality, and sexual performance begin to surface. Some individuals go on to feel that they are contagious or dangerous—a "leper" effect. There may be self-involvement, decisions to be celibate, or "antisexual," moralistic behavior. Depression, feelings of helplessness, or guilt may increase over time with some patients, who may express the concern "Why me?" (Luby and Gillespie 1981). This scenario is similar to the reactions of patients toward life-threatening diagnoses such as cancer.

One study reported that adolescents with a history of STDs had lower self-esteem than those without such a history (Orr et al. 1989). Elevated levels of psychological disturbance among patients in STD clinics have also been noted (Ikkos et al. 1987). In some individuals, the sequelae of an STD such as herpes may include a reactivation of underlying psychopathology. The extent to which these reactions occur, as well as their severity and duration, vary among individuals. An awareness of the psychological reactions that may occur, however, will aid in helping patients develop the skills to cope with these diseases.

A number of studies of herpes report elevated levels of psychological distress with adverse effects on sexuality, self-image, and love relationships. These effects may last for many months after the diagnosis or initial episode of the disease (J. R. Hillard et al. 1989). The concern has been expressed with regard to herpes that it affects young people "at a critical phase of psychosocial development as they are attempting to develop lasting attachments" (Luby and Klinge 1985, p. 496). Attempts to define individuals or populations who are at greater risk of

significant and long-lasting psychiatric distress have not been particularly successful, and thus all individuals who contract herpes (and by
extension, other STDs) should be considered to be at risk for persistent psychological symptoms (J. R. Hillard et al. 1989).

In Utero Exposure to Diethylstilbestrol

The association between in utero exposure to diethylstilbestrol (DES),
a synthetic estrogen, and vaginal clear cell adenocarcinoma was first
described in 1971 (Herbst et al. 1971). DES has not generally been
prescribed during pregnancy since that date. It was thought to decrease the risk of pregnancy loss and miscarriage, although it was ultimately shown to be ineffective for this indication. Many thousands of
women were therefore exposed to DES before birth, although fortunately, vaginal adenocarcinoma remains rare, with an estimated risk
in exposed women of 1/1,000 or less (Berek and Hacker 1989). Vaginal, uterine, and cervical structural abnormalities have also been associated with in utero exposure to DES, and such exposure has been
correlated with infertility and pregnancy loss, including preterm delivery (Herbst et al. 1981). The prognosis for a good pregnancy outcome
in DES-exposed women is generally good, with reports suggesting that
about 80% will have a live-born child (Herbst and Holt 1990).

Mothers who took DES during previous pregnancies must deal
with feelings of anxiety, guilt, and anger, particularly if their daughters also have reproductive problems. The daughters, too, may be anxious about their own future fertility and may have feelings of anger
toward their mothers and the medical profession that treated them
with medications having long-lasting sequelae. One study has suggested that, contrary to the investigators' expectations, the predominant response of 80% of the daughters was an attitude of trust and
alliance with both their mothers and their doctors; only a minority
reacted with a predominance of hostility or fear (Burke et al. 1980).
The cultivation of a collaborative physician-patient relationship may
be particularly important with DES-exposed women and their mothers, in an effort to minimize adverse emotional sequelae.

GYNECOLOGIC PROCEDURES

Preoperative Preparation for Gynecologic Surgery

Psychological preparation is an important part of the preoperative preparation for any type of surgery, but particularly so for gynecologic procedures (Youngs and Wise 1980). A woman's first reaction to the diagnosis of gynecologic problems is dependent on the severity of the medical problem, its potential or imagined sequelae (threatening her life or her fertility), the extent of the required treatment (office biopsy, ambulatory surgery, or major surgery), and the woman's own individual psychological makeup and reactions to stress in general. The practicing psychiatrist can address gynecologic concerns most effectively by having a basic understanding of the most frequently encountered gynecologic problems, their management, and the potential issues that commonly surface.

In any situation involving gynecologic pathology and the recommendation for operative intervention, informed consent is critical (Rockwell and Pepitone-Rockwell 1979). The acronym "BRAIDED" has been proposed as a mnemonic for the basic components of informed consent (Hatcher et al. 1990). The patient should be provided with a clear understanding of the following:

1. The expected *benefits* of the procedure
2. The potential *risks* of the surgery
3. The *alternatives* (both medical and surgical) to the procedure
4. That *inquiries* about the physician's recommendations are the patient's right and responsibility
5. That *decisions* to withdraw from the choice made are the patient's right
6. An *explanation* of the indications for and the type of surgery planned
7. Finally, *documentation* should be made of the preceding components.

Although some physicians consider the informed consent process a mere formality, discussing these aspects of a surgical procedure is essential to a patient's understanding and acceptance of any surgery and will minimize the potential for subsequent misunderstanding that might even result in a lawsuit. Although this medicolegal aspect of informed consent may be foremost in some physicians' consideration, the benefits to subsequent communication, understanding, and trust between the physician and the patient should not be underestimated.

Psychological preparation prior to surgery in relation to cognitive coping techniques has been addressed (Ridgeway and Mathews 1982). The logistics of surgery—how long the hospitalization is expected to last, and the average period of recovery or time off work— are important to convey to every patient. Specifics about pre- and postoperative procedures may be helpful for some patients (Ridgeway and Mathews 1982). The ability to predict which women would benefit most from which type of preoperative preparation would be useful, but most of the studies that address coping styles have been unable to identify predictive factors.

Involving the patient's family or partner in discussions of surgery may be helpful if the woman chooses to do so. The patient's resources and coping skills in previous situations should be assessed. The fact that surgery is a stress requiring the mobilization of personal resources, including family and friends, should be emphasized (Youngs and Wise 1980). At this point, the gynecologist may recognize women who are judged to be at higher risk for adverse psychological sequelae and refer them for evaluation, counseling, or therapy (Stellman 1990). If the degree of anxiety is judged by the gynecologist to exceed that usually noted, surgery should be deferred if possible, pending a referral for psychiatric evaluation (Schwab 1971).

The process of preoperative preparation includes a discussion of the specific pathology and indications for the surgery. The type of surgery should be described in terms that are understandable but not condescending. The consideration of procedures such as oophorectomy should involve a discussion of the expected benefits, risks, and alternatives, as well as the effect on physiology in terms of the production of ovarian steroid hormones. The need for hormone replacement therapy should be addressed. With a hysterectomy, it is important that the woman understand the basics—that she will experience no more menses, and that she will not be able to have children subsequently.

Dilation and Curettage

Disturbances in menstrual regularity, sometimes accompanied by excessively heavy flow, are common at the extremes of reproductive life, particularly in the perimenopausal years prior to the cessation of menses. Because the risks of uterine fibroids and endometrial pathology (including hyperplasia, polyps, and malignancy) increase with age, histologic sampling of the endometrium is warranted for abnormal bleeding in women over the age of approximately 40 or who have other risk factors, such as obesity, chronic anovulation, or polycystic ovarian disease. In the past, endometrial sampling typically required dilation and curettage (D & C).

With the advent of endometrial sampling techniques that allow an office endometrial biopsy for the diagnosis of causes of abnormal bleeding, fewer patients require D & C (Grimes 1982). The evidence for the efficacy of D & C as a therapeutic technique is not well established, despite its widespread use (Grimes 1982). An additional diagnostic tool that may be utilized in lieu of, or in addition to, D & C is hysteroscopy, in which the endometrial cavity is visualized directly with fiber optics. Women tend to cope better with the less invasive technique of office endometrial biopsy than with D & C, which is typically performed in an operating room under general anesthesia.

Sterilization

Many psychological issues related to fertility and feminine identity are aroused by the prospect of permanent sterilization. Female sterilization is now the most frequently chosen contraceptive option among married and formerly married women (Mosher 1990). Female sterilization may be performed in the immediate postpartum period or as an interval outpatient procedure. Techniques of tubal occlusion include the use of suture, cautery, plastic rings, or clips.

Women considering sterilization should be counseled about the alternative methods of contraception, including male sterilization, which has a significantly lower risk of morbidity and mortality. Women often express the belief that, since they have assumed the health risks and discomforts of pregnancy and childbirth, their partner should assume his share of responsibility with a vasectomy. Some women, however, remain protective of the concerns that their partner may express regarding a vasectomy as a threat to his potency, virility, and manhood. Many women are pragmatic in their desire to end the potential for childbearing and to assume the responsibility for permanent sterilization as they previously did for reversible methods of contraception. A woman who has been in a physically abusive relationship with an obsessively jealous and controlling man may experience an increase in abuse or conflict over a decision for sterilization, as abusive men may attempt to preserve their control over their partners by forbidding sterilization procedures.

Sterilization should be considered permanent; less permanent but long-lasting methods of contraception, such as implantable subdermal devices containing levonorgestrel or an intrauterine device, may be appropriate alternatives for women who are not ready to choose sterilization. Regret surrounding sterilization procedures is infrequent, ranging from less than 1% to 3% (Huggins and Sondheimer 1984), but certain groups appear to be at higher risk for subsequent regret. Women who are younger at the time of the procedure, who were ambivalent or pressured into the decision, who later changed partners, who made the decision for socioeconomic reasons, or who had the procedure at the time of an induced abortion or immediately postpartum may be more likely to regret having had a sterilization procedure (Huggins and Sondheimer 1984). Some young, childless women express a strong desire for sterilization and should not arbitrarily be denied the procedure. The woman's motivation and expectations regarding sterilization should be carefully explored to ascertain that the decision is not hastily made or based on misinformation, transient psychological distress or conflict, or unrealistic expectations of benefits (as, for example, the expectation that a faltering relationship will be saved).

Laparoscopy

Laparoscopy is a surgical procedure that is usually performed on an outpatient basis and involves the use of fiber optics to visualize the pelvic and abdominal organs to confirm causes of pelvic pain such as adhesions or endometriosis. Laparoscopy may also be considered to be therapeutic when techniques such as laser ablation of endometriosis or lysis of adhesions are performed under laparoscopic visualization.

Increasingly, laparoscopy or pelviscopic surgery is replacing traditional open laparotomy surgical procedures, with a resultant decrease in length of hospital stay, pain, and cost for the patient. In addition, adverse psychological sequelae of these less extensive surgeries may be lessened, although this issue has not been addressed systematically. Laparoscopy is now frequently used to diagnose and remove ectopic pregnancies. Currently, other pelviscopic techniques, such as ovarian cystectomy, oophorectomy, or myomectomy are performed by only a limited number of gynecologists.

Surgery for Urinary Incontinence or Pelvic Relaxation

As a consequence of damage to the supporting structures of the uterus and vagina from childbirth, and often with the superimposition of changes related to aging, many women develop some degree of pelvic and vaginal relaxation, including cystocele, urethrocele, rectocele, enterocele, and uterine prolapse. A significant degree of pelvic and vaginal relaxation is not typically seen in nulliparous women. Anatomic findings may be asymptomatic, or symptoms may be extremely limiting and distressing, such as stress urinary incontinence. Surgery to correct symptomatic pelvic relaxation is almost always a purely elective procedure; that is, the decision for surgery should be dictated by the woman herself, based on the degree of functional disruption of activities that are important to her or the extent of social disability that may occur as a result of urinary incontinence. Women should be made aware that incontinence is not an inevitable consequence of aging and that an evaluation of the specific cause(s) will often lead to therapies, including surgery, that are helpful or curative.

The types of surgery for vaginal or pelvic relaxation vary, depending on the anatomic alterations involved. An anterior and posterior colporrhaphy are frequently performed to correct a cystocele and rectocele, respectively, and are usually performed in conjunction with vaginal hysterectomy to correct accompanying uterine prolapse. If anatomic stress urinary incontinence is a factor, retropubic bladder neck suspension may be performed. Sexual dysfunction may occur after vaginal vault procedures due to vaginal shortening or alteration of the vaginal axis (Amias 1975; Bachmann 1990b; Masters and Johnson 1966; Sloan 1978).

Expectations of the results of surgery should be discussed prior to the procedure, as no surgery for stress urinary incontinence is 100% successful. In addition, it is important for the woman to understand that, although it is not likely, it is possible for her voiding problems to be worse as a result of surgery. It is also possible that the problem will recur and that a second surgical procedure may become necessary.

Hysterectomy

In the past, hysterectomy defined the field of gynecologic surgery. Hysterectomy rates have declined since 1970 (Easterday et al. 1983), although a number of factors, including physician gender, community practice patterns, training, and acceptance of alternatives to hysterectomy, effect marked variations in the rate (Bachmann 1990a). Hysterectomy involves the removal of the uterus, inclusive of the uterine cervix, and may be performed transvaginally or transabdominally.

The procedure known as supracervical or subtotal hysterectomy with removal of the uterine corpus, leaving the cervix in situ, was much more commonly performed prior to the recognition of the risks of cervical malignancy and premalignancy. In more recent years, supracervical hysterectomy has been performed solely in situations such as excessive hemorrhage or severe pelvic pathology, in which it was judged that further attempts to remove the cervix would involve a life-threatening risk. There has been some resurgence of interest in the supracervical procedure, however, proponents of the procedure arguing that retaining the cervix offers a number of advantages (Cutler 1988; Kikku et al. 1983).

Women may be confused about the type of hysterectomy proposed by their gynecologist. The confusion arises because the medical term *total hysterectomy*, meaning removal of the entire uterus, including the cervix, is interpreted to mean removal of the uterus and ovaries: a *total hysterectomy with bilateral salpingo-oophorectomy*. In fact, the literature relating to adverse reactions to hysterectomy is obfuscated by reports that do not take into account this distinction. In a premenopausal woman, removing the ovaries results in surgical menopause, which is usually rapid in onset and symptomatically severe.

Gynecologists are divided as to the benefits versus the risks of removal of the ovaries at the time of hysterectomy (Garcia and Cutler 1984). The argument in favor of an oophorectomy is that ovarian conservation entails the risk of subsequent ovarian cancer. Of the gynecologic cancers, ovarian cancer is the most insidious in onset, often eluding detection until it is quite advanced in stage. Of all cases of ovarian cancer, 60%–75% present in advanced stages (Knapp and Berkowitz 1986). It is often argued that the 2%–5% risk of developing ovarian cancer or requiring a second surgery for residual ovarian disease warrants an oophorectomy at the time of hysterectomy, particularly if the woman is approaching menopause (Mattingly 1977; Terz et al. 1967). The average age at menopause is 51 years, a fact relatively unknown among the lay public, who frequently assume that menopause arrives in the mid-40s. The age of, variously, 45 or even 40 years is commonly cited as the age beyond which many physicians would recommend a prophylactic oophorectomy.

The counterargument is that many normal ovaries would need to be removed in order to significantly reduce the death rate from ovarian cancer, and that normal ovaries continue to produce valuable hormones prior to, or even beyond, menopause (Underwood 1976). Ovarian steroid hormones significantly affect many body functions and not only influence the health of the female genital organs—the vagina and urethra—but also play a critical role in the preservation of bony mass and the prevention of osteoporosis, as well as reducing the risks of cardiovascular disease (Barrett-Connor and Bash 1991). Thus, their removal without adequate hormonal replacement has important adverse health consequences.

Hormone replacement therapy can often be accomplished with oral or parenteral (transdermal patch) estrogen and progestin. Such treatment involves the potential for side effects, however, as well as the problem of ongoing compliance (Speroff et al. 1991). Although it has been assumed that the postmenopausal ovary is not hormonally active, there are some data showing the continued secretion of ovarian androgens, which may support the well-being and general health (including the libido) of postmenopausal women (Garcia and Cutler 1984).

Alternatives to hysterectomy.   The current climate in the United States involves an increased skepticism about the necessity not only of oophorectomy, but also of hysterectomy itself. Alternatives to hysterectomy, such as myomectomy and endometrial ablation, either by laser or by electrical means, are being proposed. Although some of these procedures may ultimately prove to be appropriate medical management, the final word, based on definitive, long-term follow-up studies, is not yet in.

Myomectomy as an alternative to hysterectomy for women with uterine fibroids is gaining in popularity, even among women who have completed their childbearing and who would traditionally not have been considered for such a procedure. Some women note that the sensation of uterine contractions accompanying orgasm are pleasurable, and for these women, myomectomy may be appropriate. Other women feel that the monthly reassurances of menses are important to them. Studies suggest that about one-third of women who have a myomectomy have recurrent fibroids and that the need for a subsequent hysterectomy is 20%–25% (Mattingly 1977).

Endometrial ablation as an alternative to hysterectomy involves destruction of the endometrium by a technique performed through the cervix, using either an electric current or a laser. The advantages include a significant reduction in length of hospital stay and the potential for minimizing the morbidity that may be associated with hysterectomy (Bachmann 1990a; Easterday et al. 1983). The goal of endometrial ablation is to completely destroy the endometrium, thus eliminating menses. Currently, endometrial ablation is not often performed, although with future studies documenting the actual magnitude of its associated risks and complications, it may prove to be a useful technique.

Patients who request alternative surgical procedures deserve accurate information about hysterectomy as well as the alternative procedures (Bachmann 1990a). The reasons for avoiding a hysterectomy may be based on misconceptions or fears about the procedure.

Psychologic reactions to hysterectomy.   For many women, removal of the uterus has unique medical, emotional, and sexual significance (Bachmann 1990b; Polivy and Roeske 1978). The relationship to childbearing potential, femininity, and completeness are factors for many women (Polivy 1974). Although the loss of menses may be perceived as a specific benefit of the surgery, particularly if the indications include abnormal or excessive bleeding or pain, other women may feel that menses represent a familiar and comforting rhythm or monthly cycle. There may also be the idea that menstruation cleanses the body (Bachmann 1990b). Misconceptions about anatomy and sexual functioning are common, with women expressing the concern that a hysterectomy actually involves removal of the vagina, rendering sexual activity impossible postoperatively. Concerns about decreased sexual attractiveness as a woman or to one's partner may also be culturally related (Bachmann 1990a).

The issue of sexual responsiveness after hysterectomy has been addressed in several studies (Dennerstein et al. 1977; Zussman et al. 1981). The physical effects of hormone deficiency from oophorectomy contribute to symptoms of vaginal dryness, dyspareunia, and decreased genital sensation. Controversy exists, however, regarding the effect of hysterectomy on sexual function in the absence of oophorectomy or estrogen deficiency (Bachmann 1990b).

There is a current move championing supracervical or subtotal hysterectomy, with the view that the cervix itself triggers orgasm or affects the capacity to experience orgasm (Cutler 1988), although relatively few data exist (Kikku et al. 1983). It is also argued that retaining the cervix reduces the likelihood of painful coitus (Sloan 1978). These arguments are not well accepted among gynecologists who believe that careful surgical attention to minimizing loss of vaginal length will prevent subsequent dyspareunia.

In contrast to the suggestion that hysterectomy results in adverse effects on sexual functioning, a number of studies have shown either no change or a beneficial effect (Dennerstein et al. 1977; Lalinec-Michaud and Engelsmann 1985). Historically, the concept was advanced that the removal of the uterus could precipitate mental illness or depression. In 1890, Kraft-Ebing described his observation that psychoses were more frequently caused by hysterectomy than any other type of surgery. The concept of a posthysterectomy depression was widely believed (Ananth 1978; Hollender 1960). Several review articles have now questioned the concept that a posthysterectomy depression occurs frequently (Bachmann 1990b; Newton and Baron 1976; Patterson and Craig 1963; Polivy 1974). Psychological distress has recently been reported to be less frequent after hysterectomy, with decreased symptomatology (Ryan et al. 1989). It is likely that social changes in women's roles, recent changes in gynecological practice resulting in more stringent indications for hysterectomy, and the move to recognize, acknowledge, and respect the patient as a partner in decision making have contributed to a lower frequency of adverse sequelae than had been reported previously.

Some studies have compared the risk of postoperative depression or referral for psychiatric services and hospitalization after hysterectomy with the risks after other surgical procedures, such as cholecystectomy (Ananth 1978; Bachmann 1990b; Hampton and Tarnasky 1974; Polivy 1974). Some of these studies suffer from significant flaws, including small numbers, whereas some contain very few actual data and are based on impressions gained from psychiatric and psychological interviews. Some studies are retrospective, with problems of recall and bias, and many were published in the 1960s, when the indications for and frequency of the procedure were different. Some studies have varying and often short (as little as 6 weeks) follow-up periods, whereas other studies have long (3–5 years) follow-up periods but also problems with conclusions of causality. Many studies lack control subjects for age or parity; the meaning of a hysterectomy for a 20-year-old nulligravid woman is likely to be different than it is for a 60-year-old woman. Menopausal status is also often not controlled for in these studies.

Education and social class may also affect a woman's reactions to any type of surgery. Many studies have failed to control for whether the hysterectomy procedure included an oophorectomy. In addition, some studies do not separate subjects by the indications for hysterectomy; a hysterectomy for malignant disease evokes more anxiety and legitimate concerns of mortality than does a hysterectomy for benign indications (Drellich et al. 1956; Walton 1979). Studies may not control for the route of the procedure (vaginal versus abdominal); surgical morbidity varies by the type and route of the procedure (Easterday et al. 1983). Psychiatric morbidity may also vary. The definition of adverse psychological sequelae is often not clear; vague terms such as "emotional problems" and "depression" are used loosely in some studies. There are also problems concerning cultural and social assumptions about women's primary role and the functions of childbearing.

From the literature, it does appear that there are some women who appear to be at high risk for adverse psychologic reactions or psychiatric sequelae from hysterectomy (Ananth 1978). This includes, most notably and consistently, women who have had previous psychiatric problems, psychiatric care, or depression (Martin et al. 1980; Moore and Tolley 1976; Polivy 1974; Salter 1985). This group appears to have a several-fold increased risk over women without such a history. It also appears that there may be an optimal level of preoperative anxiety (Drellich et al. 1956). An attitude of casual unconcern may suggest a significant level of denial, which will ultimately result in symptomatology (Ridgeway and Mathews 1982).

Women who have a hysterectomy at a young age are at increased risk for adverse reactions (Kaltreider et al. 1979). This may be due to disruption of sexual/gender self-concepts that were not yet well established or a wish to bear more children. An emergency procedure is an additional risk factor, as there may be little time to prepare psychologically for the hysterectomy (Tang 1985).

Poor social support may also be a predictor of adverse psychological sequelae (Wolf 1970). As with any stress, there is a need for support from family, friends, and partner. Marital problems preoperatively may be a predictor of postoperative problems (Polivy 1974). Low socioeconomic status and less well-educated women also seem to have higher risks of adverse reactions, perhaps related to misconceptions and fears (Wolf 1970).

Women with a history of multiple surgeries and those with chronic pelvic pain constitute another high-risk group (Bachmann 1990b). It has been stated that "some women have psychic conflicts sailing under a gynecologic flag" (Rogers 1950, p. 322), and Barker (1968) reported that if there is no pathologic diagnosis from the surgical specimen, there is a higher risk for adverse psychological sequelae. It has also been stated, however, that "women are not as concerned about unnecessary hysterectomies as defined by others as they are about unwanted hysterectomies as defined by themselves" (Burchell 1977, p. 117).

Preoperative preparation for hysterectomy, with a focus on those women who may be at higher risk, may prove helpful in minimizing the likelihood of adverse psychological reactions (Coppen et al. 1981; Stellman 1990). The patient's own anticipation of the effects of surgery should be explored; negative expectations about hysterectomy in particular have been correlated with deterioration in sexual functioning (Dennerstein et al. 1977).

Hysterectomies have been categorized as being emergent, mandatory, urgent, advisable, or elective (Easterday et al. 1983). Particularly for advisable surgery, which constitutes the majority of hysterectomies, participation in the decision-making process will facilitate an appropriate or adaptive response. Hysterectomies performed for prevention of problems or for premalignant disease should be clearly indicated. With a hysterectomy, there are a number of quality-of-life considerations that a woman takes into account (Easterday et al. 1983; Polivy and Roeske 1978) and that are influenced by her own psychological and emotional health and her own past experiences. Often she is in the best position to weigh these factors, but she may need guidance from her gynecologist or a therapist.

With any surgery, but particularly with a hysterectomy, it is important to explain the risks and benefits of the procedure and to state clearly which symptoms will be alleviated. Realistic expectations should be fostered. Premenopausal women in whom a hysterectomy without oophorectomy is planned should be advised to expect some persistence of cyclic symptoms (premenstrual syndrome or late luteal phase dysphoria) related to ovarian hormone production, if these symptoms were present before.

LIAISON BETWEEN PSYCHIATRIST AND OBSTETRICIAN-GYNECOLOGIST

Direct communication between therapist and gynecologist is important, as miscommunications sometimes arise if physicians rely solely on the patient for information about the gynecologic diagnosis or recommendations for its treatment. When hospitalization is planned, psychiatric follow-up during the inpatient stay may be helpful.

Psychiatric care may be even more critical than gynecologic care in the weeks or months after surgery. Gynecologists may feel that their care has been completed by the time of the standard 4- to 6-week postoperative office visit, but this may not be sufficient follow-up for individuals who are at risk for depression or other severe psychiatric sequelae.

A planned surgery may sometimes prompt the gynecologist to refer a new patient for assistance with a preoperative preparation, but unfortunately it is more common for the psychiatrist to be consulted when problems arise postoperatively. Prevention and attempts to alleviate the psychiatric risks are always preferable to consultation after a problem becomes severe (Schwab 1971).

The psychiatrist or psychologist with an ongoing relationship with a patient may need to ensure that preoperative preparation for any planned gynecologic procedure is adequate. The therapist will want first to gain an appreciation of the patient's understanding and expectations, and then to explore the underlying meaning to the individual woman. The patient may have misconceptions about the procedure that need to be dispelled. Ideally, the gynecologist will have given the patient accurate information about the nature of the diagnosis and the recommended treatment; the psychiatrist may, however, need to address basic issues of anatomy, physiology, pathology, and therapy, or to speak with the gynecologist if it appears that the patient has significant misunderstandings. Although assumptions about the patient's underlying concerns may prove to be false, common concerns such as loss of sexual function, reproductive capability, or femininity may be suggested and explored as an initial effort to understand the issues for the individual woman.

Psychiatric problems after a gynecologic procedure should be evaluated in a manner similar to that for problems presenting after other life events (Dennerstein and van Hall 1986). Depression should be evaluated and appropriate treatment initiated with psychotherapy, antidepressants, or other medications, if indicated. The potential for suicide should be assessed. Supportive therapy is often most useful in conjunction with the use of antidepressants. The issue of hysterectomy or other surgery as a precipitating factor and its significance to the patient should then be more fully explored during the course of treatment (Dennerstein and van Hall 1986).

REFERENCES

Amias AG: Sexual life after gynecological operations, I. BMJ 2:608–609, 1975

Ananth J: Hysterectomy and depression. Obstet Gynecol 52:724–730, 1978

Bachmann GA: Hysterectomy: a critical review. J Reprod Med 35:839–862, 1990a

Bachmann GA: Psychosexual aspects of hysterectomy. Women's Health Issues 1:41–49, 1990b

Barker MG: Psychiatric illness after hysterectomy. BMJ 2:91–95, 1968

Barrett-Connor E, Bash TL: Estrogen and coronary heart disease in women. JAMA 265:1861–1867, 1991

Becker TM, Stone KM, Alexander ER: Genital human papillomavirus infection: a growing concern. Obstet Gynecol Clin North Am 14:389–396, 1987

Bell TA: Chlamydia trachomatis infections in adolescents. Med Clin North Am 74:1225–1233, 1990

Bell T, Hein K: Adolescents and sexually transmitted diseases, in Sexually Transmitted Diseases, 1st Edition. Edited by Holmes K, Mardh PA, Sparling P, et al. New York, McGraw-Hill, 1984, pp 73–84

Berek JS, Hacker NF: Practical Gynecologic Oncology. Baltimore, MD, Williams & Wilkins, 1989

Biro FM, Hillard PA: Genital human papillomavirus infection in adolescents. Med Clin North Am 74:1235–1249, 1990

Biro FM, Rosenthal SL, Wildey LS, et al: Self-reported health concerns and sexual behaviors in adolescents with cervical dysplasia. J Adolesc Health 12:391–394, 1991

Burchell R: Decision regarding hysterectomy. Am J Obstet Gynecol 127:113–117, 1977

Burke L, Apfel RJ, Fisher S, et al: Observations on the psychological impact of diethylstilbestrol exposure and suggestions on management. J Reprod Med 24:99–102, 1980

Centers for Disease Control: Progress toward achieving the 1990 objectives for the nation for sexually transmitted diseases. MMWR 39(4):53–57, 1990

Coppen A, Bishop M, Beard RJ, et al: Hysterectomy, hormones and behaviour: a prospective study. Lancet 1:126–128, 1981

Cutler WB: Hysterectomy: Before and After. New York, Harper & Row, 1988

Darrow WW, Pauli ML: Health behavior in sexually transmitted diseases, in Sexually Transmitted Diseases, 1st Edition. Edited by Holmes K, Mardh PA, Sparling P, et al. New York, McGraw-Hill, 1984, pp 65–73

Dennerstein L, van Hall E: Psychosomatic Gynecology: A Total Approach to Women's Health Problems. Park Ridge, NJ, Parthenon, 1986

Dennerstein L, Wood C, Burrows GD: Sexual response following hysterectomy and oophorectomy. Obstet Gynecol 49:92–96, 1977

Drellich MG, Bieber I, Sutherland AM: The psychological impact of cancer and cancer surgery, VI: adaptation to hysterectomy. Cancer 9:1120–1126, 1956

Droegemueller W, Herbst AL, Mishell DR, et al (eds): Comprehensive Gynecology. St. Louis, MO, CV Mosby, 1987

Easterday CL, Grimes DA, Riggs JA: Hysterectomy in the United States. Obstet Gynecol 62:203–212, 1983

Garcia CR, Cutler WB: Preservation of the ovary: a reevaluation. Fertil Steril 42:510–514, 1984

Grimes DA: Diagnostic dilation and curettage: a reappraisal. Am J Obstet Gynecol 142:1–6, 1982

Hampton PT, Tarnasky WG: Hysterectomy and tubal ligation: a comparison of the psychological aftermath. Am J Obstet Gynecol 119:949–952, 1974

Hatcher RA, Guest F, Stewart F, et al: Contraceptive Technology: 1990–91. New York, Irvington, 1990

Herbst AL, Holt LH: Clinical aspects of in utero DES exposure, in Obstetrics and Gynecology, Vol 4. Edited by Sciarra JJ. Philadelphia, PA, Lippincott, 1990, pp 1–13

Herbst AL, Ulfelder H, Poskanzer DC: Adenocarcinoma of the vagina: association of maternal stilbestrol therapy with tumor appearance in young women. N Engl J Med 284:878–881, 1971

Herbst AL, Hubby MM, Aziz F, et al: Reproductive and gynecologic surgical experience in diethylstilbestrol-exposed daughters. Am J Obstet Gynecol 141:1019–1028, 1981

Hillard JR, Hillard PA, Kitchell C, et al: Natural history of psychological reaction to genital herpes: a prospective study of woman university students. Journal of Psychosomatic Obstetrics and Gynaecology 10:147–156, 1989

Hillard PJA, Biro FM, Wildey LS, et al: Cervical dysplasia and human papillomavirus: evaluation in an adolescent dysplasia clinic. Adolescent and Pediatric Gynecology 2:32–36, 1989a

Hillard PJA, Biro FM, Wildey LS, et al: The value of an adolescent dysplasia clinic. Adolescent and Pediatric Gynecology 2:43–46, 1989b

Hollender MH: A study of patients admitted to a psychiatric hospital after pelvic operations. Am J Obstet Gynecol 79:498–503, 1960

Huggins GR, Sondheimer SJ: Complications of female sterilization. Fertil Steril 41:337–355, 1984

Ikkos G, Fitzpatrick R, Frost D, et al: Psychological disturbance and illness behaviour in a clinic for sexually transmitted diseases. Br J Med Psychol 60:121–126, 1987

Judson FN: Assessing the number of genital chlamydial infections in the United States. J Reprod Med 30:269–272, 1985

Kaltreider NB, Wallace A, Horowitz MJ: A field study of the stress response syndrome: young women after hysterectomy. JAMA 242:1499–1508, 1979

Kikku P, Gronroos M, Hirvonen T, et al: Supravaginal uterine amputation vs hysterectomy: effects on libido and orgasm. Acta Obstet Gynecol Scand 62:147–152, 1983

Knapp RC, Berkowitz RS: Gynecologic Oncology. New York, Macmillan, 1986

Kraft-Ebing RV: Lehrbuch der Psychiatrie. Enke, 1890

Krebs HB: Management strategies. Clin Obstet Gynecol 32:200–213, 1982

Lalinec-Michaud M, Engelsmann G: Anxiety, fears and depression related to hysterectomy. Can J Psychiatry 30:44–47, 1985

Luby E, Gillespie D: The Helper: A Quarterly Publication of the Herpes Resource Center, Vol 3. Palo Alto, CA, American Social Health Association, 1981, pp 3–4

Luby ED, Klinge V: Genital herpes: a pervasive psychosocial disorder. Arch Dermatol 121:494–497, 1985

Martin RL, Roberts WV, Cayton PJ: Psychiatric status after hysterectomy: a one year follow-up. JAMA 244:350–362, 1980

Masters WH, Johnson V: Human Sexual Response. Boston, MA, Little, Brown, 1966

Mattingly RF (ed): Te Linde's Operative Gynecology, 5th Edition. Philadelphia, PA, Lippincott, 1977

Moore JT, Tolley DH: Depression following hysterectomy. Psychosomatics 1777:86–89, 1976

Mosher WD: Contraceptive practice in the United States, 1982–1988. Fam Plann Perspect 22:198–205, 1990

Newton N, Baron E: Reactions to hysterectomy: fact or fiction? Prim Care 3:781–800, 1976

Orr DP, Wilbrandt ML, Brack CJ, et al: Reported sexual behaviors and self-esteem among young adolescents. Am J Dis Child 143:86–90, 1989

Patterson RM, Craig JB: Misconceptions concerning the psychological effects of hysterectomy. Am J Obstet Gynecol 85:104–111, 1963

Polivy J: Psychological reactions to hysterectomy: a critical review. Am J Obstet Gynecol 118:417–426, 1974

Polivy J, Roeske NCA: Quality of life and factors affecting the response to hysterectomy. J Fam Pract 3:483–488, 1978

Ridgeway V, Mathews A: Psychological preparation for surgery: a comparison of methods. Br J Clin Psychol 21:271–280, 1982

Rockwell DA, Pepitone-Rockwell F: The emotional impact of surgery and the value of informed consent. Med Clin North Am 63:1341–1351, 1979

Rogers FS: Emotional factors in gynecology. Am J Obstet Gynecol 59:321–327, 1950

Ryan MM, Dennerstein L, Pepperell R: Psychological aspects of hysterectomy. Br J Psychiatry 154:516–522, 1989

Salter JR: Gynecological symptoms and psychological distress in potential hysterectomy patients. J Psychosom Res 29:155–159, 1985

Schwab JJ: The psychiatric consultation: problems with referral. Diseases of the Nervous System 32:447–452, 1971

Sloan D: The emotional and psychosexual aspects of hysterectomy. Am J Obstet Gynecol 1312:598–605, 1978

Speroff T, Dawson NV, Speroff L, et al: A risk-benefit analysis of elective bilateral oophorectomy: effect of changes in compliance with estrogen therapy on outcome. Am J Obstet Gynecol 164:165–174, 1991

Stellman RD: Psychological aspects of gynecologic surgery, in Gynecology and Obstetrics, Vol 6. Edited by Sciarra JJ. Philadelphia, PA, Lippincott, 1990, pp 1–6

Tang GWK: Reactions to emergency hysterectomy. Obstet Gynecol 65:206–210, 1985

Terz JJ, Barber HRK, Brunschwig A: Incidence of carcinoma in the retained ovary. Am J Surg 113:511–515, 1967

Townsend DE, Richart RM: Cryotherapy and carbon dioxide laser management of cervical intraepithelial neoplasia: a controlled comparison. Obstet Gynecol 61:75–78, 1983

Underwood PB: Ovarian conservatism. South Med J 69:405–408, 1976

Walton LA: The stress of radical pelvic surgery: a review. Gynecol Oncol 7:25–35, 1979

Wolf SR: Emotional reaction to hysterectomy. Postgrad Med 47:165–170, 1970

Youngs DD, Wise TN: Psychological sequelae of elective gynecologic surgery, in Psychosomatic Obstetrics and Gynecology. Edited by Youngs DD, Ehrhardt AA. New York, Appleton-Century-Crofts, 1980, pp 255–264

Zussman L, Zussman S, Sunley R, et al: Sexual response after hysterectomy-oophorectomy: recent studies and reconsideration of psychogenesis. Am J Obstet Gynecol 140:725–729, 1981

Chapter 15

Gynecologic Oncology

Cheryl F. McCartney, M.D.

❖ ❖ ❖ ❖ ❖ ❖ ❖ ❖ ❖ ❖ ❖ ❖ ❖

Gynecologic malignancy changes a woman's life permanently. Whether she survives or eventually dies of her disease, cancer becomes part of her identity. For her remaining life, she must face the possibility of premature death. She may need to cope with disfigurement and/or dysfunction. Her relationships with her partner, family, friends, and co-workers are at risk. The crisis of cancer strengthens some of these bonds, but weakens others.

Experiencing the stresses of cancer can make a woman appreciate her life more fully, but it also may provoke psychiatric disorders that diminish her life quality. Women with a history of maladaptive coping strategies, previous severe psychiatric disorders, or low levels of social support are at high risk for the development of disabling psychiatric disorders. Vulnerability to depression is greatest in women whose cancers are far advanced at diagnosis, progress to a point of poor prognosis, or require severely disfiguring treatments (such as exenteration or vulvectomy).

One of the most important safeguards against distress for women cancer patients is a physician-patient relationship characterized by empathy, open communication, and mutual respect. This relationship with her doctors, which is amplified by the oncology staff, continues to be important even after treatment is complete. She wants to

I appreciate the helpful contributions of Sarah S. Auchincloss, M.D., Adjunct Attending Psychiatrist, Memorial Sloan Kettering Cancer Center, Assistant Attending Psychiatrist, New York Hospital.

trust that she can always count on their expertise and concern if cancer returns.

Thus, the psychiatrist's role in cancer care goes beyond consultation with individual referred patients and their families. The psychiatrist strengthens the physician-patient relationship by conveying the patient's needs, priorities, and values to the oncologist while, in a reciprocal fashion, discussing the implications of the oncologist's message with the patient. As part of the oncology team, the psychiatrist supports the development of procedures to prevent patients' emotional distress and teaches caregivers to recognize patients' psychiatric disorders. Because the care of cancer patients can be stressful and draining for caregivers, the psychiatrist also offers support to the oncology staff while teaching them to recognize and prevent burnout in themselves. The psychiatrist helps to reorient the goal of cancer care from cure, which may be impossible for all patients, to peaceful resolution of the cancer crisis. Success in reaching this goal results in lasting satisfaction for the family and oncology staff.

EMOTIONAL RESPONSE TO CANCER

Universal Issues Across the Time Course of Illness

The cancer experience unfolds during a series of nodal points in the illness. A patient perceives an abnormality, seeks medical evaluation, learns of her diagnosis, and agrees to a plan for treatment. This treatment may include surgery, radiation therapy, and/or chemotherapy. After the active phase of the prescribed treatment, which can continue for several months, she is medically monitored. If the cancer persists, or recurs after a disease-free interval, further therapy is offered, with the revised goal of prolonging survival, rather than cure. Eventually, such a patient succumbs to the cancer. She must cope with physical deterioration and with her approaching death. Fortunately, however, treatment succeeds for many patients. Although a survivor repeatedly receives good news at her checkups, she contends with ongoing concerns about the return of her disease.

Before diagnosis. Fear of cancer may lead women to refuse screening tests, deny signs of illness, and delay seeking a diagnosis (Hackett et al. 1973). Alternatively, women anticipating gynecologic surgery for benign conditions worry that their "real" problem is cancer (Steptoe et al. 1986).

At diagnosis. Modern oncologists believe in disclosing the truth to patients about the discovery of cancer, its prognosis, and planned treatment (Cassileth and Steinfeld 1987). Commonly, the patient's initial response is a typical stress response syndrome, which lasts about 1 week. With feelings of fear and helplessness, she alternates between obsessive thoughts about the cancer and denial of its existence. She may feel numb, experience difficulty concentrating and sleeping, and express irritability or anger. In addition to the anxiety and fatigue seen in women newly diagnosed with benign gynecologic conditions, cancer patients also experience depressed mood and confusion (Andersen et al. 1989b; Cain et al. 1983). These symptoms are particularly troublesome, because they impair the patient's ability to process the complex information being conveyed to her about her illness at the time that she needs to make important decisions about treatment. Once active treatment begins, the patient focuses narrowly on "getting through" it. Moderate anxiety can be adaptive at this stage. It heightens the patient's awareness of caregivers' instructions and her vigilance for abnormal symptoms that could signal harmful treatment side effects or progression of disease (Andersen and Tewfik 1985). (Psychological issues for dying patients and survivors are described in subsequent sections of this chapter.)

Individual Modifiers of Patients' Emotional Response

The most important influence on a patient's psychological adjustment to her cancer is the seriousness of the illness and the magnitude of the treatment. The psychiatric consultant should seek education from the referring gynecologic oncologist about the prognosis of the patient's cancer and about the details of the treatment that is proposed or in progress. It is important to know about expected alterations in her body (such as alopecia, shortening of the vagina, diversion of the bowel into a colostomy, excision of the clitoris) and consequences for function (such as diarrhea, fatigue, vaginal bleeding, pain, diminished sexual responsiveness). Psychiatric disorders are more common and more severe with greater disfigurement and dysfunction.

Cancer's challenge to normal adult development varies with a woman's age and stage in the life cycle. Hospitalization and debilitating treatments restrict the adolescent's normal striving for independence from parents. Loss of fertility and changed sexual function interfere with a young adult's confidence in searching for a mate. Disability may disrupt her efforts to launch a career. A woman in midlife has already begun to recognize that her lifetime will be finite. Her grown children may provide support, but divorce or death may have removed her mate. Work is an alternative source of self-esteem when her body image is diminished. Older women have already begun to anticipate death but are less adaptable to changes in surroundings and bodily functions.

As in any other crisis, individual personality characteristics affect the cancer patient's ability to cope with stress. Kobasa and Puccetti (1983) introduced the concept of hardiness, an attitude that a person has influence over what occurs in life, a sense of commitment to self, and a sense of challenge in the face of a changing environment. Hardiness serves a stress-buffering role in cancer, resulting in fewer physical symptoms and less psychological distress (Ostroff et al. 1990). In contrast, maladaptive coping strategies can lead to heightened anxiety, pain, and a sense of being overwhelmed.

Social support from a woman's mate, family, friends, co-workers, community members, religious affiliates, and caregivers enhances her physical recovery, psychological well-being, and social functioning (Bloom 1986). Her husband's and children's ability to support her may be compromised if they are unsuccessfully struggling with worries about her illness or with their changed roles at home necessitated by her absence (Lichtman and Taylor 1986). In addition, Cassileth et al. (1985) found that the responses of spouses and close family members to illness closely parallel those of the patient. Thus, psychological intervention with the family has dual benefits: it restores their emotional comfort and improves their ability to support the patient.

Other patients are another valuable source of education and emotional support. Both individually and in support groups, these women reassure, counsel, and offer practical suggestions. Outcome studies show that support groups improve cancer patients' coping skills, mood, and vigor while decreasing their anxiety, fatigue, and confusion (Cain et al. 1986; Fawzy et al. 1990a; Spiegel 1990).

Gynecologic cancer ends a woman's fertility and compromises her sexuality. If she desires more children or believes that the ability to conceive affects her sexual attractiveness, her sense of loss will be profound. The occasional woman who is pregnant when cancer is discovered may have to endure the loss of her fetus as well as her potential future fertility during curative therapy for cancer. Previous success in maintaining a stable sexual relationship, whether heterosexual or homosexual, may help to facilitate a woman's adjustment to the alterations in sexual function that will occur. Previous sexual dysfunction may heighten her vulnerability to posttreatment sexual impairment. The pain of past sexual traumas, such as incest or rape, may be revived during gynecologic cancer treatment. Sources of self-esteem, such as career, can buffer the injury to self-worth due to loss of fertility and changes in sexuality.

PSYCHIATRIC DISORDERS IN GYNECOLOGIC CANCER PATIENTS

About half of all cancer patients have psychiatric disorders (Derogatis et al. 1983). The majority are adjustment disorders that are easily and quickly treatable with crisis intervention psychotherapy, behavioral techniques, and/or small doses of psychotropic medication. Without treatment, these disorders can have consequences beyond emotional distress. Mood problems can cause delayed reporting of symptoms, refusal of treatment, deterioration of important relationships, and delayed return to pre-illness role because of loss of motivation for self-care and pessimistic outlook. Depression and anxiety increase the perception of pain. In severe depression or delirium, suicide is a risk. Mental disorders can diminish a patient's ability to care for herself and to follow instructions.

Insufficient detection of these psychiatric problems is the biggest barrier to effective treatment (Derogatis et al. 1976; McKegney and Beckhardt 1982). Psychiatric liaison programs improve oncologists' identification of disorders, increase their requests for psychiatric consultations, and improve the collaborative working relationship between the cancer care team and the psychiatrist (McCartney et al. 1989).

Anxiety and panic symptoms often occur at turning points of illness: diagnosis, recurrence, treatment failure, and even at termination of successful curative treatment when patients fear the loss of close monitoring by medical staff. Gynecologic cancer treatment may evoke memories, and the associated anxiety, of past traumatic events. Anxiety may also occur in response to some usual diagnostic and treatment interventions, such as needle phobias arising during intravenous chemotherapy or claustrophobia during magnetic resonance imaging. Fear of chemotherapy itself, and of the nausea and vomiting that is chemically induced by it, can evoke anxiety. This anxiety can then intensify the posttreatment nausea and vomiting (Andrykowski 1990). Patients may become conditioned to hospital-associated stimuli (such as disinfectant odor), which then trigger both anticipatory nausea and anxiety. There is promise that this conditioning cycle may be diminished with a new antiemetic, ondansetron hydrochloride (Zofran injection). Clinical experience suggests that it offers improved primary prevention of nausea symptoms (Gelb 1991).

The differential diagnosis of all psychological symptoms in the cancer population should include a search for organic causes. Organic anxiety disorder can result from poorly controlled pain, hypoxia, pulmonary embolism, sepsis, delirium, hypoglycemia, bleeding, or heart failure. Akathisia, a side effect of neuroleptic drugs used as antiemetics, can be mistaken for anxiety. Corticosteroids can cause anxiety. Withdrawal from alcohol, drugs of abuse, or therapeutic drugs to which the patient is tolerant also causes anxiety symptoms.

After attention to any organic causes, treatment includes psychotherapy, behavioral techniques, and short-acting benzodiazepines (Massie 1989). Similar measures effectively decrease anticipatory nausea associated with chemotherapy.

Prevalence studies in hospitalized gynecologic cancer patients indicate that about 20%–25% have major depressive disorders (Cain et al. 1983; Evans et al. 1986). Women with the highest risk for depression are those with a history of mood disorder, those with advanced stages of cancer, and those with poorly controlled pain (Bukberg et al. 1984; Cain et al. 1983; Massie and Holland 1990). Psychological symptoms of guilt, helplessness, hopelessness, worthlessness, loss of interest, and inability to experience pleasure are more useful criteria than are the physical symptoms of anorexia, sleep disturbance, fatigue, decreased sexual desire, and inability to concentrate (Massie and Holland 1990), because the physical symptoms may also be due to cancer itself.

Organic causes of depression include disturbances in metabolic, nutritional, endocrinologic, and neurologic function. Cancer patients whose depression is due to fever or anemia will experience rapid relief when these conditions are corrected. Drugs that are often used in this population and that can cause organic depressive disorder are methyldopa, reserpine, propranolol, barbiturates, diazepam, and amphotericin B. The steroids prednisone and dexamethasone can cause severe mood changes ranging from mania to suicidal depression. Chemotherapeutic agents that are used in gynecologic oncology and that may have depressive side effects are vincristine, vinblastine, procarbazine, interferon (Massie and Holland 1990), hexamethylmelamine (now known as altretamine) (Silberfarb 1983), and ifosfamide (Zalupski and Baker 1988) (Table 15–1). Although some of these drugs can be discontinued if depressive side effects occur, psychiatrists must often help patients to tolerate the unpleasant effects of chemotherapeutic agents because of their potential life-preserving effects.

Treatment of depression includes crisis intervention psychotherapy to look at the meaning of cancer within the context of the patient's life and to help her activate effective coping mechanisms (S. Greer 1989; Massie and Holland 1990). Antidepressants are also very effective, but at lower doses than in a medically healthy population. An advantage of using tricyclic antidepressants is the availability of assays for drug blood levels for careful monitoring of this vulnerable group of patients. Low initial doses (e.g., 10–25 mg of imipramine or doxepin at bedtime) are appropriate, with increases as tolerated every few days. A beneficial effect of antidepressants is potentiation of pain medications. Although some patients may decline to continue the antidepressant because of intolerance to side effects, others may actually benefit from the sedation or the decreased bowel motility. For patients whose depression is complicated by anxiety, alprazolam may alleviate both symptoms. Withdrawn patients with advanced disease may benefit from psychostimulants (e.g., dextroamphetamine or methylphenidate, starting at a dose of 2.5 mg at 8 A.M. and noon, increasing if needed to a maximum daily dose of 30 mg). These drugs promote a sense of well-being, stimulate appetite, and counteract the sedative side effects of narcotics while potentiating their pain relief effects.

Table 15–1. Anticancer drugs that may cause psychiatric side effects

Drug name	Delirium	Depression
Bleomycin		
Carboplatin		
Cisplatin	+	
Cyclophosphamide (Cytoxan)	+	
Dacarbazine (DTIC-Dome)	+	
Dactinomycin (actinomycin D)		
Doxorubicin (Adriamycin)		
Etoposide (VP-16)		
5-Fluorouracil	+	
Hexamethylmelamine (altretamine)	+	+
Ifosfamide	+	+
Interferon	+	+
Melphalan (Alkeran)		
Methotrexate	+	
Mitomycin-C		
Mitoxantrone hydrochloride		
Procarbazine	+	+
Taxol		
Vinblastine	+	+
Vincristine	+	+
Corticosteroids		+/Mania

Electroconvulsive therapy may be the treatment of choice for an elderly woman with multiple medical problems or for a psychotically depressed, intensely suicidal patient.

Organic mental disorders are common in cancer patients but are often overlooked by oncology staff until symptoms are severe. About 15%–20% of hospitalized cancer patients have some degree of cognitive dysfunction (Patchell and Posner 1989), and by the terminal phase of illness, about 85% have delirium (Massie et al. 1983). Drugs and medical complications of cancer are common etiologic agents for the delirium. The chemotherapeutic agents listed as possible causes of organic affective disorders can also cause delirium. Additional causal agents are methotrexate, cisplatin, cyclophosphamide (Patchell and Posner 1989), dacarbazine (Silberfarb 1983), and 5-fluorouracil (Moore et al. 1990). Central nervous system toxicity has been reported with the use of imipenem (Calandra et al. 1985), metronidazole (Snavely and Hodges 1984), and ciprofloxacin (Halkin 1988).

Dementia (and mental retardation) may be irreversible states that impair a patient's ability to make treatment decisions, to follow complex medical instructions, and to care for herself. With documentation of these disorders, patients may qualify for disability benefits to pay for supplemental caretakers and other assistance.

Substance use disorders are often intensified by the stress of cancer. Intoxication and withdrawal from alcohol and drugs of abuse can complicate treatment for the cancer patient. Partners who are impaired by substance abuse problems have trouble helping the patient when she needs it most.

PAIN

Prevalence

A common obstacle to satisfactory quality of life throughout the course of cancer is pain. About one-third of patients in active treatment and two-thirds of those with advanced cancer have pain that is severe enough to require treatment with opioid drugs. Although appropriate use of pharmacologic approaches to pain relief could probably control 70% of cancer pain (Portenoy 1988), evaluations of practice have unfortunately shown that management strategies are often inadequate (Dorrepaal et al. 1989).

Consequences

Beyond the discomfort inherent in the pain itself, pain restricts productive work and pleasurable social activities. It interrupts sleep. Spiegel and Sands (1991) suggest that pain may play a causal role in producing depression. Especially in the terminally ill, intense pain may lead to thoughts of and plans for suicide.

Treatment of Cancer Pain

After comprehensive assessment of the pain complaint, a management plan is developed. (A thorough description of evaluation and therapy can be found in Portenoy 1988.) Often, primary therapy of the tumor with chemotherapy and/or radiotherapy effectively reduces pain. Pharmacologic management should follow an "analgesic ladder," beginning with nonsteroidal antiinflammatory drugs such as aspirin or ibuprofen for mild pain. Adjuvant analgesics, such as antidepressants, can be added for their potentiation effect. For moderate pain, weak oral opioids, such as codeine, can be added to the nonsteroidal antiinflammatory drug and the adjuvant analgesic. Patients with severe pain need potent opioids, such as morphine, which can be potentiated with nonsteroidal anti-inflammatory drugs and/or adjuvant analgesics.

Ongoing monitoring of pain status is important during both the development and the maintenance of the management strategy. Switching nonsteroidal anti-inflammatory drugs may be necessary to find the one to which the patient responds best. Titrating the opioid to a favorable level (or to the level of intolerable side effects) can be accomplished by around-the-clock dosing (usually every 4 hours), with rescue doses as needed 2 hours after the regular dose. When the appropriate dose is found, fixed dosing is best. The patient is thus spared the "breakthrough" pain and the anxious wait for the next requested dose.

There is no evidence that the use of opioid analgesics for cancer pain in otherwise normal patients leads to the development of addictive behaviors. Patients can often remain comfortable on stable doses of opioids for a long time. If increased doses are needed after a period of adequate pain relief, evaluation for progression of disease or increased psychological distress is indicated. If pharmacologic management is not completely effective, other interventions can be added. Anesthetic injections, physical therapy, stimulation of afferent neural structures, and neurosurgical ablation procedures may have a role in specific cases.

PSYCHIATRIST'S ROLE WITH THE DYING PATIENT

When a patient's tumor progresses despite the curative and palliative treatments offered, the oncologist knows that the patient will die of her disease. Gentle but candid disclosure to the patient about the change in her status from "active treatment" to "terminally ill" allows her to participate maximally in planning her remaining lifetime according to her individual needs and personal values. The liaison psychiatrist can be a helpful resource for the oncologist during this emotionally stressful phase of the illness.

The following issues are important:

❖ Patients wait for the doctor to initiate a discussion about the implication of tumor growth despite cancer therapy.
❖ They want assurance that all indicated therapeutic measures were attempted so that the death can be seen as legitimate and unavoidable (Osterweis et al. 1984).
❖ Although patients want a central role in decision making about further care, they appreciate the physician's articulation of a personal recommendation (Wanzer et al. 1984).
❖ Patients want assurance that the oncology team will not abandon them during the dying process. They hope for amelioration of feared symptoms: pain, shortness of breath, and nausea and vomiting.
❖ Families appreciate a follow-up contact with the oncology team

during bereavement. They may want to ask questions about the patient's medical course or to express feelings about the relationship with the treatment team. Some may be experiencing pathological grief and may need referral for mental health treatment.

Wanzer et al. (1984) advise a decrease in aggressive treatment of the hopelessly ill patient when such treatment would only prolong a difficult and uncomfortable process of dying. They suggest that terminally ill patients decide among four possible levels of care. The choice simplifies subsequent management decisions because they are confined by the level selected: 1) emergency resuscitation, 2) intensive care and advanced life support, 3) general medical care including antibiotics, drugs, surgery, chemotherapy, artificial hydration, and nutrition, and 4) general nursing care and comfort measures.

The "do not resuscitate" decision is often deferred because patients and families have magical beliefs about what emergency resuscitation can achieve, despite a woman's terminal condition. Havlir et al. (1989) described the advantages of discussing code status in patients' homes. Patients were well enough to participate actively, family members benefited by hearing the patients' thoughts and wishes, and house staff were relieved of the responsibility of conducting such a difficult conversation with an acutely ill patient with whom they were only newly acquainted (Havlir et al. 1989). The decision not to resuscitate paves the way for the patient to prepare a legally binding living will, which expresses her desires even if she later becomes incompetent to speak for herself.

The National Hospice Study comparing conventional with hospice care showed at least comparable outcomes on measures of function and quality of life (Greer et al. 1986; Wallston et al. 1988). This program offers comprehensive palliative and supportive care to dying patients in their home settings. A multidisciplinary team assists and trains family members. The emphasis is on symptom control and psychosocial counseling.

Personal growth, new insights, and efforts to resolve troubled relationships often accompany the losses of the dying process. The woman wants to review her life, express appreciation to loved ones and caregivers, and say her goodbyes. Oncology staff can help dying patients to plan realistically for activities that will provide pleasure and peace in their limited life spans. Consideration can be given to decisions about legacies and funeral arrangements. The dying mother of young children must plan for their ongoing care after her death, as well as prepare them to accept their terrible loss. To leave them a message about her love and her values, she may want to provide letters, audiotapes, videotapes, and/or photo albums.

In a study of psychiatric consults from a gynecologic oncology service, McCartney et al. (1989) found that two-thirds of all consults are requested within 6 months of patients' deaths. Psychiatric disorders are most frequent and most severe in terminal illness, as noted above. Furthermore, oncologists recognize that the focus of treatment must shift to emotional concerns and comfort measures when surgery, radiotherapy, and chemotherapy are no longer indicated. Along with providing crisis intervention psychotherapy, behavioral techniques, and psychotropic drugs that may be indicated for the patient, the psychiatrist often needs to expand the focus of the consult to include interventions with the family, liaison between the patient and oncology caregivers, and, at times, attention to the stress of the caregiving team in response to their work with cancer patients.

It is appropriate for a psychiatrist to evaluate all patients who express suicidal ideas. Such thoughts occur not only in patients who are clinically depressed, but also in patients who have significant pain, progressive disease with irreversible disability, and/or delirium. With effective management of these problems, patients' desires for suicide or euthanasia have been found to diminish (Breitbart 1989; Coyle et al. 1990). Coyle et al. (1990) do acknowledge that suicidal thoughts are likely to persist in a subset of terminally ill patients who suffer from severe symptoms that are extremely difficult to control.

There is ongoing debate among oncology professionals about the role of physicians in assisting patients to commit suicide. Orentlicher (1989) argues that nothing should compromise the image of the physician as helper and healer. He expresses concern that if a physician indicates sympathy to the patient's suicidal thoughts, this attitude will undermine the patient's confidence in the physician's commitment to any level of care (Orentlicher 1989). Alternatively, Quill (1991) recently reported an interaction with his own terminally ill patient, for

whom he prescribed barbiturates. He educated her about their use to
induce sleep, and "made sure that she knew the amount needed to
commit suicide" (p. 693). He believed that he knew her well, that she
had made a rational decision, and that she was facing severe suffering
(Quill 1991). In any case, a physician's willingness to listen, to hear
out the meaning of the losses associated with the patient's cancer, her
worst fears, and most desperate plans, without expressing any value
judgment, is often very comforting to the patient.

PSYCHOLOGICAL ISSUES FOR CANCER SURVIVORS

The completion of treatment with favorable results is another cancer
milestone. The patient's new status of "survivor" is accompanied by
worries and adjustments as well as by relief (Welch-McCaffrey et al.
1989). The patient is constantly vigilant for any physical signs of recurrence, especially at times of follow-up examinations. Most patients'
fears of recurrence and death diminish gradually during the disease-
free years after treatment. Often, her confrontation with death leads a
woman to a psychosocial reorientation in which she appreciates her
remaining life more profoundly.

The relationship with the oncology team is intense during active
treatment. A patient feels reassured by the regular interactions with
staff and the frequent feedback about her condition. She needs to be
prepared for the insecurity she may feel when this continual monitoring ends and should be offered opportunities to call with questions
between scheduled follow-up visits that may be months to a year in the
future.

The survivor must also cope with any physical compromise that
she had agreed would be an acceptable cost of treatment. Her adjustment to this new body image, an element of her self-esteem, may
challenge her emotional resources. She may face anatomic modifications ranging from a large surgical scar to a colostomy or vulvectomy.
Functional alterations, such as short bowel syndrome, infertility, and
sexual dysfunction, are often a consequence of treatment. Even if
these changes would not interfere with her ability to work after recovery, myths and misconceptions about cancer held by employers may

result in employment and insurance problems, such as dismissal, demotion, reduction of work-related benefits, and denial of application for health insurance coverage at a new job.

A survivor also experiences changes in social support. Her marriage may become stronger or may be disrupted due to the stress of the cancer crisis. Cella (1987) describes a sorting-out process with friends, during which the survivor becomes closer with some, pulls away from others, and loses some relationships because the well person withdraws due to discomfort about cancer, fear of contagion, or a wish to reassure herself that she is not vulnerable. A single woman survivor often has a special problem with social isolation. Fearing rejection by a new love object because of her cancer, she guards herself against possible new involvements. A useful reference for caregivers and cancer survivors is the recent publication by Mullan and Hoffman (1990).

SEXUALITY

Sexuality, an important quality-of-life issue in gynecologic cancer, is often overlooked because caregivers neglect to ask about sexual function. Oncologists may forget to ask about sex because they must focus on the complexities of treatment and on thorough follow-up searches for recurrence. Other caregivers may be uncomfortable discussing sex or may assume that older or partnerless women would not want to talk about it. Patients are interested, but hesitate to initiate a conversation about sex, deferring to caregivers to raise the issue (Auchincloss 1989).

The extent of sexual disruption increases proportionally with the severity of disease and the magnitude of treatment. For example, about 30%–40% of early cervical and endometrial cancer patients have sexual problems. Sexual activity is completely stopped by 80%–90% of patients who undergo radical vulvectomy or pelvic exenteration for central recurrence of cervical cancer (Andersen 1987; Andersen et al. 1989a). Although cancer-related sexual dysfunction does not necessarily damage marital happiness or stability, these problems are an ongoing cost to the quality of life that challenges the coping strategies of patients and partners. Sexual problems often arise as a concern of patients during the first year after treatment ends and may persist for subsequent years, exacting a significant toll on the relationship until they are identified and addressed.

Evaluation of sexual problems in cancer patients should include an assessment of the somatic, psychological, and interpersonal aspects of sexual function. Somatic effects include the illness and treatment impact on the organs of intercourse and on the woman's overall health. Surgery to pelvic structures may result in a shortened or narrowed vagina. Pelvic irradiation obliterates venous plexuses and arteries surrounding the vagina, interfering with lubrication and elasticity. As fibrosis occurs, the pelvic organs may become fixed and the vagina less able to expand. The loss of ovarian function with surgery, radiation, or chemotherapy causes loss of estrogen, which results in vaginal dryness. Any treatment may thus be associated with dyspareunia or postcoital bleeding.

Other aspects of treatment may also cause impairment. Function is altered and self-esteem is affected by fecal and urinary diversion through ostomies. The external genitalia are excised in vulvectomy, causing blunted genital sensitivity and possible introital stenosis. In addition to the direct, local, physical impact of treatment, sexual desire is greatly reduced by general physical debilitation and the effects of therapeutic drugs or pain. The patient may be coping with the symptoms of treatment-related onset of menopause, which may affect sexual desire and response as well.

Sexual function is also affected by psychological stresses. Fear of recurrence can cause hypervigilance for physical signs that might signal cancer (such as bleeding or pain). The meaning given to the cancer by the woman may cause her to lose sexual desire. Loss of the uterus has been felt by some women to render them unfeminine and even less worthy as people. Guilt about past sexual activities (masturbation, premarital or extramarital sex, sexually transmitted disease, abortion) and trauma from past sexual abuse can be evoked by treatments to sexual body sites. Depression reduces sexual desire.

Interpersonal issues also contribute to sexual adjustment. The partner's attitude toward the role of sexuality in the relationship and his or her enduring support for rebuilding a sexual life are important determinants of outcome. Cultural expectations about fertility, body integrity, and women's "proper" interest in sex affect a patient's attitude about resuming sex after cancer.

The goals of therapy for cancer-related sexual dysfunctions must be guided by the patient's and partner's receptiveness to the intervention. To all patients, caregivers should convey the messages that everyone has a sex life, everyone can keep a partner sexually happy, problems with sex are not uncommon in connection with cancer treatment, and such problems are treatable. Rather than focus on performance, patients' attention should be redirected to gradual resumption of sexual expression in a relaxed, comfortable manner, with a focus on pleasure. Healing occurs most easily in a supportive, nondemanding atmosphere. Certainly, permission to be sexual, education about sexuality and its modifications secondary to cancer, and specific suggestions about technique are important interventions (Schover and Jensen 1988). Problems with vaginal dryness may be effectively treated with lubricants (e.g., Astroglide) and vaginal moisturizers (Replens), which are formulated especially for low-estrogen states.

Painful sex may indicate recurrence. Even if its cause is benign, such pain causes rapid and persistent loss of sexual desire. Thus, any pain during sex should be medically evaluated, the cause treated, and alternatives established to any practice that causes discomfort. The oncology professional should be aware that because the cancer treatment has been stressful, costly, and lengthy, patients may be willing to attend only a few sessions of psychological-behavior therapy. Still, this may offer lasting benefit. Excellent resources for mental health professionals about this type of evaluation and treatment are the references listed by Auchincloss (1989) and Schover and Jensen (1988). For patients, a booklet by Schover (1988), "Sexuality and Cancer: For the Woman Who Has Cancer, and Her Partner," is available through the American Cancer Society.

NEW DIRECTIONS IN PSYCHOONCOLOGY

Researchers are developing valid and reliable measures of the global concept of quality of life to enable them to assess the effects of cancer and its treatments on patients' overall sense of satisfaction, well-being, and contentment (Schipper 1990). Such measures will be helpful for pretreatment preparation of patients. Studies can be designed to compare the relative comfort and acceptability of treatments with equal survival value and to identify treatments that should be modified because of high quality-of-life costs (McCartney and Larson 1987).

The effect of psychosocial variables on clinical outcome is another exciting new topic (Cassileth et al. 1989; Fawzy et al. 1990b; Richardson et al. 1990; Spiegel et al. 1989). Reviewing existing studies, Stein et al. (1991) determined that "it is premature to consider any therapeutic effects of the treatment of depression on immunocompetence and disease" (p. 176). Thus, caregivers should correct any patient's erroneous and demoralizing conclusion that her cancer progressed because she could not sustain a positive attitude. They concluded that "Nonetheless, the value of psychosocial interventions on the quality of life and mental state of seriously ill persons should not be underestimated" (p. 176).

REFERENCES

Andersen BL: Sexual functioning complications in women with gynecologic cancer. Cancer 60:2123–2128, 1987

Andersen BL, Tewfik HH: Psychological reactions to radiation therapy: reconsideration of the adaptive aspects of anxiety. J Pers Soc Psychol 48:1024–1032, 1985

Andersen BL, Anderson B, deProsse C: Controlled prospective longitudinal study of women with cancer, I: sexual functioning outcomes. J Consult Clin Psychol 57:683–691, 1989a

Andersen BL, Anderson B, deProsse C: Controlled prospective longitudinal study of women with cancer, II: psychological outcomes. J Consult Clin Psychol 57:692–697, 1989b

Andrykowski MA: The role of anxiety in the development of anticipatory nausea in cancer chemotherapy: a review and synthesis. Psychosom Med 52(4):458–475, 1990

Auchincloss SS: Sexual dysfunction in cancer patients: issues in evaluation and treatment, in Handbook of Psychooncology. Edited by Holland JC, Rowland JH. New York, Oxford University Press, 1989, pp 383–413

Bloom JR: Social support and adjustment to breast cancer, in Women With Cancer. Edited by Andersen BL. New York, Springer-Verlag, 1986, pp 204–229

Breitbart W: Suicide, in Handbook of Psychooncology. Edited by Holland JC, Rowland JH. New York, Oxford University Press, 1989, pp 291–299

Bukberg J, Penman D, Holland JC: Depression in hospitalized cancer patients. Psychosom Med 46(3):199–212, 1984

Cain EN, Kohorn EI, Quinlan DM, et al: Psychosocial reactions to the diagnosis of gynecologic cancer. Obstet Gynecol 62:635–641, 1983

Cain EN, Kohorn EI, Quinlan DM, et al: Psychosocial benefits of a cancer support group. Cancer 57:183–189, 1986

Calandra GB, Brown KR, Glad LC, et al: Review of adverse experiences and tolerability in the first 2516 patients treated with imipenem/cilastatin. Supplement: Proceedings of a symposium (June 7, 1985). Carbapenems: a new class of antibiotics. Am J Med 78(6A):73–78, 1985

Cassileth BR, Steinfeld AD: Psychological preparation of the patient and family. Cancer 60:547–552, 1987

Cassileth BR, Lusk EJ, Strouse TB, et al: A psychological analysis of cancer patients and their next-of-kin. Cancer 55:72–76, 1985

Cassileth BR, Walsh WP, Lusk EJ: Psychosocial correlates of cancer survival: a subsequent report 3 to 8 years after cancer diagnosis. J Clin Oncol 4:541–542, 1989

Cella DF: Cancer survival: psychosocial and public issues. Cancer Invest 5(1):59–67, 1987

Coyle N, Adelhardt J, Foley KM, et al: Character of terminal illness in the advanced cancer patient: pain and other symptoms during the last four weeks of life. Journal of Pain and Symptom Management 5(2):83–93, 1990

Derogatis LR, Abeloff MD, McBeth CD: Cancer patients and their physicians in the perception of psychological symptoms. Psychosomatics 17:197–201, 1976

Derogatis LR, Morrow GR, Fetting J, et al: The prevalence of psychiatric disorders among cancer patients. JAMA 249(6):751–757, 1983

Dorrepaal KL, Aaronson NK, van Dam FS: Pain experience and pain management among hospitalized cancer patients: a clinical study. Cancer 63(3):593–598, 1989

Evans DL, McCartney CF, Nemeroff CB, et al: Depression in women treated for gynecological cancer: clinical and neuroendocrine assessment. Am J Psychiatry 143:447–452, 1986

Fawzy FI, Cousins N, Fawzy NW, et al: A structured psychiatric intervention for cancer patients, I: changes over time in methods of coping and affective disturbance. Arch Gen Psychiatry 47(8):720–725, 1990a

Fawzy FI, Kemeny ME, Fawzy NW, et al: A structured psychiatric intervention for cancer patients, II: changes over time in immunological measures. Arch Gen Psychiatry 47(8):729–735, 1990b

Gelb LN: New anti-nausea medication approved. FDA Medical Bulletin 21(1):6, 1991

Greer S: Can psychological therapy improve the quality of life of patients with cancer? Br J Cancer 59(2):149–151, 1989

Greer DR, Mor V, Morris JN, et al: An alternative in terminal care: results of the national hospice study. Journal of Chronic Diseases 39:9–26, 1986

Hackett TP, Cassem NH, Raker JW: Patient delay in cancer. N Engl J Med 289:14–20, 1973

Halkin H: Adverse effects of the fluoroquinolones. Reviews of Infectious Diseases 10 (suppl):258–261, 1988

Havlir D, Brown L, Rousseau GK: Do not resuscitate discussions in a hospital-based home care program. J Am Geriatr Soc 37(1):52–54, 1989

Kobasa SC, Puccetti MC: Personality and social resources in stress resistance. J Pers Soc Psychol 45:839–850, 1983

Lichtman RR, Taylor SE: Close relationships and the female cancer patient, in Women With Cancer. Edited by Andersen BL. New York, Springer-Verlag, 1986, pp 233–256

Massie MJ: Anxiety, panic, and phobias, in Handbook of Psychooncology. Edited by Holland JC, Rowland JH. New York, Oxford University Press, 1989, pp 300–309

Massie MJ, Holland JC: Depression and the cancer patient. J Clin Psychiatry 51 (suppl):12–19, 1990

Massie MJ, Holland J, Glass E: Delirium in terminally ill patients. Am J Psychiatry 140(8):1048–1050, 1983

McCartney CF, Larson DB: Quality of life in patients with gynecologic cancer. Cancer 60:2129–2136, 1987

McCartney CF, Cahill P, Larson DB, et al: Effect of a psychiatric liaison program on consultation rates and on detection of minor psychiatric disorders in cancer patients. Am J Psychiatry 146(7):898–901, 1989

McKegney FP, Beckhardt RM: Evaluative research in consultation-liaison psychiatry. Gen Hosp Psychiatry 4:197–218, 1982

Moore DH, Fowler WC, Crumpler LS: 5-Fluorouracil neurotoxicity. Gynecol Oncol 36:152–154, 1990

Mullan F, Hoffman B: Consumer Reports: An Almanac of Practical Resources for Cancer Survivors: Charting the Journey. Mt. Vernon, New York, Consumers Union, 1990

Orentlicher D: Physician participation in assisted suicide. JAMA 262(13):1844–1845, 1989

Osterweis M, Solomon F, Green M: Assisting the bereaved: roles of health professionals and institutions, in Bereavement: Reactions, Consequences, and Care. Edited by Osterweis M, Solomon F, Green M. Washington, DC, National Academy Press, 1984, pp 215–236

Ostroff J, Lesko L, Mashberg D: Hardiness as a mediator of physical and psychological well-being of chronic myelocytic leukemia (CML) patients (abstract A1185). Proceedings of the annual meeting of the American Society of Clinical Oncology, 1990

Patchell RA, Posner JB: Cancer and the central nervous system, in Handbook of Psychooncology. Edited by Holland JC, Rowland JH. New York, Oxford University Press, 1989, pp 327–341

Portenoy RK: Practical aspects of pain control in the patient with cancer. Cancer 38(6):327–352, 1988

Quill TE: Death and dignity: a case of individualized decision making. N Engl J Med 324(10):691–694, 1991

Richardson JL, Zarnegar Z, Bisno B: Psychosocial status at initiation of cancer treatment and survival. J Psychosom Res 34(2):189–201, 1990

Schipper H: Quality of life: principles of the clinical paradigm. Journal of Psychosocial Oncology 8:171–184, 1990

Schover LR: Sexuality and Cancer: For the Woman Who Has Cancer, and Her Partner. New York, American Cancer Society, 1988

Schover LR, Jensen SB: Sexuality and Chronic Illness: A Comprehensive Approach. New York, Guilford, 1988

Silberfarb PM: Chemotherapy and cognitive defects in cancer patients. Annu Rev Med 34:35–46, 1983

Snavely SR, Hodges GR: The neurotoxicity of antibacterial agents. Ann Intern Med 101:92–104, 1984

Spiegel D: Facilitating emotional coping during treatment. Cancer 66(6): 1422–1426, 1990

Spiegel D, Sands S: Pain and depression in cancer patients. Paper presented at session #16, CME Syllabus and Proceedings Summary, American Psychiatric Association 144th annual meeting. Washington, DC, May 1991

Spiegel D, Bloom JR, Kraemer HC, et al: Effect of psychosocial treatment on survival of patients with metastatic breast cancer. Lancet 2:888–891, 1989

Stein M, Miller AH, Trestman RL: Depression, the immune system, and health and illness. Arch Gen Psychiatry 48:171–177, 1991

Steptoe A, Horti J, Stanton S: Concern about cancer in women undergoing elective gynaecological surgery. Soc Sci Med 23(11):1139–1145, 1986

Wallston KA, Burger C, Smith RA, et al: Comparing the quality of death for hospice and non-hospice cancer patients. Med Care 26(2):177–182, 1988

Wanzer SH, Adelstein SJ, Cranford RE, et al: The physician's responsibility toward hopelessly ill patients. N Engl J Med 310(15):955–959, 1984

Welch-McCaffrey D, Hoffman B, Leigh SA, et al: Surviving adult cancers, II: psychosocial implications. Ann Intern Med 111(6):517–524, 1989

Zalupski M, Baker LH: Ifosfamide. J Natl Cancer Inst 80:556–566, 1988

Chapter 16

Women and AIDS

Mary Ann Chiasson, Dr.P.H.
Carola Marte, M.D.
Pauline Thomas, M.D.
Dooley Worth, Ph.D.

❖ ❖ ❖ ❖ ❖ ❖ ❖ ❖ ❖ ❖ ❖ ❖ ❖ ❖

W hat began in 1981 with a few isolated case reports of unexplained opportunistic infections and unusual cancers in homosexual men is now recognized as a global pandemic. The World Health Organization estimates that 8–10 million adults have already been infected with human immunodeficiency virus (HIV), the organism that causes acquired immunodeficiency syndrome (AIDS). Approximately one-third of those infected are women (Chin 1990). This chapter focuses on the effect of HIV infection and AIDS on women in the United States.

AIDS

Modes of Transmission

Epidemiologic investigations have shown that HIV can be transmitted through the exchange of infected blood or other body fluids during sexual intercourse, the sharing of needles or other drug injection equipment by parenteral drug users, or blood or blood component transfusion, or from mother to fetus. All evidence collected to date indicates that transmission does not occur through casual contact with infected individuals (Friedland and Klein 1987).

313

Sexual transmission of HIV from male to male, male to female, female to male, and female to female has been reported. Among heterosexuals, risk factors associated with male-to-female transmission are anal intercourse, bleeding from trauma during sex, not using condoms, multiple sexual contacts, immunodeficiency in the HIV-infected partner, and oral contraceptive use. In Africa, where heterosexual transmission accounts for most AIDS cases, an increased risk of HIV infection through female-to-male transmission is present in uncircumcised men with a recent history of a genital ulcer (Holmberg et al. 1989).

Overall, the rate of heterosexual transmission is estimated to be about 0.2% per exposure (Hearst and Hulley 1988), which is much lower than the 22%–25% risk of transmission of *Neisseria gonorrhoeae* from a single sexual exposure (Holmes et al. 1970). The rate of transmission varies considerably, however, and some persons become infected after a single or few sexual exposures, whereas others remain uninfected after hundreds of exposures (Holmberg et al. 1989).

Epidemiology

In the United States, 158,287 adults and adolescents meeting the AIDS case surveillance definition were reported through December 1990 (Centers for Disease Control 1991b). Women comprise 10% of the AIDS cases reported to date, but from 1988 to 1989 AIDS cases increased by 29% in women, compared with an increase of 18% in men (Centers for Disease Control 1990a). Increasing AIDS-related mortality has accompanied the increasing AIDS caseload in women. AIDS became one of the 10 leading causes of death in women ages 15–44 years in the United States in 1987 (Chu et al. 1990).

Women of reproductive age (ages 15–44 years) account for 85% of all female AIDS cases. Thus, in addition to the major impact AIDS has had on the morbidity and mortality of women in the United States, there is a direct link between the epidemic in women and that in children. Maternal-fetal transmission of HIV accounts for about 83% of the 2,786 pediatric AIDS cases reported in the United States.

Poor black and Hispanic women have been disproportionately affected by the AIDS epidemic. They account for 72% of all female

AIDS cases, although they account for only 19% of the female population of the United States (Centers for Disease Control 1990a).

Distribution in Women by Mode of Transmission

An analysis of the risk behaviors of AIDS patients reported to the Centers for Disease Control shows that intravenous drug use accounts for 51% of the 15,493 cases of AIDS in females. An additional one-third of female AIDS cases are attributed to heterosexual contact: 11% of these women are from countries where heterosexual transmission accounts for most AIDS cases, and 89% report sex with a man at risk for AIDS, primarily intravenous drug users (70%) and bisexual men (11%). Recipients of blood products account for 9% of the AIDS cases in females, and the remaining 7% are of undetermined risk (Centers for Disease Control 1991b).

MEDICAL UPDATE

Diagnosis and HIV Antibody Testing

Most individuals develop antibodies to HIV 6–12 weeks after infection. HIV testing is done by a sequence of immunoassays. A sensitive but less specific screening test, the enzyme-linked immunosorbent assay (ELISA), is repeated if positive and is followed by the more specific Western blot. Anxiety over the possibility of "silent" infection (i.e., infection despite seronegativity) may lead some individuals to seek repeated testing.

HIV infection is now recognized to be a chronic condition with a spectrum of disease ranging from symptom-free to devastating illness. The median time from infection to a diagnosis of AIDS in men is estimated to be 10 years. It is not known whether the natural history of HIV infection in women differs. Most infected individuals eventually progress to illness and AIDS. Only 19% of a cohort of 341 men known to have seroconverted between 1977 and 1980 were without signs or symptoms of AIDS in 1990 (Rutherford et al. 1990).

AIDS is a clinical diagnosis and was originally defined as the presence of certain opportunistic diseases or unusual tumors in the absence of other causes of cellular immunodeficiency. Pneumocystis carinii pneumonia (PCP) is the most common illness by which AIDS is defined in men and women. In 1987 the Centers for Disease Control expanded the AIDS case definition to include dementia, wasting syndromes, and several additional infections and conditions (Centers for Disease Control 1987). Most were formerly defined as ARC (AIDS-related-conditions), a term that has remained in unofficial usage.

Gynecologic Disease

Most HIV-related gynecologic conditions are more prevalent and/or more severe manifestations of known diseases (Allen 1990). Unusually persistent vaginal candidiasis, genital herpes (sometimes painfully ulcerated in severely immunodepressed individuals), and pelvic inflammatory disease are often more difficult to treat successfully than in uninfected women.

Gynecologic disease related to human papillomavirus is of particular concern. Cervical dysplasia appears to be more prevalent in HIV-infected women (Centers for Disease Control 1990b; Provencher et al. 1988). Recent evidence suggests that in some cases cervical carcinoma in HIV-infected women may be aggressive and progress to fatality before the affected woman reaches a diagnosis of AIDS (Maiman et al. 1990). Regular pelvic examinations, therefore, and prompt follow-up of abnormal Pap tests are important for HIV-infected women.

Neuropsychiatric Aspects

HIV can invade the nervous system directly or predispose an infected individual to opportunistic infections or malignancies (Brew et al. 1988; Levy 1988). Although the virus may enter into the central nervous system at the time of initial infection, it is rare that symptoms of HIV dementia occur before other manifestations of HIV disease. Cognitive symptoms, especially difficulty with concentration and memory, are often the earliest sign of dementia.

Since many of the nonspecific symptoms associated with neurologic disease can be caused by mass lesions such as cerebral toxoplasmosis, tuberculosis, or lymphoma, it is important for clinicians to maintain a high index of suspicion and not delay neurologic workup because of a presumptive diagnosis of a psychiatric condition. For instance, an apparent reactive depression may be the first symptom of a neurologic infection. An important diagnostic criterion is whether the condition is stable or progressive. In addition, changes in mental status may be a side effect of antiretroviral therapy.

Family Planning and Reproductive Choices

For women who are HIV infected, decisions about childbearing are understandably difficult. It is important that all pregnant women have access to HIV counseling and testing. It is equally important that all HIV-infected women receive counseling about the full range of reproductive choices and information about perinatal transmission (Sunderland 1990). HIV-infected women who are known to be pregnant require sensitive and noncoercive counseling and support for their choices.

Treatment

Antiviral therapy and prophylaxis against PCP have made a great difference in the prognosis of individuals with more advanced immune suppression (Harris 1990; Lemp et al. 1990). Initiation of antiviral therapy is based on assays of T4 lymphocytes. The T4 lymphocyte is the cell primarily invaded by HIV, although monocytes and macrophages are also infected. Since 1987, zidovudine (formerly azidothymidine, or AZT) has been prescribed for individuals diagnosed with AIDS, HIV-related symptoms, or fewer than 200 T4 cells/μl of blood, resulting in improved survival time and fewer opportunistic infections (Fischl 1990). Clinical trials of new antiviral medications and combination treatment regimens are now under way.

AZT has also been recommended for an earlier stage of disease, that is, when T4 cell counts are fewer than 500/μl (National Institutes of Health 1990). Although the data show a delay in the onset of symptoms and opportunistic infections, the question of statistically improved survival has not yet been resolved. Also unresolved is the question of viral resistance to AZT. The optimal time for initiating AZT therapy in asymptomatic patients with 200–500 T4 cells/μl is not known at this time, and clinicians vary on how strongly they urge AZT for those at the higher end of the range.

Prophylaxis for PCP, either with inhaled pentamidine or oral sulfa agents, is prescribed when T4 cell counts are fewer than 200/μl or 20% of total lymphocytes (Centers for Disease Control 1989b). Trials are now being conducted of toxoplasmosis prophylaxis by sulfa regimens that would prevent both PCP and toxoplasmosis. Prophylactic regimens for other common opportunistic organisms, for example, atypical mycobacteria, are also being investigated.

PSYCHOSOCIAL ISSUES

HIV Antibody Testing

Women are increasingly being targeted for HIV testing, particularly pregnant women and prostitutes. It is therefore important to examine the psychosocial implications of such testing. Too often women are encouraged to be tested because of the possible effects on others (e.g., infants and men).

Being tested and waiting for test results is a period of high anxiety for most women, a period in which they may actually increase their risk taking. Anxiety does not necessarily stop when the test results are received.

Negative test results.   Most women who receive a negative test result are greatly relieved—some too much so. If they had repeated exposure to HIV, they may conclude that they are "immune" to the virus. Others disbelieve their test results and may go so far as to develop false symptoms (Worth 1990). The women most likely to respond with disbelief are those whose male sex partners are seropositive.

Women in discordant couples who test HIV seronegative are faced with a unique set of problems. Someone else's behavior has put them at risk. Their relationship to this behavior is often based on various types of dependency (e.g., legal, sexual, economic, emotional). Some women in this situation feel that "it would be easier to be seropositive." This would allow them to avoid feelings of guilt if they wish to leave their relationship due to their fear of infection, of not being able to have children with their partners, of having to renegotiate their relationship, of their partner's death, of surviving alone, of being a single parent, or of not being able to handle the burdens imposed by a caretaking role.

Positive test results. The fears of seropositive women in discordant couples are very different. They are ordinarily focused on their partner's leaving them to be sick and to die alone. Blachman (1988) and others suggest that this is not an unrealistic fear for heterosexual women and that infected or symptomatic women are more likely to be abandoned by their male partners than the reverse.

Single seropositive women have special problems. They tend to isolate themselves and to consider themselves "tainted." They may stop dating, believing it is unethical to become involved with someone and not disclose that they are infected, but fearing that such disclosure would result in never again having the possibility of an intimate relationship—a devastating possibility for a woman in her 20s or 30s (Eric et al. 1989; D. Worth, unpublished ethnographic research data, The Women's AIDS Group Program, Stuyvesant Polyclinic/New York City Department of Health, 1987).

Living With HIV Infection and AIDS

HIV-seropositive women often experience feelings of total loss of control over their lives and their bodies. This results in loneliness, helplessness, hopelessness, and anger. Anger manifests itself as both bouts of depression and acting out. Some women direct their anger at men in general, because it is men who have introduced them to drugs, who continue to put them at risk through unprotected sex, and who may have "betrayed" them by having sex with other men. Anger is also directed at societal norms that encourage women to become "risk managers" for their relationships (that is, being expected to control their partners' sexual behavior). Still another target of the anger of these women may be those who are supposed to help them, particularly male health care providers with whom women find it difficult if not impossible to discuss sexual questions and who may treat them in ways that increase their sense of victimization by uncaring, impersonal health and social service institutions. Unfortunately, the treatment of women in ways that decrease their self-esteem is not limited just to male health care providers.

Women's anger is not always externalized, as it is often deemed socially or culturally unacceptable for women to express anger. Instead, many women berate themselves for having engaged in behavior that led to infection or for having stayed in relationships that were destructive—relationships based on sharing drugs, lies, and/or abusive behavior.

Internalized anger damages self-esteem, leaving women feeling that they do not have the right to protect themselves sexually and adding to their fear of rejection if they insist on it. Diminished self-esteem also makes women vulnerable to resuming or increasing their drug use (Sorrel and Springer 1989). Underlying such anger is fear of abandonment, death, and dying. This fear encompasses a woman's anticipation of her own death (particularly of dying alone) or the death of a significant other or child.

It should be stressed that often such anger is an initial stage in a woman's reaction to infection. Many women, including women who are active users of intravenous drugs, are galvanized after their first reaction to live their lives to the fullest, seizing control of their health and attempting to alter their risk-taking behavior (Eric et al. 1989).

Mental Health Needs

The psychological needs of women who are infected, or whose partners are, differ from those of men. Women need to know that it is acceptable for them to put their own needs first. This is often a particular problem with female partners of users of intravenous drugs; they seldom are able to put themselves first in this way, because they are socialized to assume the role of caretaker to others from earliest childhood (Wermuth and Ham 1989).

Women need to know that they are cared about for themselves.

This is crucial for female users of intravenous drugs, who are severely socially stigmatized and are often offered services only as "mothers of vulnerable children." This reinforces their perception that they themselves are not worth helping (Mitchell 1988).

Psychosocial counseling for women at risk of HIV infection, although it touches on many traditional issues, must take on issues not ordinarily dealt with in women's mental health programs (e.g., the need for bereavement counseling for young adults, sexual behavior modification, and overcoming addiction). Women need to be offered resources to help them learn to face new issues and feelings. "Survivor's guilt," anger, depression, suicidal ideation, and multiple bereavement processes can be ameliorated by seeking mental health services (Blachman 1988; Dobko and Benedik 1989; Wofsy 1988).

Spiritual and social support also play important roles in providing support to women attempting to change their life-styles. The effect of spiritual beliefs and social support on survival needs often determines how women make critical choices about living with HIV infection and illness (Grant and Anns 1988).

In addressing the specific needs of women, mental health providers need to reorient themselves, recognizing the importance of spiritual and social support and training in AIDS and chemical dependency; reevaluating standard measures for looking at the behavior of substance-abusing women; and introducing cross-cultural or culture-specific counseling (Mondanaro 1989).

Obstacles to Behavior Changes

Female intravenous drug users make up the majority of women with HIV infection and AIDS. In many cases they are the partners of other active intravenous drug users. Ultimately, female intravenous drug users who wish to reduce their risk but are in such relationships are faced with a choice of reducing their risk or continuing their relationship. Although there is support for women to reduce risk, very little support exists for women who need to leave their relationships and who need housing, income, police protection, drug treatment, etc. To fully support women who are at highest risk of HIV infection and AIDS, we need to both reexamine how we deliver mental health services to women and create supportive social networks for women who wish to leave relationships that are tied to risk taking.

HIV AND PREGNANCY

Epidemiologic Considerations

Two issues are of particular concern to the pregnant woman who is infected with HIV: 1) her chances for a healthy child and 2) the potential implications to her own health of the interaction between the infection and body stresses related to the pregnancy. The chances for a healthy child are also of concern in the management of the pregnant woman who is not currently positive for HIV antibodies but who is engaging in behavior that places her at risk. If she becomes infected during pregnancy, her child may be infected as well. For the HIV-infected woman who is taking antiretroviral therapy, the potential adverse effects of antiviral agents on the developing fetus are also of concern.

Regardless of whether a woman seeks medical care early enough in the pregnancy to consider the option of induced abortion, her prenatal and postpartum management can be influenced by the probability that she may transmit HIV to her infant. Data from a variety of studies in the United States and Europe place the rate of HIV transmission from mother to child at 12%–35% (European Collaborative Study 1992; Oxtoby 1990; Tovo 1992). These odds can be discussed with women seeking medical care in the first half of pregnancy, but they may not accurately define the risk for every woman. Some data indicate that the risk of transmission may be greater for women with advanced HIV illness, as measured by either clinical status or levels of T helper cells (European Collaborative Study 1992; Gabiano et al. 1992; Ryder et al. 1989). These data are not proven by large numbers and are not sufficiently refined at the time of this writing to allow generation of a risk algorithm for the individual woman.

Some data indicate that women who are symptomatic with HIV illness are more likely to deliver prematurely (Mok et al. 1989). This is thought to be due to the effects of chronic opportunistic illness in the mother, rather than to any direct influence of HIV. Premature birth in itself has not been shown to contribute to risk of infection in the infant (European Collaborative Study 1992; Oxtoby 1990).

The determination of infection status in the infant remains problematic and is a source of stress postpartum to parents and health care workers (Rogers et al. 1990). Infants born to HIV-infected mothers test positive for HIV antibody for up to 15 months after birth whether they are actually infected or not, owing to the active passage of maternal immunoglobulin across the placenta in utero. Using research methods such as polymerase chain reaction, HIV-specific immunoglobulin A, and virus culture, it is now technically possible to confirm infection status by 6 months of age. These methods are not universally available, however, and no technique has yet been proven to be sufficiently sensitive and specific in infants under age 6 months (Centers for Disease Control 1991a; Falloon et al. 1989). At present in the United States, many HIV infections in infants are detected only when the infant begins to manifest clinical illness consistent with HIV (Oxtoby 1990). Lack of infection is established only at the point that the infant loses maternal antibody, on average by age 10 months, but not infrequently as late as age 15 months (Rogers et al. 1990).

Despite the difficulties in confirming a diagnosis of HIV infection in the young infant, special medical attention is now recommended for those potentially infected. Although the efficacy of antiretroviral therapy in infants is still under study, guidelines have been recently published for antibiotic prophylaxis against PCP in children, based on CD4 lymphocyte levels (Centers for Disease Control 1991a). Monitoring of CD4 lymphocytes is recommended for infants born to HIV-positive women. A high degree of efficacy of prophylaxis for PCP has now been well demonstrated. Other aspects of medical management include fever management, nutrition, frequency and type of medical evaluation, and immunizations that may be especially tailored for the infant born to an HIV-infected woman. Information on the possibility that careful medical management and new therapies may prolong the child's life should be discussed with the HIV-infected pregnant woman and should be included in counseling pregnant women about the advisability of being tested for HIV. Diagnosis of HIV infection in the pregnant woman not only can enhance her own medical care, but also provides the earliest possible alert to the pediatrician who will be managing her child's care.

Medical Update and Treatment

Data are not available to formulate definitive guidelines for treatment of HIV-infected pregnant women. The current standard of care is to combine thorough perinatal care with equally scrupulous HIV care. With the exception of antiviral therapy, prophylaxis and treatment for HIV disease is comparable to that for women who are not pregnant (Minkoff 1987; Nanda 1990). Although T4 cell counts may decrease during pregnancy, current data suggest that pregnancy does not alter the natural history or hasten the progression of HIV disease.

The safety of AZT during pregnancy is now in an early phase of evaluation. Because of the potential risk of mutagenicity or congenital malformation (so far not observed in practice), AZT is usually suggested only after the first trimester. Whether AZT during pregnancy can reduce perinatal transmission is also being investigated. It is particularly important for pregnant women to understand the possible risks and benefits to both themselves and the fetus.

Special concerns during pregnancy include diagnosis and treatment of sexually transmitted diseases and opportunistic infections, to which the fetus as well as the mother are vulnerable. Startling increases in the incidence of both maternal and congenital syphilis, in addition to the apparent recrudescence of treated syphilis in some HIV-infected individuals, underscore the importance of syphilis screening during pregnancy and at parturition (Centers for Disease Control 1989a; Hook 1989; Musher et al. 1990).

Prophylaxis against PCP is also recommended, although possible harm to the fetus has not been studied. Congenital anomalies associated with maternal prophylaxis have not been reported, and the severity of acute PCP is cited by clinicians who favor prophylaxis. Screening for opportunistic infections that can harm the fetus and the mother, such as toxoplasmosis and cytomegalovirus infection, is recommended. Tuberculosis is increasingly prevalent in HIV-infected persons, and it is recommended that both positive tests for purified protein derivative and active disease be treated as in women who are not pregnant.

REFERENCES

Allen MH: Primary care of women infected with the human immunodeficiency virus. Obstet Gynecol Clin North Am 17:557–569, 1990

Blachman M: Seropositive women: clinical issues and approaches. Focus 3:2–3, 1988

Brew B, Sidtis J, Petito CK, et al: The neurologic complications of AIDS and human immunodeficiency virus infection, in Advances in Contemporary Neurology. Edited by Plum F. Philadelphia, PA, FA Davis, 1988, pp 1–49

Centers for Disease Control: Revision of the CDC surveillance case definition for acquired immunodeficiency syndrome. MMWR 36 (suppl 1):3–15, 1987

Centers for Disease Control: Congenital syphilis—New York City, 1986–1988. MMWR 38:825–829, 1989a

Centers for Disease Control: Guidelines for prophylaxis against Pneumocystis carinii pneumonia for persons infected with human immunodeficiency virus. MMWR 38 (suppl 5):1–9, 1989b

Centers for Disease Control: AIDS in women—United States. MMWR 39:845–846, 1990a

Centers for Disease Control: Risk for cervical disease in HIV-infected women—New York City. MMWR 39:846–849, 1990b

Centers for Disease Control: Guidelines for prophylaxis against Pneumocystis carinii pneumonia for children infected with human immunodeficiency virus. MMWR 40(RR-2):1–13, 1991a

Centers for Disease Control: HIV/AIDS Surveillance Report. January 1991b, p 6

Chin J: Challenges of the nineties. World Health, November–December 1990, pp 4–6

Chu Sy, Beuhler JW, Berkelman RL, et al: Impact of the human immunodeficiency virus epidemic on mortality in women of reproductive age, United States. JAMA 264:225–229, 1990

Dobko T, Benedik B: The medical and emotional support needs of women with HIV. Paper presented at the 5th International AIDS Conference, Montreal, Canada, June 1989

Eric K, Drucker E, Worth D, et al: The women's center: a model peer support program for high risk IV drug and crack using women in the Bronx. Paper presented at the 5th International AIDS Conference, Montreal, Canada, June 1989

European Collaborative Study: Risk factors for mother-to-child transmission of HIV-1. Lancet 339:1007–1112, 1992

Falloon J, Eddy J, Wiener L, et al: Human immunodeficiency virus infection in children. J Pediatr 114:1–30, 1989

Fischl MA: Treatment of HIV infection, in The Medical Management of AIDS, 2nd Edition. Edited by Sande MA, Volberding PA. Philadelphia, PA, WB Saunders, 1990

Friedland GH, Klein RS: Transmission of the human immunodeficiency virus. N Engl J Med 317:1125–1135, 1987

Gabiano C, Tovo PA, deMartino M, et al: Mother-to-child transmission of human immunodeficiency virus type 1: risk of infection and correlates of transmission. Pediatrics 90:369–374, 1992

Grant D, Anns M: Counseling AIDS antibody-positive clients: reactions and treatment. Am Psychol 44:72–74, 1988

Harris JE: Improved short-term survival of AIDS patients initially diagnosed with Pneumocystis carinii pneumonia, 1984 through 1987. JAMA 263:397–401, 1990

Hearst N, Hulley SB: Preventing the heterosexual spread of AIDS: are we giving our patients the best advice? JAMA 259:2428–2432, 1988

Holmberg SD, Horsburgh CR Jr, Ward JW, et al: Biologic factors in the sexual transmission of human immunodeficiency virus. J Infect Dis 160:116–125, 1989

Holmes KK, Johnson DW, Trostle HJ: An estimate of the risk of men acquiring gonorrhea by sexual contact with infected females. Am J Epidemiol 91:170–174, 1970

Hook EW: Syphilis and HIV infection. J Infect Dis 160:530–534, 1989

Lemp GF, Payne SF, Neal D, et al: Survival trends for patients with AIDS. JAMA 263:402–406, 1990

Levy JA: The biology of the human immunodeficiency virus and its role in neurological disease, in AIDS and the Nervous System. Edited by Rosenblum ML, Levy RM, Bredesen DE. New York, Raven, 1988, pp 327–345

Maiman M, Fruchter RG, Serur E, et al: Human immunodeficiency virus infection and cervical neoplasia. Gynecol Oncol 38:377–382, 1990

Minkoff HL: Care of pregnant women infected with human immunodeficiency virus. JAMA 258:2714–2717, 1987

Mitchell J: Women, AIDS and public policy. AIDS Public Policy 3:50–52, 1988

Mok JQ, Hague RA, Yap P, et al: Vertical transmission of HIV: a prospective study. Arch Dis Child 64:1140–1145, 1989

Mondanaro J: Chemically Dependent Women: Assessment and Treatment. Lexington, MA, DC Heath, 1989

Musher DM, Hamill RJ, Baughn RE: Effect of human immunodeficiency virus (HIV) infection on the course of syphilis and on the response to treatment. Ann Intern Med 113:872–881, 1990

Nanda D: Human immunodeficiency virus infection in pregnancy. Obstet Gynecol Clin North Am 17:617–626, 1990

National Institutes of Health: State-of-the-art conference on azidothymidine therapy for early HIV infection. Am J Med 89:335–344, 1990

Oxtoby MJ: Perinatally acquired human immunodeficiency virus infection. Pediatr Infect Dis J 9:609–619, 1990

Provencher D, Valme B, Averette HE, et al: HIV status and positive Papanicolaou screening: identification of a high-risk population. Gynecol Oncol 31:184–188, 1988

Rogers MF, Ou CY, Kilbourne B, et al: Advances and problems in the diagnosis of HIV infection in infants, in Pediatric AIDS—The Challenge of HIV Infection in Infants, Children and Adolescents. Edited by Pizzo PA, Wilfert CM. Baltimore, MD, Williams & Wilkins, 1990, pp 159–174

Rutherford GW, Lifson AR, Hessol NA, et al: Course of HIV-1 infection in a cohort of homosexual and bisexual men: an 11 year follow up study. BMJ 301:1183–1188, 1990

Ryder RW, Nsa E, Hassig SE, et al: Perinatal transmission of the human immunodeficiency virus type 1 to infants of seropositive women in Zaire. N Engl J Med 320:1637–1642, 1989

Sorrel S, Springer E: The argument against HIV antibody testing in chemical dependency treatment programs. J Psychoactive Drugs 21:419–421, 1989

Sunderland A: Influence of human immunodeficiency virus education on reproductive decisions. Obstet Gynecol Clin North Am 17:585–594, 1990

Tovo PA, deMartino M, Gabiano C, et al: Prognostic factors and survival in children with perinatal HIV-1 infection. Lancet 339:1249–1253, 1992

Wermuth L, Ham L: Perceptions of AIDS risk among women sex partners of IV drug users in San Francisco. Paper presented at the 5th International AIDS Conference, Montreal, Canada, June 1989

Wofsy C: Women and the acquired immuno-deficiency syndrome: an interview. West J Med 149:687–690, 1988

Worth D: Women at high risk of HIV infection: behavioral, prevention and intervention aspects, in Behavioral Aspects of AIDS and Other STDs. Edited by Ostrow D. New York, Plenum, 1990

SECTION III

GENERAL ISSUES

Chapter 17

REPRODUCTIVE CHOICES AND DEVELOPMENT: PSYCHODYNAMIC AND PSYCHOANALYTIC PERSPECTIVES

Malkah T. Notman, M.D.
Carol C. Nadelson, M.D.

❖ ❖ ❖ ❖ ❖ ❖ ❖ ❖ ❖ ❖ ❖ ❖ ❖

Reproductive choices profoundly affect an individual's life. Some are made almost automatically, as part of becoming an adult and identifying with one's parents. Others are made inadvertently, influenced by unconscious factors. Even if these choices are conscious and deliberate, however, they express deep-seated attitudes, beliefs, and expectations about oneself, one's gender role, and one's relationship to society.

In the last several decades, many social changes have influenced the size of families and the timing of pregnancies. Increased work opportunities and the necessity for many women to work have affected decisions about having children. These choices, then, are also the result of social forces, as well as of the individual meanings of pregnancy and parenting. Wishes to have children are very powerful for both men and women, but for women, who have until recently defined themselves more in relation to family than to work, these wishes more closely express the central fulfillment of many aspects of gender role and aspirations.

Wishes to conceive and carry a pregnancy and to deliver a baby do not necessarily reflect a grasp of the real tasks of parenting, with all of its accompanying changes and responsibilities. Instead, they can represent a sense of fulfillment of one's identity as a man or a woman.

Even for those who choose not to have children, knowing one has the capacity to do so is an important part of one's adult gender identity. Expectations about being able to have and care for children are part of growing up.

The importance of producing children to a society varies to some extent among cultures with differing economic conditions and values. In all cultures, however, women's roles as mothers and nurturers of young children remain central, although there is an enormous range in the other roles and activities that each culture assigns to men and women (LeVine 1991). In most cultures, women are the primary caretakers of infants and children, whether they also work in the fields or in factories or stay at home.

The "reproductive clock" and the knowledge that fertility is time limited also form a background context for many women's development and choices in a way that it does not for men. Women are aware of their reproductive potential early in their lives. A woman's sexual behavior is always affected by the possibility of pregnancy, whether she is always thinking about it consciously or not. This possibility creates both a promise and a vulnerability.

The cessation of fertility at menopause also has a different impact on women in different cultures and in different life circumstances, but it is universal in marking an end to childbearing potential. Recent technology that has extended the possibility of pregnancy beyond normal menopause by the use of egg donation and hormonal treatment may change the time frame for some women, but it is unlikely that childbearing will extend to the geriatric age group. The reality that reproduction is finite thus influences other choices. Most women are very aware of the biological clock as it affects their career and marital choices and their wishes to experiment with work and life-styles. Sometimes it is denied and then becomes a pressing issue when they reach a particular birthday, such as 30 or 35 (Nadelson 1989; Notman 1973; Notman 1979).

In the early 1970s, when career opportunities for women were first expanding, some women were postponing childbearing or considering it an elective choice. This was particularly true for those women who had educational and career possibilities. Later childbearing became more common and, aside from teenage mothers, the age for first pregnancies rose. Having a first baby later was also made more feasible by better general health and improved technology, which resulted in older, healthy, primiparous women being found to be at no greater risk for pregnancy complications than younger women (Bunker et al. 1976; Friedman 1978). As women who had delayed childbearing became older, many found themselves under increasing pressure to have children. Those women became concerned about infertility, and many sought help from new technologies to meet the "baby hunger" that they experienced.

The development of these new technologies has had complex effects. Although some women have perceived these advances as an effort by a predominantly male medical establishment to control women and demonstrate heroic medical achievements, most women have felt grateful to be offered the possibility of fertility that had seemed foreclosed. Despite the many possible causes of fertility problems, women have traditionally been seen as responsible for them. They have felt burdened, and guilty even when the defect was not theirs.

Decisions About Marriage

Despite recent social changes, marriage is still perceived by many as the central adult role for women in contemporary society. Other activities, such as work, have been regarded as temporary or as subordinate to and dependent on family functions (Bernard 1975; Kuhlen and Johnson 1952). This has not been as true for men. Nevertheless, the effect of marriage on women may be more negative than we usually believe it to be. Bernard (1973) and others (Gove and Tudor 1973) have documented that marriage improves mental health and satisfaction for men but not for women. Some data indicate that more married women than unmarried women are depressed, whereas more unmarried men than married men are depressed. One risk factor reported for depression is having children under age 3 at home without the support of other adults (Brown and Harris 1978).

There has always been considerable pressure for women to marry. In the past, their social and economic status depended upon the status of the men who were responsible for them, that is, their fathers and husbands. The decision for a woman was usually not whether to marry, but whom and when to marry. The loss of self-esteem and damage to her pride and her family's reputation when a woman remained unmarried led to the familiar desperation of women who became "old maids." This was not so for an unmarried man—a bachelor (Bernard 1991; Nadelson and Notman 1981). These attitudes remain to some extent, although more women choose not to marry and many more choose to divorce than in the past when women had no way of being economically independent.

Four decades ago, when Kuhn (1955) studied a group of men and women who had not married, their reasons for doing so were often expressed negatively: hostility toward marriage or toward members of the opposite sex, dependency on parents, poor health, feelings of physical unattractiveness, unwillingness or inability to assume responsibility, social inadequacy, the perception of marriage as a threat to career goals, economic problems, and geographic, educational, or occupational isolation that limited the chances of meeting an eligible mate (Nadelson and Notman 1981). Two decades later, a shift was noted; being single was more often considered a positive choice. Both men and women spoke of increased freedom and enjoyment of life, opportunities to meet people, economic independence, and a chance for personal development (Stein 1976). In addition, people have spoken more openly about not wanting children, about their homosexuality, or about their childhood experiences with their parents' marital unhappiness or divorce as contributors to their decision not to marry (Nadelson and Notman 1981).

Unconscious and neurotic factors, such as strong dependency needs; difficulty forming a stable, secure identity; or an intolerable fear of isolation or loneliness, also influence the motivation to marry. The desire for children is a strong motivator for marriage. Within a marriage, as indicated previously here, many conscious and unconscious factors influence the decision to have children. Some people have little interest in actually being with children or in taking on parental roles. Others believe that they cannot be good parents. Some explicitly prefer the freedom of childlessness or want to invest their energy in careers. Sometimes, despite a strong wish for children, women fear pregnancy. Others struggle with unresolved, difficult, and ambivalent relationships with their mothers that affect their confidence in becoming mothers themselves (Notman and Nadelson 1981; Veevers 1979).

Some studies, including one by Kaltreider et al. (1979), have found an association between the choice for childlessness and a woman's poor relationship with her mother. Some of the women studied have been found to identify primarily with their fathers. In this era of recombined or reconstituted families, there are also many couples in which one partner has had children in a previous marriage and does not want more, leaving the other partner without children of his or her own. Some women who choose not to have children have feared that becoming a mother would inevitably draw them back to regressive or devalued positions. Women electing to remain childless may identify with negative aspects of their mothers' conflicts and experiences.

Although voluntary childlessness has been regarded as pathological or selfish by many, it is somewhat more acceptable than it was a generation ago. Voluntary childlessness as an alternative choice has been studied in recent years (Veevers 1979). Some of the determinants of these decisions have been described above. Some couples decide at the outset not to have children; others postpone the decision until a future time that does not arrive. Sometimes poor socioeconomic conditions; personal circumstances such as careers in dance, athletics, or other demanding professions; an ideology that negates childbearing; or a lesbian sexual orientation have precluded children. Veevers (1979) noted that "with the exception of race, childlessness tends to be influenced . . . by the major socioeconomic determinants known to influence fertility in general . . . education, urbanity, socioeconomic status . . . religious beliefs" (p. 208).

Women who are childless because they do not marry or are infertile may feel bereft and need to mourn what parenthood meant to them. Part of the process of working through these feelings involves shifting their orientation and looking for other experiences to fulfill these needs. If they are infertile, they also face the narcissistic injury that may accompany that realization, which can threaten their sense of femininity and even their perception of fully being an adult, since adulthood is so often closely associated with parenthood (Mazor 1978).

GENDER IDENTITY AND DEVELOPMENT

It is useful at this point to review ideas about gender development and its relationship to reproduction. Reproduction has been an important part of female identity. In early psychoanalytic writings about male and female development, gender identity, or the awareness of one's sex, was thought at one time to be established when the young child becomes aware of the genitals and of the differences between males and females. This, according to Freud's (1905) early formulations, took place relatively later in childhood than is now thought to be the case. Now it is known to start even before birth with the parents' expectations and beliefs about gender and their baby.

In Freud's view, girls and boys develop similarly until about the age of 3, when they become aware of their genital differences. During the first 3 years of life, according to Freud, the little girl does not know about the existence of her vagina. She comes to know about it later. Her full development of femininity was thought to take place with puberty. Freud thought that the early developments of the girl and boy were similar, along "masculine" lines. Then, when the boy notices that the girl has no penis, he becomes anxious at the thought that he might lose his own penis. The little girl, who has noticed that the boy has something she does not have, becomes envious, wants one, and blames her mother for not having supplied it for her. Because she feels she is lacking something important, she feels defective.

It is now recognized that the greater power and value that society gives to males plays an important role in this sense of defectiveness and in the importance of the penis. In the late 19th and early 20th centuries in Freud's culture, however, it was thought to be self-evident that the girl's "lack" of a penis was really something missing, rather than a different anatomical way of being. Classical Freudian theory also held that the little girl was left with lifetime penis envy, and that this was an organizing and driving force in her development. In this view, the girl thinks of her mother—and of all women—as defective because they also lack a penis (Freud 1905). Contemporary psychoanalytic thinking informed by developmental observations and research recognizes that, although penis envy exists in some women, it is not the central organizer of development (Grossman and Stewart 1976).

In earlier psychoanalytic theory, the girl's feeling that she was missing a penis was thought to be responsible for her disappointment in her mother, her subsequent turning from her mother to her father as her love object, and the initiation of her Oedipus complex. According to this theory, she is also drawn to her father for other complex reasons, such as her expanded interests and his affection and character. The little girl then develops erotic feelings toward her father and competitive and rivalrous feelings toward her mother. In this period, the girl also becomes interested in having a baby by her father, as a substitute for the penis she could not have. Thus, she both identifies and competes with her mother, expressed in the wish to "marry daddy when I grow up." This view, however, also places the little girl at risk of alienating her mother, whom she also loves and needs, so she defers her wish for a baby until she grows up and finds her own husband. This resolves the immediate dilemma in favor of the identification with her mother. The idea that the original wish for a baby arose as a substitute for a penis did not fully recognize the girl's early identification with her mother as the bearer of babies nor her aspirations to be like an adult woman as a motivating force.

Classical psychoanalytic theory hypothesized that the boy, confronted by the possibility of losing his penis and becoming like a girl, thought of castration as a punishment for forbidden wishes and hence developed intense anxiety. According to this theory, this anxiety acts as a strong pressure for him to relinquish his erotic sexual feelings toward his mother and his rivalrous, aggressive, competitive wishes toward his father. Since the boy also loves and needs his father, he resolves his conflict by identification with his father and postponement of his wishes for his mother, planning instead to seek a woman "just like" his mother when he is older. The boy's relatively abrupt move out of his oedipal period based on his castration anxiety was contrasted with the more gradual developmental shift for the girl. Accompanying the identifications with the parents that result from the oedipal resolution, the girl and boy also internalize parental values and morality in the form of the superego (Freud 1924).

Contemporary theory about development casts a different light on some of these formulations. Research and clinical data suggest that a more complex process occurs. Children develop their gender identity from birth onward. Prenatal hormones also exert an influence. Girls follow a different developmental path than do boys from the beginning. Both the boy's and the girl's early development occurs within the context of a close relationship to the mother, who is usually the primary caretaker. For the girl, the relationship with the parent of the same sex facilitates a different kind of mutual identification than for the boy. The mother identifies with the girl and sees herself in the girl baby, and the girl gradually identifies with the mother. This identification remains a powerful force throughout life. This does not mean the relationship is wholly positive or without conflict. The girl's gender identity develops from an identification with her mother and also with her mother's "feminine" roles and activities, in whatever way the particular culture presents these. Her turning toward her father also is supported by her identification with her mother, who, after all, preceded her in this (Clower 1991; Freud 1933; Notman et al. 1991; Person 1980).

The little boy also has an early close relationship with his mother. She is different from him, however, and in order to consolidate his male gender identity, he needs a male identification figure. He distances himself from the early relationship to his mother to some extent and from his "babyish" or childish ways. This shift is a crucial one for the boy. Because of the need to move away from his early feminine identification, he has to relinquish his ties not only with his mother, but also with what he perceives to be feminine ways and must build some emotional barriers against his early attachments (Chodorow 1978). It is also thought that envy of the capacity to have babies is found in little boys. In their development toward masculinity, they must abandon this possibility (Fast 1984; McDougall 1989).

Early gender identity, by which is meant the knowledge that one is male or female, is now thought to be established by about age 1½ years (Stoller 1976). Although the development of gender identity continues throughout childhood and is consolidated in a more permanent way in adolescence, it does not depend entirely on the awareness of genital differences, although one's body image does play an important role in one's sense of who one is. It also incorporates the multiple identifications and learning that take place from early life, including the powerful effects of socialization. Gender identity also includes the cognitive awareness of what behavior and attitudes "go with" being female or male and the way these roles are shaped in a given culture (Notman 1991; Silverman 1981; Stoller 1976). Some cultures have preadolescent and adolescent rituals to mark the transition into the more adult roles. For males, these can involve abrupt separation from their mothers and from other women and initiation into the company and behaviors of men.

Gender identity development also includes ideas about reproductive capacity, which are more elaborated for the girl. Ideas about her ability to have children are both concrete and the subject of fantasy for her, because her reproductive capacities are not real but only potential until she reaches sexual maturity. In fact, one aspect of the adult female body, the breasts, does not appear until puberty. The boy has a somewhat different experience than the girl in that, although his genitals change in size and shape, all of his genitalia are visible and present at birth.

Older controversies about the course and determinants of gender development concerned the extent to which it depends on the awareness of genital differences, the role of hormones, and the importance of the shift to genital drives and experiences from early, pregenital ones. For example, for a long time, the questions as to whether the little girl is aware of the existence of her vagina and whether she perceives the clitoris to be an inferior penis were important issues. It is now thought that the girl is aware of the existence of her vagina early in life and that her sense of her femininity does not depend so heavily on this specific knowledge (Clower 1976; Lerner 1976). The sense of inferiority that women describe in their feelings about their bodies is strongly determined by cultural attitudes and also, when it is present, by identification with mothers who feel depressed or defective. It is clear that not all women feel negative about their gender or their bodies.

Certain psychological characteristics that have been described as more prominent in men than in women, such as the importance of establishing boundaries, categories, and rigid classifications (Chodorow 1989), have been linked with the man's need to continually mark the distance and difference from his strong, maternal, preoedipal ties and identifications. Research findings support the existence of male-female personality differences in this culture (Gilligan

1982; Russo 1991). Women are found to be more affiliative and more invested in maintaining relationships, whereas men are more "instrumental" and "independent," that is, action oriented and oriented to "doing" (Block 1976; Chodorow 1989; Freud 1925).

Both mothers and fathers behave differently toward their female children than toward their male children from earliest infancy (Block 1976; Moss 1967). These behaviors transmit cultural patterns that promote and consolidate gender differences. Personality differences between men and women are also shaped by these processes, as well as by biological factors.

The importance of pregnancy and motherhood as a source of emotional maturation for the mother was emphasized in earlier psychoanalytic literature (Benedek 1970; Bibring et al. 1961; Notman and Lester 1988). Current views support this as a factor but also include the importance of parenthood for both parents (Anthony and Benedek 1970; Cath et al. 1989). It is, of course, possible to become a parent and not experience the maturational effect by remaining remote, preoccupied, and unaffected, or by becoming overwhelmed. For women who do not become pregnant or mothers, there are other pathways for reworking their identification with their mothers.

SEXUALITY

Along with other classical psychoanalytic views about women's development and psychology, the concepts of passivity, dependency, and masochism as the "feminine trio" led to a view of female sexuality that did not include activity or gratification. Set in the Victorian culture, it did not take into account historical or cross-cultural evidence. Women were seen as accepting of sexual activity in order to please their partner or to become pregnant, although Freud (1931) recognized female sexual desire and the importance of sexual gratification.

Another change from earlier writings on sexuality concerns the idea that there is a difference between a vaginal orgasm and a clitoral orgasm, and that the capacity for vaginal orgasm was associated with the attainment of greater developmental maturity. This is no longer the prevailing view in the face of the studies of sexual response by Masters and Johnson (1970) and the work of Kaplan and others. (Kaplan 1974; Kirkpatrick et al. 1981). Normal sexual functioning involves the sexual relationship and both partners. It is therefore not usually appropriate to discuss disorders such as frigidity or premature ejaculation outside the context of the other partner's response.

That there has been a "revolution" in sexual attitudes and behaviors has been recognized. The availability of contraceptives has made unintended pregnancy less of a risk than it was formerly, and views about female sexuality have changed. Contraception has also made possible the separation of sexuality from reproduction. Sexual pleasure as a goal for women and sexual activity outside of marriage have become more acceptable. Although there has been new attention to sexual functioning as an important area of gratification and health, there do appear to be some differences in men's and women's attitudes and experiences of sexuality. For women particularly, sexual functioning is preferably linked with a relationship that offers intimacy and that satisfies needs other than those of sexual gratification only (Person 1980). For men particularly, sexual performance consolidates gender identity. It is not clear how much the physiological differences in male and female sexual response cycles affect the psychological experiences.

HOMOSEXUALITY

Just as patterns of heterosexual behavior vary, so do patterns of homosexual behavior. Some lesbians living in committed relationships choose to have children by adoption or artificial insemination. Some have arranged for known donors, whereas others have chosen anonymous donors. Different kinds of relationships have been emerging as these families develop. There is as yet no definite data about how these families fare, but other studies (Kirkpatrick et al. 1981) of homosexual parents do not indicate that a high degree of pathology exists in their children.

There are also differences in the dynamics of male and female homosexuality. Some capacity to respond erotically under some circumstances to individuals of the same sex is probably universal. Whereas for some individuals a homosexual orientation seems the only possible way, for others, there seems to be more of a choice. Individuals with homosexual orientations sometimes marry and have children and then later act upon these homosexual feelings and "come out," usually breaking up the marriage. Some have homosexual relationships during a marriage. Sometimes the feelings of emotional and sexual attraction to individuals of the same sex are unconscious until some experience or life circumstance mobilizes them. Sometimes they are conscious but not acted upon until a later time.

CONTRACEPTION

The effectiveness of contraception depends on both the effectiveness of the individual method of contraception and how well the method fits the life-style and preferences of the person who is using it. Many effective contraceptive methods do not take into account individual preferences, so that they may not be used as intended. Thus, they may be less effective in practice than a less-foolproof method to which there is less resistance. For example, a woman who hesitates to touch or explore her genitals may be inhibited in using a diaphragm. In order for a contraceptive decision to be made, it is also important to take into account the nature of the sexual relationship between the two people.

The only available reversible method of contraception for men is the condom, which has the additional benefit of protection from sexually transmitted diseases, especially acquired immunodeficiency syndrome (AIDS). Since it needs to be used with, and interrupts, each act of intercourse, however, some couples find it awkward to use. It is perceived to interfere with spontaneity, romance, and sensation. For a man who has anxieties about sexual performance, these problems can forestall condom use. Condoms are also less effective than other means of contraception because they can break or fall off, a possibility that creates anxiety.

Vasectomy was advocated some years ago but is currently used less often. It is sometimes, but not reliably, reversible with microsurgical techniques. The decision for sterilization is often made because a couple feels that they are in a stable marriage and have the number of children they want. They may later regret their decision when a subsequent marriage or the death of a child evokes new desires for parenthood. Some women have also chosen more permanent methods, such as tubal ligation or even hysterectomy. These have been used after a woman has had children or, less often, to prevent pregnancies. This is done for complex reasons that are sometimes adaptive and sometimes self-destructive. Hysterectomy is also used for contraception, explicitly or not, by some women who have religious prohibitions against the use of birth control.

Another important consideration in assessing which contraceptives to use is the individual's capacity for planning, the individual's degree of impulsiveness, the availability of various methods, and unconscious resistances. A person's life circumstances can also contribute to the appropriateness of a particular method. For example, a young girl living with parents who do not know and would not approve of her sexual activity is likely to have trouble with a diaphragm, since she has to keep it hidden, which may be difficult.

Oral contraceptives, although generally safe and effective, seem less acceptable to some women who are not in stable relationships. These women do not want to take medication continually when sex can be sporadic, especially since there are side effects and uncertain long-term effects. Medical contraindications against the use of oral contraceptives also need to be considered. There are also reported instances in which instructions have been given to take the pill regularly, but the woman continues to use it sporadically or only in relation to each sexual experience (Lidz 1978).

Barrier methods, such as the diaphragm and spermicidal creams or jellies, require planning with the expectation of intercourse and the willingness to interrupt sexual activity, which can be particularly difficult for adolescents. For many young women, the use of a method such as the diaphragm implies that she expects to have sex, which can be difficult for her to acknowledge. As noted above, the diaphragm must be inserted into the vagina, and this requires a willingness to touch the genitals.

Diaphragms and oral contraceptives must be prescribed by a physician. Many young people do not have access to medical resources, either for economic reasons or because they live in a community where it would become known or where there are barriers to getting medical help for themselves independently of their families.

Some men may consciously want to use contraceptives but may have unconscious resistances related to the link between masculinity and potency and the ability to impregnate a woman. Interference with pregnancy is thus experienced as a threat to masculinity. A man may also resent having to pay attention to contraception because he sees it as "a woman's job" and the resulting pregnancies as her concern (Notman and Nadelson 1978).

Unconscious wishes for a pregnancy may also interfere with a woman's use of contraceptives. Becoming pregnant may be an unconscious way of reacting to a loss or a disappointment (Notman and Lester 1988). Women who experience conflicts about a career choice can become pregnant in an unconscious attempt to avoid the conflict.

CONSULTATION-LIAISON PSYCHIATRY

The psychiatrist working in obstetrics and gynecology has several roles, including a consultative one in which patients with psychiatric symptoms such as depression, psychosis, and behavior disorders, as well as functional disorders and psychosomatic illnesses, are evaluated. Liaison activities include teaching and offering a psychiatric perspective for understanding obstetric-gynecologic problems. This requires assimilating and integrating information from several fields, including obstetrics-gynecology, endocrinology, and psychiatry.

A growing body of recent information in areas such as contraception, pregnancy, induced abortion, sterilization, rape, menopause, and sexual functioning has challenged widely held myths and provided new insights and information, expanding the liaison role of psychiatrists (Nadelson et al. 1985). Formal consultation in these areas is not often sought, since the problems are not always defined as psychiatric and, in fact, may occur in "normal" patients, such as pregnant women. Problems may also involve the relationship between physician and patient, for example, noncompliance with medication or a regimen or differences between the patient and physician in priorities and wishes.

Because the area of reproduction and sexuality is so clearly a highly emotionally charged one and the obstetrician-gynecologist physician is also vulnerable to emotional responses to sexuality and reproduction, he or she may avoid investigating these concerns with patients, just as others do. Many emotionally related problems may be avoided by the physician and may be referred to the office nurse, to the hospital social worker, or to less experienced or knowledgeable people. "Delegating the feelings" is supported by attitudes deriving from early training in medical school, where students generally have been taught about sexuality and reproduction only incidentally, while studying other subjects, and in a neutral way, to increase "objectivity." Therefore, information about sex and reproduction may not be integrated in such a way that it specifically addresses the kinds of problems faced by physicians in practice. The practitioner does not have ready answers.

The obstetrician-gynecologist functions as the primary care physician for many women, is often the exclusive physician for women during their reproductive years, and provides care for women during a number of critical life phases. Attention to sexuality and the emotional aspects of gynecologic problems is therefore especially important. The liaison psychiatrist can play an important role in this area. The gynecologist must also become accustomed to new realities, including the possibility of sexually transmitted diseases in a wide cross-section of patients, requests for contraceptive services and sexual counseling for unmarried couples, and gynecologic care of patients identifying themselves as bisexual or lesbian. The fact that many women postpone pregnancy until their education and training are completed or their careers established means that the older pregnant woman is seen more often. Furthermore, a number of women, many of whom are nulliparous and in their early 20s, seek surgical sterilization.

The new reproductive technologies have raised clinical as well as ethical issues for which the gynecologist may be unprepared. The physician may often be asked to perform a permanent procedure, to act merely as a technician who has no part to play in the decision made by the patient. The role and responsibility of the physician, the patient, and, indeed, of society are being questioned from ethical, political, medical, psychological, and economic perspectives. The liaison psychiatrist must be aware of these changed social realities and may be in a position to integrate and interpret their implications, especially for the physician whose major focus may be on the medical priorities.

REFERENCES

Anthony EJ, Benedek T (eds): Summing up, in Parenthood: Its Psychology and Psychopathology. Boston, MA, Little, Brown, 1970, pp 599–603

Benedek T: The psychobiology of pregnancy, in Parenthood: Its Psychology and Psychopathology. Edited by Anthony EJ, Benedek T. Boston, MA, Little, Brown, 1970, pp 137–151

Bernard J: The Future of Marriage. New York, Bantam Books, 1973

Bernard J: Women, Wives, and Mothers: Values and Options. Chicago, IL, Aldine, 1975

Bernard J: Ground rules for marriage: perspectives on the pattern of an era, in Women and Men: New Perspectives on Gender Differences. Edited by Notman MT, Nadelson CC. Washington, DC, American Psychiatric Press, 1991, pp 89–115

Bibring G, Dwyer T, Huntington D, et al: A study of the psychological processes in pregnancy and of the earliest mother-child relationship. Psychoanal Study Child 16:9–72, 1961

Block J: Assessing sex differences: issues, problems, and pitfalls. Merrill Palmer Quarterly, Vol 22, October 1976

Brown GW, Harris T: Social Origins of Depression. New York, Free Press, 1978

Bunker JP, Donohue VC, Cole P, et al: Elective hysterectomy—pro and con. N Engl J Med 295:264–268, 1976

Cath S, Gurwitt A, Ginsberg L: Fathers and Their Families. Hillsdale, NJ, Analytic Press, 1989

Chodorow N: The Reproduction of Mothering: Psychoanalysis and the Sociology of Gender. Berkeley, University of California Press, 1978

Chodorow N: Feminism and Psychoanalytic Theory. New Haven, CT, Yale University Press, 1989

Clower V: Theoretical implications in current views of masturbation in latency girls. J Am Psychoanal Assoc 24:109–125, 1976

Clower VL: The acquisition of mature femininity, in Women and Men: New Perspectives on Gender Differences. Edited by Notman MT, Nadelson CC. Washington, DC, American Psychiatric Press, 1991, pp 75–88

Fast I: Gender Identity: A Differentiation Model. Hillsdale, NJ, Analytic Press, 1984

Freud S: Three essays on the theory of sexuality (1905), in The Standard Edition of the Complete Psychological Works of Sigmund Freud, Vol 7. Translated and edited by Strachey J. London, Hogarth Press, 1953, pp 135–243

Freud S: The dissolution of the Oedipus complex (1924), in The Standard Edition of the Complete Psychological Works of Sigmund Freud, Vol 19. Translated and edited by Strachey J. London, Hogarth Press, 1961, pp 171–179

Freud S: Some psychical consequences of the anatomical distinction between the sexes (1925), in The Standard Edition of the Complete Psychological Works of Sigmund Freud, Vol 19. Translated and edited by Strachey J. London, Hogarth Press, 1961, pp 248–258

Freud S: Female sexuality (1931), in The Standard Edition of the Complete Psychological Works of Sigmund Freud, Vol 21. Translated and edited by Strachey J. London, Hogarth Press, 1961, pp 223–243

Freud S: Femininity (1933), in The Standard Edition of the Complete Psychological Works of Sigmund Freud, Vol 22. Translated and edited by Strachey J. London, Hogarth Press, 1964, pp 112–135

Friedman E: The physiological aspects of pregnancy, in The Woman Patient, Vol 1: Medical and Psychological Interfaces. Edited by Notman MT, Nadelson CC. New York, Plenum, 1978, pp 55–71

Gilligan C: In a Different Voice: Psychological Theory and Women's Development. Cambridge, MA, Harvard University Press, 1982

Gove WR, Tudor JF: Adult sex roles and mental illness. American Journal of Sociology 78:812–835, 1973

Grossman W, Stewart W: Penis envy: from childhood wish to developmental metaphor. J Am Psychoanal Assoc 24:193–212, 1976

Kaltreider N, Wallace A, Horowitz M: A first study of the stress response syndrome: young women after hysterectomy. JAMA 242:1499, 1979

Kaplan HS: The New Sex Therapy. New York, Brunner/Mazel, 1974

Kirkpatrick M, Smith C, Roy R: Lesbian mothers and their children: a comparative survey. Am J Orthopsychiatry 51:543–551, 1981

Kuhlen R, Johnson G: Changes in goals with adults of increasing age. Journal of Consulting Psychology 12:1–4, 1952

Kuhn M: How mates are sorted, in Family, Marriage and Parenthood. Edited by Becker H, Hill R. Boston, MA, DC Heath, 1955

Lerner H: Parental mislabeling of female genitals as a determinant of penis envy and learning inhibitions in women. J Am Psychoanal Assoc 24:269–283, 1976

LeVine RA: Gender differences: interpreting anthropological data, in Women and Men: New Perspectives on Gender Differences. Edited by Notman MT, Nadelson CC. Washington, DC, American Psychiatric Press, 1991, pp 1–8

Lidz R: Conflicts between fertility and infertility, in The Woman Patient, Vol 1: Medical and Psychological Interfaces. Edited by Notman M, Nadelson C. New York, Plenum, 1978, pp 131–137

Masters W, Johnson V: Human Sexual Inadequacy. Boston, MA, Little, Brown, 1970

Mazor M: The problem of infertility, in The Woman Patient, Vol 1: Medical and Psychological Interfaces. Edited by Notman MT, Nadelson CC. New York, Plenum, 1978, pp 137–160

McDougall J: The dead father. Int J Psychoanal 70:205–219, 1989

Moss H: Sex, age and state as determinants of mother-infant interaction. Merrill Palmer Quarterly 13:19–36, 1967

Nadelson CC: Issues in the analyses of single women in their thirties and forties in the middle years, in New Psychoanalytic Perspectives. Edited by Oldham S, Liebert R. New Haven, CT, Yale University Press, 1989, pp 105–122

Nadelson CC, Notman MT: To marry or not to marry: a choice. Am J Psychiatry 138:1352–1356, 1981

Nadelson CC, Notman MT, Ellis EA: Psychosomatic aspects of obstetrics and gynecology, in Psychosomatic Illness Review. Edited by Dorfman W, Cristofar L. New York, Macmillan, 1985, pp 162–179

Notman MT: Pregnancy and abortion: implications for career development of professional women. Ann N Y Acad Sci 208:205–210, 1973

Notman MT: Midlife concerns of women: implications of the menopause. Am J Psychiatry 136:1270–1274, 1979

Notman MT: Gender development, in Women and Men: New Perspectives on Gender Differences. Edited by Notman MT, Nadelson CC. Washington, DC, American Psychiatric Press, 1991, pp 117–127

Notman MT, Lester E: Pregnancy: theoretical considerations. Psychoanalytic Inquiry 8:139–159, 1988

Notman MT, Nadelson CC (eds): The Woman Patient, Vol 1: Medical and Psychological Interfaces. New York, Plenum, 1978

Notman MT, Nadelson CC: Changing views of femininity and childbearing. Hillside Journal of Clinical Psychiatry 3:187–202, 1981

Notman MT, Klein R, Jordan JV, et al: Women's unique developmental issues across the life cycle, in American Psychiatric Press Review of Psychiatry, Vol 10. Edited by Tasman A, Goldfinger SM. Washington, DC, American Psychiatric Press, 1991, pp 556–577

Person E: Sexuality as a mainstay of identity: psychoanalytic perspectives, in Women: Sex and Sexuality. Edited by Stimpson C, Person E. Chicago, IL, University of Chicago Press, 1980, pp 36–61

Russo NF: Reconstructing the psychology of women: an overview, in Women and Men: New Perspectives on Gender Differences. Edited by Notman MT, Nadelson CC. Washington, DC, American Psychiatric Press, 1991, pp 43–61

Silverman M: Cognitive development and female psychology. J Am Psychoanal Assoc 29:581–605, 1981

Stein P: Single in America. Englewood Cliffs, NJ, Prentice-Hall, 1976

Stoller RJ: Primary femininity. J Am Psychoanal Assoc 24:59–78, 1976

Veevers J: Voluntary childlessness: a review of issues and evidence. Man and Family Review 2:1–26, 1979

Chapter 18

FEMALE SEXUAL DISORDERS

R. T. Segraves, M.D., Ph.D.
K. B. Segraves, Ph.D.

❖ ❖ ❖ ❖ ❖ ❖ ❖ ❖ ❖ ❖ ❖ ❖ ❖ ❖

Sexual function is influenced by complicated and interactive biological and psychological factors. Thus, the diagnosis of sexual dysfunction is complicated because of the numerous diverse etiologies that must be considered. The differential diagnosis of sexual disorders is not widely understood by psychiatrists. Because of the possibility of interaction between biological and psychological factors, the evaluation of many disorders of female sexual function by necessity involves the close collaboration between specialists in obstetrics-gynecology and those in psychiatry. The psychiatric clinician will focus on a careful sexual and psychiatric history, attempting to ascertain the specific nature of the problem (e.g., affective disorder, marital discord, or transient stress) and whether it appears to be secondary to other psychiatric disease. The evaluation by the gynecologist will be equally meticulous and will attempt to rule out diverse physical etiologies, including vulvovaginitis, hormonal changes associated with menopause or perimenopause, and endometriosis.

Although the field of gynecology has shown an increasing awareness of the need to assess sexual function, most gynecologists recognize the need to collaborate with psychiatrists in this assessment. It is indeed the rare psychiatrist or gynecologist who is capable of independent assessment and treatment of the full spectrum of female sexual disorders. The requisite knowledge base crosses subspecialty boundaries and is still evolving. In the evaluation of erectile problems in males, there are several standard protocols that can be followed. These would probably include nocturnal penile tumescence studies, penile blood pressure, and serum testosterone and prolactin determination, as well as pudendal nerve conduction studies. Similar protocols for the evaluation of female sexual problems are not available. For example, the role of androgen therapy in postmenopausal women with low sexual desire is controversial. Similarly, the usefulness of vaginal photoplethysmography in evaluating female arousal disorders is unclear, and pudendal nerve conduction studies are rarely utilized in the evaluation of female patients with anorgasmia. This chapter examines various topics at the interface of psychiatry and gynecology concerning female sexual response.

NOMENCLATURE

A review of the historical development of the nomenclature utilized to describe female sexual disorders will be helpful in highlighting the rapidly changing terminology in this area of psychiatry. Some consensus regarding terminology resulted from Masters and Johnson's (1966) description of four stages of sexual responses (excitement, plateau, orgasm, and resolution) and definitions of three separate female psychosexual disorders: dyspareunia, vaginismus, and orgasmic dysfunction (primary and secondary). For approximately 10 years, the diagnostic system introduced by Masters and Johnson was utilized by most clinicians and clinical investigators. A major change in diagnostic nomenclature resulted from two sex therapists—Lief (1977), who identified the phenomena of low sexual desire, and Kaplan (1977, 1979), who introduced a three-stage model of sexual response: desire, excitement, and orgasm. Kaplan's concepts clearly influenced DSM-III (American Psychiatric Association 1980). In this manual, there are separate diagnoses for inhibited orgasm. In the revised manual, DSM-III-R (American Psychiatric Association 1987), a sexual aversion disorder was included. The other major changes were changes in terminology. For example, inhibited sexual excitement was now labeled hypoactive sexual desire disorder. Therefore, what may previously have been diagnosed as frigidity or general sexual unresponsiveness may now be diagnosed as hypoactive sexual desire disorder. Obviously, the rapid changes in terminology make it extremely difficult to combine findings from literature only 10–15 years ago with the findings of contemporary investigations.

Most investigators stress the importance of accurately diagnosing the phase of the sexual response cycle that is impaired. Kaplan (1983a) postulates that the earlier the impairment in the sexual response cycle, the worse the psychopathology and prognosis. This hypothesis, however, has not been subjected to empirical investigation.

PREVALENCE

It is difficult to obtain true estimates of the incidence and prevalence of female sexual disorders in the general population, as few studies have employed random sampling of the population, standardized sexual interviews, or operationalized definitions of syndromes (Nathan 1986; Spector and Carey, in press). The changing nosology mentioned in the preceding section also contributes to the difficulty in combining the available data base.

A number of studies have indicated that these disorders are quite common in general medical and gynecological clinics (Burnap and Golden 1967; Catalan et al. 1981; Ende et al. 1984; Levine and Yost 1976). For example, Ende et al. (1984) reported that 27% of women attending a general medical practice reported lack of sexual desire, and 25% reported lack of orgasm. In a study of sexual problems in a gynecologic clinic, Levine and Yost (1976) found that 17% of the women reported difficulty achieving orgasm in partner-related activity.

Studies reporting the frequency with which different syndromes appear in treatment settings have reported high frequencies of orgasm disorders (Bancroft and Coles 1976; Renshaw 1988) and desire disorders (Hawton et al. 1986; Lief 1985; LoPiccollo 1980; Schover and LoPiccollo 1982). Most investigators have reported female arousal disorder to be somewhat rarely encountered in clinical practice (Nathan 1986). Vaginismus and dyspareunia both appear to have a prevalence rate close to 5% (Renshaw 1988).

The largest modern study of the relative prevalence of female sexual disorder was the result of a large multisite pharmaceutical study

(R. T. Segraves and Segraves 1991; K. B. Segraves and Segraves 1991). Of 532 women seeking treatment for sexual problems, 475 (89%) had a primary diagnosis of hypoactive sexual desire disorder. Only 40 women had a primary diagnosis of female arousal disorder, and only 17 had orgasm disorders as a primary diagnosis. One of the most remarkable findings of this study was the frequency with which patients had multiple diagnoses. Of the women with a primary diagnosis of hypoactive sexual desire disorder, 41% had either an arousal or orgasm disorder as well, and 18% had disorders of all three phases of the sexual response cycle.

DIFFERENTIAL DIAGNOSIS

It is important to emphasize that both biological and psychological factors may coexist in the genesis of sexual disorders. Thus, rather than attempt to diagnose whether the problem is organic or psychogenic in etiology, the clinician should focus on which factor is the major contributor to the problem and which factor is correctable. In general, problems that are situational or partner-specific will be predominantly psychogenic in etiology (Moore 1989). Similarly, lifelong problems often have a large psychogenic component (Kaplan 1983b). In clinical practice, the presumption of a predominantly psychogenic etiology for a sexual problem is often made when a biological etiology has been excluded by gynecologic examination.

Dyspareunia

Dyspareunia is a commonly encountered complaint in gynecologic practice and most often has a primary organic etiology (Smith and Buck 1983; Wabrek and Wabrek 1975). Although a variety of physical factors may cause dyspareunia (Kaufman 1983a; Moore 1989), the three most common organic causes are vaginitis, pelvic infections, and senile vaginitis (Smith and Buck 1983). The most common psychological cause of dyspareunia is lack of sexual arousal (Sarrel and Sarrel 1989), which may have numerous etiologies. All cases of dyspareunia should be considered as having a biological component until proven otherwise.

Vaginismus

Vaginismus is caused by involuntary contractions of the perivaginal muscle (Van de Wiel et al. 1990). These involuntary contractions may result from any cause of severe pelvic pain, such as endometriosis and pelvic inflammatory disease, or from a psychological fear of penetration (Green 1983; Kaplan 1983b). Although many forms of vaginismus occur with any attempt at vaginal penetration (e.g., coitus, pelvic examination, tampons), some cases may occur only with coitus and not during a pelvic examination. Thus, the absence of vaginal contractions during a pelvic examination does not rule out this diagnosis.

Hypoactive Sexual Desire Disorder

Concern regarding disorders of sexual desire have assumed a position of increased importance in the field of sex therapy and are some of the most perplexing and prevalent of the sexual disorders (Leiblum and Rosen 1988; Rosen and Leiblum 1989). One of the first steps in differential diagnosis is to determine whether the problem is primary or appears secondary to another disorder. For example, decreased sexual desire may be a response to other sexual dysfunction (Levine 1989), chronic illness (Bullard 1988; Schover and Jensen 1988), or depressive illness (Levine 1989) or a side effect of medication (R. T. Segraves 1988a). A second step in differential diagnosis is to determine whether the problem is global or situational. If a patient reports decreased sexual desire in her relationship but normal sexual fantasies and frequent masturbation, the clinician would suspect relationship deterioration as a probable etiology. Lifelong patterns of low sexual desire are generally assumed to be psychogenic in etiology, although it is quite possible that some patients have lifelong patterns of low sexual desire secondary to constitutional factors. The role of hormonal influences in the genesis of hypoactive sexual desire disorders is unclear (R. T. Segraves 1988b). Although some investigators have reported beneficial effects from androgen therapy in patients who have undergone surgical menopause (i.e., oophorectomy), it is unclear whether assessment of androgen levels should become part of the routine assessment of women with desire disorders.

Female Sexual Arousal Disorder

Information concerning female arousal disorder is limited (Moore
1989; Nathan 1986; R. T. Segraves and Segraves, in press), and this
diagnosis is infrequently made in psychiatric practice. In one multisite
study of 532 female patients with sexual disorder, only 8% had this
diagnosis. Most of the patients with this diagnosis also had problems
with desire and/or orgasm as well. Less than 2% had female sexual
arousal disorder as a solitary diagnosis.

According to DSM-III-R, the diagnosis of female arousal disorder
can be made if there is a failure of subjective sexual arousal or a failure
of vaginal lubrication. It is not uncommon for a discrepancy to exist
between subjective and objective measures of sexual arousal (Heiman
1980) and for some women to experience vaginal lubrication without
conscious awareness of subjective sexual arousal (Hoon and Hoon
1978; Steinman et al. 1981). In clinical practice, psychogenic arousal
disorders usually present as a failure of subjective sexual arousal. A
complaint of failure of lubrication in the presence of increased subjective arousal is most often due to estrogen deficiency (Bancroft 1983).
Diabetes mellitus may also be associated with a decreased lubrication
response to sexual stimulation (Kaufman 1983b).

Inhibited Female Orgasm

A careful sexual history is paramount in the differential diagnosis of
inhibited female orgasm. First, it is necessary to establish whether the
disorder is lifelong or acquired.

Lifelong inhibited female orgasm is rarely due to organic factors
(Kaplan 1983b) and may spontaneously remit in the early years of
marriage (Kinsey et al. 1953). It is widely accepted that the ability to
have an orgasm can be attained with learning and practice (Moore
1989). There is minimal evidence relating anorgasmia with psychiatric
disease.

Acquired inhibited female orgasm may be due to a variety of psychological and biological factors. If the problem is situational (e.g.,
anorgasmic with husband but easily orgasmic with masturbation or an
alternative partner), the clinician should immediately suspect rela-

tionship deterioration. Global acquired inhibited female orgasm may be due to affective disorder, anxiety disorder, or overwhelming transient stress.

In most of the cases mentioned here, sexual desire and arousal will also be affected. If the patient reports a decreased capacity to become orgasmic despite normal libido and normal sexual arousal, one should consider the possibility of organic etiologies. A variety of physical causes for anorgasmia exist (R. T. Segraves and Segraves, in press). One first would attempt to rule out correctable causes such as pharmacological side effects (R. T. Segraves 1985). A variety of neurological conditions, such as spinal cord lesions (Berard 1989), multiple sclerosis (Lilius et al. 1976; Lundberg 1978), and surgery injuring the neurological innervation of the genitals (Consolo et al. 1989), may result in the inability to reach orgasm. Current evidence is contradictory concerning the prevalence of anorgasmia in women with diabetes mellitus (Kolodny 1971; Schreiner-Engel et al. 1987). Although it has been proposed that weak pubococcygeal muscles may decrease sexual responsivity (Kegel 1956), there is little evidence to support this contention (Chambless et al. 1984).

PSYCHOTHERAPEUTIC TREATMENT

Treatment for sexual complaints has and continues to evolve, beginning from a strict psychoanalytic intrapsychic approach, to a basic behavioral approach involving prescribing a "set" of homework exercises (regardless of the complaint), to the present approach, which relies on an individualized multiple perspective. Sexual functioning is dependent on multiple intrapsychic factors, such as culture, values, beliefs, assumptions, and expectations, as well as environmental factors. The biological components (chronic health conditions, hormones, medication) and developmental events (menstruation, pregnancy, childbirth, and aging), although poorly understood in females, point to the complexity of sexual functioning.

Today, therapists draw from multiple theoretical orientations when designing treatment approaches. Patients today present with what look like more complicated complaints. One explanation for this is the way in which we now define sexual complaints. Another possible explanation is that most women now seeking treatment have tried various techniques suggested in self-help books and recommended by the popular press. Gone are the days when a woman would present with the problem of anorgasmia and masturbation training would quickly reverse the problem.

Today, a woman may present with the complaint of hypoactive sexual desire. When the therapist explores the problem, this woman reports no problem with arousal or orgasm. The interview reveals no medications or medical conditions that might help to explain the problem. The woman reports she is in a "good" and stable relationship and cannot identify any external stressors that might relate to her complaint. Another example is of a woman with the complaint of secondary anorgasmia. This woman's history reveals that she was molested by an uncle when she was 10. The woman is a computer analyst, has been married for the past 12 years, and has a 9-year-old daughter. This woman describes her marriage as stable and her husband as loving and nonabusive. Still another example is of a woman presenting with the complaint of an unconsummated, 12-year, "stable and caring" relationship. Simply prescribing "sensate focus" exercises to the women described by these examples would be a disservice. Indiscriminately assigning set exercises may exacerbate some sexual problems by emphasizing the negative associations to the behaviors or may increase anxiety due to the performance component of the exercise. Such a treatment approach may diminish self-esteem or exacerbate partner conflict.

Therapists who treat the sexual complaints of women are made painfully aware of the paucity of available research concerning the sexual functioning of women. Women who present for treatment of sexual concerns necessitate both creative thinking and tenacity on the part of the therapist. A careful and comprehensive biopsychosocial assessment can aid in preparing effective treatment approaches. Identifying the predominant sexual phase that is involved in the complaint and the associated phases that may be secondarily affected is important in designing effective treatment plans.

For example, a woman may report that she is unable to reach orgasm during extensive and what she determines to be adequate stimulation. Given the number of effective treatment approaches for anorgasmia, the therapist might be tempted to begin treatment. Further questioning, however, might reveal that this patient engages in sexual behavior when she experiences no sexual desire or drive. She reports the need to use artificial lubricant, as she reports being "dry" during foreplay. The woman denies having any pain during intercourse. When questioned, she reports that she is never conscious of "wanting" to engage in sexual activity of any kind. She is a "willing and compliant" participant in sexual activity initiated by her partner because, by her report, she cares very much for her husband and for their relationship.

Here, the presumptive diagnosis is anorgasmia secondary to hypoactive desire disorder. This diagnosis is generally more difficult to reverse completely. Treatment would be tailored to the presumed contributing factors, with the realization that not much is known about the possible biologic contributing factors.

The therapist might want to interview the couple to determine how each perceives and explains the problem. The woman might be asked to become more aware of her sexual thoughts and level of sexual desire, independent of her partner's. Therapy might first focus on helping the woman to identify her internal dialogue, noting what is sexually enhancing and what is a sexual "turnoff." Attempting to build on any desire-enhancing thoughts and behaviors may provide a starting point from which an attempt can be made to increase the woman's sexual awareness. This woman might benefit from "fantasy training" exercises, or an increase of exploratory exposure to romantic or erotic materials (novels that are erotic and not necessarily explicit). These activities would be mutually arrived at (between therapist and patient) and carried out without "expecting" an increase in drive, rather having her "just experience" the activity. Hence, this is done more as awareness training rather than as the creation of a performance ideal. This might be followed by exploration of her internal dialogue during sexual activity or during exposure to sexual material, identifying what her attitudes or feelings are regarding her internal dialogue. The goal would be to make the woman more aware of her own drive level, her sexual thoughts or fantasies, and her own comfort level for a range of sexual activities.

In time, the woman and her partner might benefit from "sensate-focus" exercises (pleasuring experiences) to help them learn what enhances or detracts from sexual arousal. During this treatment, the partner would benefit from knowing the treatment plan and being included in the process. The partner's cooperation and sensitivity would be important to the successful treatment of this problem. He might be asked to put his needs on hold temporarily, in an effort to promote his partner's explorations into her sexuality.

This example demonstrates the need to individualize treatment approaches. Although sensate-focus exercises have a place in the treatment of certain sexual complaints, they are presented as a part of a more comprehensive approach to the woman's presenting problem. Treatment of sexual complaints might necessitate drawing from a mass of cumulative theories and techniques (psychodynamic, systems theory, cognitive-behavioral, marital, family, stress management, communication skills training, social skills training, etc.). It is hoped that biological determinants of female sexual functioning will be identified in the near future, which will help in the design of more effective and efficient treatment approaches to female sexual complaints.

EFFECT OF PREGNANCY ON SEXUAL BEHAVIOR

With a few exceptions (Masters and Johnson 1966), most investigators have reported a gradual decline in sexual interest as pregnancy progresses (Reamy et al. 1982; White and Reamy 1982). The decline is precipitous in the third trimester (Perkins 1982) and is accompanied by a decline in coital frequency (Cohen 1985; Perkins 1982) and in noncoital sexual activity (Cohen 1985). This decline in sexual activity is more marked in nulliparous than in multiparous women and is more marked in women who demonstrated minimal sexual interest prior to pregnancy (Cohen 1985). It should be noted that the decline in sexual activity during pregnancy has been found in multiple countries (Cohen 1985).

Various explanations have been advanced for this decline in sexual activity. Massive changes in hormone levels take place during pregnancy and the postpartum period, which could contribute to the change in sexual activity. However, there is no evidence linking these endocrine changes to changes in sexual activity. Cultural and psychological factors are more likely to account for the change in sexual interest (Bancroft 1983). Religious and cultural taboos against sex during pregnancy are common (Bancroft 1983), and fears that sexual activity will cause miscarriage or complications of pregnancy, although unproven, are ingrained in many societies (Cohen 1985). Ambivalence and increased emotional lability are also common during pregnancy, and many couples who are comfortable with independent lives may greet the increased dependence induced by pregnancy with conflicted feelings. In addition to affecting a woman's sense of body image, the somatic changes during pregnancy often require modification of sexual technique. Although sexual changes during pregnancy are common, they are often managed by the obstetrician with the psychiatric consultant rarely being utilized.

EFFECTS OF GYNECOLOGIC CONDITIONS AND PROCEDURES ON SEXUAL BEHAVIOR

Involuntary Infertility

The diagnosis of infertility can result in a narcissistic crisis in one or both partners, depending on the level of personal investment in having a child. Given all of the factors involved in the discovery, evaluation, treatment, and aftermath of infertility, one might expect profound relationship changes, including changes in sexual function.

There are daily reminders of one's infertility: commercials and movies with cherub-like children cooing in their parents' faces, demonstrating "the perfect" family; announcements of the arrival or expectation of a baby among family and friends; holidays that emphasize the family, with "Mother's Day" and "Father's Day" hitting closest to the source of the pain. Infertility may cause a series of emotions to begin to surface within the couple. One or both partners can begin to feel alone, empty, anxious, depressed, ugly, sexually inadequate, unproductive, barren, and responsible for a break in the continuity of one's family (Salzer 1986).

Sexual dysfunction can be the cause or the result of a couple experiencing infertility. A thorough psychosexual history is needed to determine whether the infertility is due to a sexual problem. Although they are in a minority, some sexual problems, such as premature ejaculation, vaginismus, impotence, and retrograde ejaculation, may contribute to infertility

When the male partner is unable to penetrate the vagina because the woman experiences vaginismus, the couple may benefit from sex therapy. Here, the woman is taught to begin to insert the smallest in a set of vaginal dilators. Once she is able to do this comfortably, her husband is instructed, under her guidance, to begin by inserting first his finger, then two, until the woman is mentally and physically ready to accommodate his penis. This process often requires a great deal of time and patience on the part of both couple and therapist. Treatment of infertility by artificial insemination with the husband's sperm would be an option during this process.

Although sexual dysfunction can be the cause of infertility, more often sexual dysfunction is the result of both the evaluation and the ongoing treatment of infertility. Usually, it is the woman who seeks treatment first. In many cases, she is seen a number of times before the partner becomes involved in the infertility evaluation. The woman will often undergo diagnostic tests that can be physically invasive and painful. Both partners may experience the evaluation and treatment of infertility as a major invasion of privacy. When the male partner is involved in the workup, he has less of a physician-patient relationship, which may lead him to feel like an outsider or just a "producer of sperm." Involving both partners early in the fertility workup can minimize some of these problems.

Vaginismus or erectile failure might only occur during the ovulatory period of the cycle (Drake and Grunert 1979) or prior to specific tests. Stress that is imposed by the demand to engage in a completed intravaginal intromission can result in lack of lubrication or vaginismus in the female and erectile failure in the male. The male partner may become impotent prior to certain tests (semen analysis, postcoital test, sperm penetration assay) for which he is asked to produce an erection and to ejaculate at a certain time of a specified day, while being cognizant that his sperm will be observed and graded within a couple of hours by a member of the treatment team.

During the process of trying to conceive, there comes a time when "infertility" becomes the final diagnosis. Even with all of the new techniques and advancements, the treatment of infertility does not always lead to successful pregnancy and childbirth. A responsible treatment team needs to address this issue, both among themselves and with the couple. Current research (Sauer et al. 1990) often reinforces the couple's denial, delaying the reparative work needed to go beyond infertility. Accepting the diagnosis of infertility may result in intense mourning. This mourning takes its toll on whatever sexual functioning is left in the relationship. Sexual apathy may be predominant, along with sexual avoidance. During the struggle to conceive, sex becomes associated with reproduction. Accepting the diagnosis of being infertile often results in the couple not wanting to engage in intercourse. Intercourse is a reminder of what can never be—"so why bother?" Others may become promiscuous or want to engage in sex frequently as a means of bolstering their sense of self-esteem or desirability.

Trying to recapture the active, spontaneous, mutually enjoyable sex life the couple once experienced prior to the diagnosis of infertility is a difficult and sometimes impossible task. Some couples are never able to resume earlier pleasures. Infertility and its treatment may end in broken relationships. Other couples struggle to find new and different ways to be intimate and to engage in sexual relations that do not resonate with the times and positions that became routine during their attempts to conceive. Some couples need time to become intimate again before they can resume intercourse. Physician and therapist must be sensitive to the wide variations in responses and the time needed to rebuild.

Menopause

With menopause, there is a marked drop in estrogen production that is often accompanied by vasomotor instability (hot flashes) and vaginal atrophy (Rinehart and Schiff 1985; Schover and Jensen 1988). A small number of women report some decline in sexual activity associated with menopause (Bachmann et al. 1985). Many factors may account for the decreased sexual activity accompanying menopause, including concomitant aging and decreased sexual ability in the partner (Coop 1984), sociocultural expectations (Semmens and Semmens 1984), psychological distress associated with the symbolic meaning of menopause (Rinehart and Schiff 1985), and discomfort with menopausal symptoms (McCoy et al. 1985). Estrogen replacement therapy may help to alleviate the physical symptoms of menopause and thus contribute to an increase in coital frequency, although it is doubtful that estrogen has a direct effect on libido (R. T. Segraves 1988b).

Two recent studies suggest that the reaction to erotic stimuli may undergo only minor changes with menopause. Morrell et al. (1984) found that postmenopausal women had decreased vaginal responses to erotic stimuli as compared with premenopausal women. There were also differences in subjective arousal. Myers and Morokoff (1985) did not find a difference between pre- and postmenopausal women in their vaginal response (measured by photoplethysmography) to erotic stimuli. In view of the multiple influences on sexuality in the menopausal female, an evaluation of a complaint of decreased sexual responsivity should involve close collaboration between the psychiatrist and the gynecologist.

Hysterectomy

The evidence concerning the sexual consequences of hysterectomy is unclear. Some investigators have found no evidence of a harmful effect of hysterectomy on sexual function (Coopen et al. 1981), whereas others have reported decreases in libido after this surgical procedure (Munday and Cox 1967; Zussman et al. 1981). Clearly, research in this area is complicated by numerous factors, including the psychological meaning of this event to the patient, the partner's reaction to the event, the degree of discomfort preceding the procedure, the presence or absence of postoperative complications, and whether the procedure included bilateral oophorectomy (R. T. Segraves 1988b).

There is evidence that estrogen-androgen preparations may be especially effective in restoring libido in women who have undergone surgical menopause. The first double-blind study was reported by Greenblatt et al. (1950). Postmenopausal women were randomly allocated to one of four groups taking diethylstilbestrol, methyltestosterone, a combination of both of these drugs, or placebo. The estrogen preparation relieved hot flashes, and the androgen preparation increased libido. Most women preferred the combination therapy. Similar findings have been reported more recently in Canada (Sherwin and Gelfand 1984, 1985; Sherwin et al. 1985). It should be noted that this therapy has not been embraced by most gynecologists in the United States.

Surgery for Malignancy

In recent years, interest has focused on sexual functioning after treatment of gynecological cancer (Andersen 1987; Capone et al. 1980; Schover et al. 1987). This research has documented considerable psychological distress and accompanying sexual disinterest after disfiguring surgical procedures (Andersen 1985).

Pelvic exenteration involves surgical removal of the uterus, fallopian tubes, ovaries, urinary bladder, rectum, and vagina. Surgical reconstruction of a neovagina is often performed; however, many patients report a total cessation of sexual activity after this surgery (Andersen and Hacher 1983; Broun et al. 1972; Demsey et al. 1975; Vera 1981).

Radical vulvectomy is often followed by loss of orgasmic capacity and blunting of genital sensation (Andersen and Hacker 1983; Andersen et al. 1988; DiSala et al. 1979). Schover and von Eschenbach (1985) reported that most women are able to resume normal sexual activity after radical cystectomy.

Other Surgical Procedures

Certain surgical procedures, such as sympathectomy, abdominoperitoneal resection, retroperitoneal lymphadenectomy, and aortoiliac surgery, interrupt the sympathetic innervation of the genital organs and cause male sexual problems. One would suspect that these procedures would also interfere with female sexual responsivity. However, there is minimal evidence concerning the sexual effects of these procedures in females (Schover and Jensen 1988).

Induced Abortion

An immediate negative response to therapeutic abortion is common (Friedman 1974). However, few women experience serious psychiatric complications or long-term adverse effects on sexual behavior (Gebhard et al. 1958).

ORAL CONTRACEPTIVES AND SEXUAL BEHAVIOR

The evidence concerning a relationship between oral contraceptive use and altered sexual behavior is inconclusive (R. T. Segraves 1988b). Although several investigators have reported that oral contraceptive use may be associated with diminished libido (Leeton et al. 1978), the bulk of the available evidence does not suggest that oral contraceptive use has a direct effect on libido (Bancroft 1983; Bardwick 1973; Cullberg 1972). Some women may experience diminished libido secondary to mild dysphoria or nausea during the first several months of oral contraceptive use. If a patient presents with a solitary complaint of diminished libido after beginning oral contraceptives and this does not appear to be related to the psychological meaning of using birth control, a reasonable approach would be to confer with the gynecologist concerning whether a trial of a different agent is warranted.

PSYCHIATRIC DRUGS AND SEXUAL FUNCTION

A relatively large amount of literature exists on the effects of drugs on male sexual function (R. T. Segraves et al. 1985). In contrast, the literature concerning drug effects on female sexual function is relatively sparse (R. T. Segraves 1985). Case reports suggest that monoamine oxidase inhibitors, heterocyclic antidepressants, neuroleptics, and minor tranquilizers may be associated with anorgasmia in the female. Anorgasmia has been reported with phenelzine (Barton 1979; Moss 1983; Rabkin et al. 1985; Wyatt et al. 1971), isocarboxazid (Lesko et al. 1982), and tranylcypromine (Gross 1982). Anorgasmia has also been reported with imipramine (Couper-Smartt and Rodham 1973), clomipramine (Monteiro et al. 1987; Quirk and Einarson 1983), amoxepine (Shen and Park 1982), nortriptyline (Sovner 1983), and fluoxetine (Musher 1990). Female anorgasmia may be related to the serotonergic activity of certain antidepressants; coadministration of cyproheptadine has been reported to restore orgasmic function.

Orgasmic dysfunction has been reported with thioridazine (Shen and Park 1982), trifluoperazine (Degen 1982), and fluphenazine (Ghadirian et al. 1982). Loxapine appears to cause anorgasmia relatively infrequently.

Both alprazolam (Sangal 1985) and diazepam (Riley and Riley 1986) have been reported to cause anorgasmia. To our knowledge, anorgasmia has not been reported with buspirone.

A few general guidelines are available to help the clinician minimize sexual side effects of psychiatric drugs. The first step is to determine whether a reduced dose will ameliorate the sexual problem while still effectively managing the psychiatric disorder. If dose reduction is not possible, careful substitution of alternative agents may be necessary. Of the antidepressant agents, bupropion appears to have the fewest sexual side effects and should be employed if the patient has difficulty with other antidepressants. If the patient cannot take bupropion, desipramine has a relatively low incidence of sexual side effects. If the patient must remain on an agent that causes anorgasmia, the coadministration of cyproheptadine may alleviate the anorgasmia. If the patient must remain on a monoamine oxidase inhibitor, the patient can be reassured that the side effect of anorgasmia may spontaneously remit after 2–3 months of continuous pharmacotherapy.

Of the antipsychotic agents, anorgasmia has been reported to be quite common with thioridazine. This drug should thus be avoided unless other clinical situations mandate its use. The available information suggests that loxapine and haloperidol may be relatively free of sexual side effects (R. T. Segraves 1988b). If a minor tranquilizer is required, buspirone would be preferred to one of the benzodiazepines.

CONCLUSIONS

From this overview of sexual disorders at the boundary between obstetrics-gynecology and psychiatry, the reader should be reminded of how little definitive information is available and thus of the frequent need for a collaborative team approach to diagnosis and treatment planning. Human sexuality is an excellent opportunity for the psychiatrist, as a physician with training in both physical and psychological medicine, to make a significant contribution to patient care.

REFERENCES

American Psychiatric Association: Diagnostic and Statistical Manual of Mental Disorders, 3rd Edition. Washington, DC, American Psychiatric Association, 1980

American Psychiatric Association: Diagnostic and Statistical Manual of Mental Disorders, 3rd Edition, Revised. Washington, DC, American Psychiatric Association, 1987

Andersen BL: Sexual functioning and morbidity among cancer survivors. Cancer 55:1835–1842, 1985

Andersen BL: Sexual functioning complications in women with gynecological cancer. Cancer 60:2123–2128, 1987

Andersen BL, Hacher NF: Psychological adjustment following pelvic exenteration. Obstet Gynecol 61:331–338, 1983

Andersen BL, Turnquist D, LaPolla J, et al: Sexual functioning after treatment of in situ vulvar cancer: preliminary report. Obstet Gynecol 71:15–19, 1988

Bachmann GA, Leiblum SR, Sandler B, et al: Correlates of sexual desire in post-menopausal women. Maturitas 7:211–216, 1985

Bancroft J: Human Sexuality and Its Problems. Edinburgh, UK, Churchill Livingstone, 1983

Bancroft J, Coles L: Three year's experience in a sexual problems clinic. BMJ 1:1575–1577, 1976

Bardwick J: Psychological factors in the acceptance and use of oral contraceptives, in Psychological Perspectives on Populations. Edited by Fawsett JT. New York, Basic Books, 1973, pp 133–152

Barton TL: Orgasmic inhibition by phenelzine. Am J Psychiatry 136:1616–1617, 1979

Berard EJJ: The sexuality of spinal cord injured women: physiology and pathophysiology: a review. Paraplegia 27:99–112, 1989

Broun RS, Haddox J, Posada A, et al: Social and psychological adjustment following pelvic exenteration. Am J Obstet Gynecol 114:162–171, 1972

Bullard DG: The treatment of desire disorders in the medically ill and physically disabled, in Sexual Desire Disorders. Edited by Leiblum SR, Rosen RC. New York, Guilford, 1988, pp 348–386

Burnap DW, Golden JS: Sexual problems in medical practice. Journal of Medical Education 42:673–680, 1967

Capone MA, Good RS, Westie KS, et al: Psychosocial rehabilitation of gynecologic oncology patients. Arch Phys Med Rehabil 61:128–132, 1980

Catalan J, Bradley M, Gallwey J, et al: Sexual dysfunction and psychiatric morbidity in patients attending a clinic for sexually transmitted diseases. Br J Psychiatry 138:292–296, 1981

Chambless DL, Sultan FE, Stern TE: Effect of pubococcygeal exercise on coital orgasm in women. J Consult Clin Psychol 52:114–118, 1984

Cohen AW: Human sexuality during normal pregnancy, in Human Sexuality: Psychosexual Effects of Disease. Edited by Farber M. New York, Macmillan, 1985, pp 55–76

Consolo A, Bragaglia RB, Petrucci C, et al: Survival and complications after radical surgery for carcinoma of the rectum. J Surg Oncol 41:27–32, 1989

Coop J: Menopause: associated problems. BMJ 289:970, 1984

Coopen A, Bishop M, Beard RT, et al: Hysterectomy, hormones and behavior. Lancet 1:126–128, 1981

Couper-Smartt J, Rodham R: A technique for surveying side-effects of tricyclic drugs with reference to reported sexual effects. J Int Med Res 1:473–476, 1973

Cullberg J: Mood changes and menstrual symptoms with different progestogen/estrogen combinations. Acta Psychiatr Scand Suppl 236:9–86, 1972

Degen K: Sexual dysfunction in women using major tranquilizers. Psychosomatics 23:959–961, 1982

Demsey GM, Buchsbaum HJ, Morrison J: Psychosocial adjustment to pelvic exenteration. Gynecol Oncol 3:325–334, 1975

DiSala PJ, Creasman WT, Rich WM: An alternative approach to early cancer of the vulva. Am J Obstet Gynecol 133:825–829, 1979

Drake TS, Grunert GM: A cyclic pattern of sexual dysfunction in the infertility investigation. Fertil Steril 32:542–545, 1979

Ende J, Rockwell S, Glasgow M: The sexual history in general medicine practice. Arch Intern Med 144:558–561, 1984

Friedman CM: The decision-making process and the outcome of therapeutic abortion. Am J Psychiatry 131:1332–1337, 1974

Gebhard DH, Pomeroy WB, Martin CE, et al: Pregnancy, Birth and Abortion. New York, Harper & Row, 1958

Ghadirian AM, Chouinard G, Annable L: Sexual dysfunction and plasma prolactin levels in neuroleptic-treated schizophrenic outpatients. J Nerv Ment Dis 170:463–467, 1982

Green T: Vaginismus, in Clinical Management of Sexual Disorders. Edited by Meyer JK, Schmidt CW, Wise TN. Baltimore, MD, Williams & Wilkins, 1983, pp 340–344

Greenblatt RB, Barfield WE, Garner JF, et al: Evaluation of an estrogen, androgen, estrogen-androgen combination and a placebo in the treatment of the menopause. Journal of Clinical Endocrinology 10:1547–1558, 1950

Gross MD: Reversal by bethanechol of sexual dysfunction caused by anticholinergic antidepressants. Am J Psychiatry 139:1193–1194, 1982

Hawton K, Catalan J, Martin P, et al: Prognostic factors in sex therapy. Behav Res Ther 24:377–385, 1986

Heiman JR: Female sexual response patterns: interactions of physiological, affective and contextual cues. Arch Gen Psychiatry 37:1311–1316, 1980

Hoon EF, Hoon PW: Styles of sexual expression in women: clinical implications of multi-variate analysis. Arch Sex Behav 7:105–116, 1978

Kaplan HS: Hypoactive sexual desire. J Sex Marital Ther 3:3–9, 1977

Kaplan HS: Disorders of sexual desire. New York, Brunner/Mazel, 1979

Kaplan HS: The comprehensive evaluation of the psychosexual disorders, in The Evaluation of Sexual Disorders: Psychological and Medical Aspects. Edited by Kaplan HS. New York, Brunner/Mazel, 1983a

Kaplan HS: The data, in The Evaluation of Sexual Disorders: Psychological and Medical Aspects. Edited by Kaplan HS. New York, Brunner/Mazel, 1983b

Kaufman SA: The gynecological evaluation of female dyspareunia and unconsummated marriage, in The Evaluation of Sexual Disorders: Psychological and Medical Aspects. Edited by Kaplan HS. New York, Brunner/Mazel, 1983a

Kaufman SA: The gynecological evaluation of female excitement disorders, in The Evaluation of Sexual Disorders: Psychological and Medical Aspects. Edited by Kaplan HS. New York, Brunner/Mazel, 1983b

Kegel AH: Sexual functions of the pubococcygeous muscle. Western Journal of Surgery 60:521–524, 1956

Kinsey AC, Pomeroy WB, Martin CE: Sexual Behavior in the Human Female. Philadelphia, PA, WB Saunders, 1953

Kolodny RC: Sexual dysfunction in diabetic females. Diabetes 20:557–559, 1971

Leeton J, McMaster R, Worsley A: The effects on sexual response and mood after sterilization of women taking long term oral contraceptives: results of a double-blind crossover study. Aust N Z J Obstet Gynecol 18:194–197, 1978

Leiblum SR, Rosen RC: Introduction: changing perspective on sexual desire, in Sexual Desire Disorders. Edited by Leiblum SR, Rosen RC. New York, Guilford, 1988, pp 1–20

Lesko LM, Stotland NL, Segraves RT: Three cases of female anorgasmia associated with MAOIs. Am J Psychiatry 139:1353–1354, 1982

Levine SB: Hypoactive sexual desire and other problems of sexual desire, in Treatments of Psychiatric Disorders: A Task Force Report of the American Psychiatric Association, Vol 3. Washington, DC, American Psychiatric Association, 1989, pp 2264–2279

Levine SB, Yost MA: Frequency of sexual dysfunction in a general gynecological clinic: an epidemiological approach. Arch Sex Behav 5:229–238, 1976

Lief HI: Inhibited sexual desire. Medical Aspects of Human Sexuality 7:94–95, 1977

Lief HI: Evaluation of inhibited sexual desire: relationship aspects, in Comprehensive Evaluation of Disorders of Sexual Desire. Edited by Kaplan HS. Washington, DC, American Psychiatric Press, 1985, pp 59–76

Lilius HG, Valtonen EJ, Wikstrom J: Sexual problems in patients suffering from multiple sclerosis. Journal of Chronic Diseases 29:643–647, 1976

LoPiccollo L: Low sexual desire, in Principles and Practice of Sex Therapy. Edited by Leiblum SR, Pervin LA. New York, Guilford, 1980, pp 29–64

Lundberg PO: Sexual dysfunction in patients with multiple sclerosis. Sexuality and Disability 1:218–222, 1978

Masters WH, Johnson VE: Human Sexual Response. Boston, MA, Little, Brown, 1966

McCoy N, Cutler W, Davidson JM: Relationship among sexual behavior, hot flashes, and hormone levels in premenopausal women. Arch Sex Behav 14:385–394, 1985

Monteiro WO, Noshirvani HF, Marks IM: Anorgasmia from clomipramine in obsessive-compulsive disorder: a controlled trial. Br J Psychiatry 151:107–112, 1987

Moore C: Female sexual arousal disorder and inhibited female orgasm, in Treatments of Psychiatric Disorders: A Task Force Report of the American Psychiatric Association, Vol 3. Washington, DC, American Psychiatric Association, 1989, pp 2279–2290

Morrell MJ, Dixen JM, Carter SC, et al: The influence of age and cycling status on sexual arousability in women. Am J Obstet Gynecol 148:66–71, 1984

Moss HB: More cases of anorgasmia after MAOI treatment. Am J Psychiatry 140:266, 1983

Munday RN, Cox LW: Hysterectomy for benign lesions. Med J Aust 2:759–763, 1967

Musher JS: Anorgasmia with the use of fluoxetine. Am J Psychiatry 147:948, 1990

Myers L, Morokoff P: Physiological and subjective sexual arousal in pre- and postmenopausal women. Poster presented at the annual meeting of the American Psychological Association, Los Angeles, CA, August, 1985

Nathan SG: The epidemiology of the DSM III psychosexual dysfunctions. J Sex Marital Ther 12:267–282, 1986

Perkins RP: Sexuality in pregnancy: what determines behavior? Obstet Gynecol 59:189–198, 1982

Quirk KC, Einarson TR: Sexual dysfunction and clomipramine. Can J Psychiatry 27:228–231, 1983

Rabkin J, Quitkin F, McGrath P, et al: Adverse reactions to monoamine oxidase inhibitors. J Clin Psychopharmacol 5:2–9, 1985

Reamy K, White S, Daniell W, et al: Sexuality and pregnancy. J Reprod Med 27:321–329, 1982

Renshaw DC: Profile of 2376 patients treated at the Loyola Sex Clinic between 1972 and 1987. J Sex Marital Ther 3:111–117, 1988

Riley AJ, Riley EJ: The effect of single dose diazepam on female sexual response induced by masturbation. Sexual and Marital Therapy 1:49–53, 1986

Rinehart JS, Schiff I: Sexuality and the menopause, in Human Sexuality: Psychosexual Effects of Disease. Edited by Farber M. New York, Macmillan, 1985, pp 77–84

Rosen RC, Leiblum SR: Assessment and treatment of desire disorders, in Principles and Practice of Sex Therapy. Edited by Leiblum SR, Rosen RC. New York, Guilford, 1989, pp 19–50

Salzer LP: Infertility: How Couples Can Cope: Survive Infertility: Strengthen Your Marriage. Boston, MA, GK Hall, 1986

Sangal R: Inhibited female orgasm as a side-effect of alprazolam. Am J Psychiatry 142:1223–1224, 1985

Sarrel PM, Sarrel LJ: Dyspareunia and vaginismus, in Treatments of Psychiatric Disorders: A Task Force Report of the American Psychiatric Association, Vol 3. Washington, DC, American Psychiatric Association, 1989, pp 2291–2299

Sauer MV, Paulson RJ, Lobo RA: A preliminary report on oocyte donation extending reproductive potential to women over 40. N Engl J Med 323:1157–1160, 1990

Schover LR, Jensen SB: Sexuality and Chronic Illness: A Comprehensive Approach. New York, Guilford, 1988

Schover L, LoPiccollo J: Effectiveness of treatment for dysfunction of sexual desire. J Sex Marital Ther 8:179–197, 1982

Schover LR, von Eschenbach AC: Sexual function and female radical cystectomy: a case series. J Urol 134:465–468, 1985

Schover LR, Evans RB, von Eschenbach AC: Sexual rehabilitation in a cancer center: diagnosis and outcome in 384 consultations. Arch Sex Behav 16:445–461, 1987

Schreiner-Engel P, Schiavi RC, Vietorisz D, et al: The differential impact of diabetes type on female sexuality. J Psychosom Res 31:23–33, 1987

Segraves KB, Segraves RT: Hypoactive sexual desire disorder: prevalence and co-morbidity in 906 subjects. J Sex Marital Ther 17:55–58, 1991

Segraves RT: Psychiatric drugs and orgasm in the human female. Journal of Psychosomatic Obstetrics and Gynaecology 4:125–128, 1985

Segraves RT: Drugs and desire, in Sexual Desire Disorders. Edited by Leiblum SR, Rosen RC. New York, Guilford, 1988a, pp 313–347

Segraves RT: Hormones and libido, in Sexual Desire Disorders. Edited by Leiblum SR, Rosen RC. New York, Guilford, 1988b, pp 271–312

Segraves RT, Segraves KB: Diagnosis of female arousal disorder. Sexual and Marital Therapy 6:9–14, 1991

Segraves RT, Segraves KB: Medical aspects of orgasm disorders, in Handbook on the Assessment and Treatment of Sexual Dysfunction. Edited by O'Donohue W, Geer JH. New York, Pergamon (in press)

Segraves RT, Madsen R, Carter SC, et al: Erectile dysfunction associated with pharmacological agents, in Diagnosis and Treatment of Erectile Disturbances. Edited by Segraves RT, Schoenberg HW. New York, Plenum, 1985, pp 23–64

Semmens JP, Semmens EC: Sexual function and the menopause. Clin Obstet Gynecol 27:717–722, 1984

Shen WW, Park S: Thioridazine-induced inhibition of female orgasm. Psychiatry Journal University of Ottawa 7:249–251, 1982

Sherwin BB, Gelfand MM: Effects of parenteral administration of estrogen and androgen on plasma hormone levels and hot flashes in the surgical menopause. Am J Obstet Gynecol 148:552–557, 1984

Sherwin BB, Gelfand MM: Differential symptom response to parental estrogen and/or androgen administration in the surgical menopause. Am J Obstet Gynecol 151:153–160, 1985

Sherwin BB, Gelfand MM, Brender W: Androgen enhances sexual motivation in females: a prospective, crossover study of sex steroid administration in the surgical menopause. Psychosom Med 47:339–351, 1985

Smith E, Buck N: Dyspareunia, in Clinical Management of Sexual Disorders. Edited by Meyer JK, Schmidt CW, Wise TN. Baltimore, MD, Williams & Wilkins, 1983, pp 205–213

Sovner R: Anorgasmia associated with imipramine but not desipramine: a case report. J Clin Psychiatry 44:345–346, 1983

Spector IP, Carey MP: Incidence and prevalence of the sexual dysfunctions: a critical review of the empirical literature. Arch Sex Behav (in press)

Steinman DL, Wincze JP, Sakheim DK: A comparison of male and female patterns of sexual arousal. Arch Sex Behav 10:529–547, 1981

Van de Wiel HBM, Jaspers JPM, Schultz WCMW, et al: Treatment of vaginismus: a review of concepts and treatment modalities. Journal of Psychosomatic Obstetrics and Gynaecology 11:1–18, 1990

Vera MI: Quality of life following pelvic exenteration. Gynecol Oncol 12:355–366, 1981

Wabrek AJ, Wabrek CJ: Dyspareunia. J Sex Marital Ther 1:234–241, 1975

White SE, Reamy K: Sexuality and pregnancy: a review. Arch Sex Behav 11:429–444, 1982

Wyatt RJ, Fram DH, Buchbinder R: Treatment of intractable narcolepsy with a monoamine oxidase inhibitor. N Engl J Med 285:987–991, 1971

Zussman L, Zussman S, Sunley R, et al: Sexual response after hysterectomy-oophorectomy: recent studies and reconsideration for psychogenesis. Am J Obstet Gynecol 104:725–729, 1981

Chapter 19

THE MALE PERSPECTIVE

William H. Miller, Jr., M.D.

❖ ❖ ❖ ❖ ❖ ❖ ❖ ❖ ❖ ❖ ❖ ❖ ❖

Although relationships with men are important in women's lives and reproductive choices, the perspective of the male partner is often ignored in the discussion of psychosomatic obstetrics and gynecology. A review finds the literature brief and theoretical, with little scientific data on the effects *of* and *on* the male.

One major basis for modern theory and practice of psychiatry is Freudian psychoanalytic thought. These theories are based on the male perspective out of a Victorian age with constricted, stereotypical beliefs concerning women's proper place in society. Older traditional psychoanalytic thinking holds that the "true" nature of women finds fulfillment only in the conventional roles of wife and mother (Chesler 1972; Lerner 1988). Despite this male-oriented psychodynamic approach and the importance it placed on reproduction, surprisingly little information is found regarding the male views on female reproductive concerns.

This chapter reviews several areas regarding the male perspective, including the decision to become a parent, issues of expectant parenthood, and the impact of the postpartum period. Men's concerns about infertility, loss of a child, and premenstrual syndrome will also be addressed.

PREGNANCY

It is not unusual for pregnancy to be an "accident." The decision to become pregnant may not be consciously made by either partner.

This is especially the case for adolescent couples, who are often engaged in sexual intercourse without planning. They may either deny or consciously seek the possibility of conception. Pregnancy can be viewed by the male as a badge of honor, validating his manhood. Often the father-to-be has given little thought to the ramifications and responsibilities that accompany pregnancy and parenthood.

On the other hand, in some subcultures, choice, rather than fate, increasingly determines whether a couple will try to become pregnant. The decision-making process raises some similar issues for men and women. The narcissistic wish to produce and identify with one's own child is universal, as is the wish to reproduce one's own image (Brazelton and Cramer 1990). Men commonly desire to have a male infant in order to bolster and confirm their own masculine identity. A son can be the fulfillment of a father's frustrated ambitions. The desire to guarantee the progression of one's family lineage—as Freud said, "our only path to immortality"—is seen in men as well as women (Freud 1905). The birth of a son is a link to the past as well as to the future, as exemplified by fathers giving sons their own names and the names of men they most admire (Brazelton and Cramer 1990). Having a child can also be motivated by oedipal rivalry with a man's own father. In addition, he has an opportunity to surpass his father by doing a better job of parenting.

These psychodynamic issues are reflected in perceived practical considerations and fears. Issues of commitment and finality regarding the relationship between the woman and the man emerge. Job security, financial stability, and loss of freedom and flexibility in one's life are major concerns facing men as well as women considering parenthood (Rubin 1980). Fathers-to-be can experience feelings of helplessness as they attempt to weigh the impact of the stress, disruption, and economic and other sacrifices of parenthood, as contrasted with the joy and satisfaction of creating and rearing one's own child (Potts 1980). High expectations and pressures to achieve financial and career-related goals can lead to hesitancy in deciding to have a child. These "practical" issues may stem from inner developmental conflicts. Dealing with these "practicalities" in the relationship and/or in psychotherapy can facilitate the process of working through narcissistic wishes and oedipal rivalries. These issues can resurface and change as the demands of parenthood change and as children grow and mature.

Social changes in careers and relationships, which delay attempts at childbearing for some women, can delay fatherhood for their male partners as well. Some men have so-called "second families" in subsequent marriages that present the responsibilities of parenting later in life. They may experience concerns about seeing these children raised prior to their own death or age-related disabilities (Rubin 1980). There may be a fear that "time is running out" to fulfill the need to continue their lineage, a male counterpart of the female "biological clock." Issues of financial stability may play a different role in the decision making. Some men, although they are financially affluent, may be severely strained by the financial burden of two sets of children. On the positive side, greater life stability in financial and work areas may offer these fathers an opportunity to play a greater role in the lives of their children. Dealing with the loss of freedom and the need to change established life patterns at this stage of life may be significant. Erikson's stage of generativity versus stagnation may be involved in the decision-making process of an older man (Erikson 1950).

When pregnancy becomes a reality, many conflicting emotions, such as feelings of both gratification and anxiety, can surface. After the pregnancy is confirmed, the mother becomes the center of attention. Her energies are focused on the changes she is experiencing, as well as on changes in her life pattern and the new responsibilities she will face (Trad 1990). The expectant father may feel excluded. Often his need for support is not recognized and addressed should he or his partner have psychiatric difficulty. It is important for the therapist to acknowledge the father's changes in responsibilities, expectations, and fantasies.

The pressures facing the expectant father create a developmental crisis (Osofsky 1982). Because the woman is physically pregnant, the father may feel isolated and alone, experiencing the pregnancy secondhand. This can lead to resentment and competition. A resultant increase in dependency needs may raise suppressed parental and sibling rivalry issues. This can result in guilt and/or acting out. Increases in extramarital affairs, substance abuse, and sexual problems are seen in men during their partners' pregnancies. These may be a result of this feeling of being displaced (Osofsky 1982).

A study by Gerzi and Berman (1981) in which married expectant fathers were compared with married men without children found significantly increased anxiety in the expectant fathers. Psychological tests and interviews demonstrated a statistically significant contribution of oedipal dynamics, sibling rivalry reactions, and guilt to this anxiety. They concluded that anxiety was aroused both by intrapsychic meanings and reality factors surrounding the pregnancy.

At least one study has shown that husbands are generally less involved in maintaining the marital relationship than are wives (Assor and Assor 1985). The regular nurturing of the relationship by women helps maintain the steady state of marriage. As the woman's focus shifts from the marriage and her partner to the pregnancy and her soon-to-be-born child, the husband may feel somewhat deprived just at the time when he needs to feel the relationship is strong. At the same time, he may need to assume different responsibilities in supporting and nurturing the marriage. This may result in resentment toward the wife and the future child.

As the pregnancy progresses, the expectant father can show increased awareness of his own body. This may reflect a repressed wish to be pregnant (Trad 1990). This identification with the wife, or perhaps with his own mother, can result in "couvade" syndrome, presenting with symptoms ranging from aches and pains to nausea, vomiting, and other gastrointestinal symptoms similar to those of pregnancy (Brazelton and Cramer 1990). A study by Clinton (1987) in which expectant fathers were objectively assessed found an increased incidence of colds, irritability, weight gain, insomnia, and restlessness. As the expectant father tries to repudiate these "feminine" feelings, resentment may again surface toward his wife and child. Empathy for the effects and ramifications of pregnancy for his wife is consistent with the resolution of these negative feelings.

Men often experience some guilt and fear during the delivery. The expectant father is guilty about the pain he "put his wife through" during childbirth and is anxious about his own lack of control during the delivery process (Trad 1990). The need to master his apprehension over labor and impending parenthood may be displaced to overconcern about the baby's health. This distress over the infant's well-being can also be a result of a reaction formation, a defense against the unresolved resentment for being displaced by the child.

The postpartum period may be a time when fathers experience symptomatology such as increased difficulties in concentration, excessive fatigue, insomnia, restlessness, headaches, and irritability. These are common complaints of the postpartum mother as well (see Chapter 7). The symptoms are significantly increased in postpartum fathers as compared with a control group (Clinton 1987). Another study found that 62% of fathers experienced a so-called "postpartum depression," though presumably not a major depression according to DSM-III-R criteria (American Psychiatric Association 1987), at some time in the 4 months after their child was born (Zaslow et al. 1981). It was felt that this was related to the fact that the infant did not live up to their antepartum expectations. On the other hand, in a study of couples participating in childbirth education classes, no overt depressive symptoms were found postpartum in the men studied (Quadagno et al. 1986). The postpartum period was an emotional period for both men and women and was experienced in similar ways. Perhaps appropriate education moderates some of the expectations new fathers have of themselves.

The unborn or newborn child can be viewed by the father as a competitor, and if he consequently withdraws from the infant and mother, marital disruption can be increasingly evident. Competition can begin early in the pregnancy. Fathers' involvement in planning the pregnancy, prenatal obstetric visits, childbirth education, and decision making can set up either collaboration or competition between parents and is a necessary part of the growing attachment to the child. Thus, earlier involvement of the father can result in the strengthening of marital bonds. Increasing support from the father may help sustain the mother during this time of dealing with her own developmental crisis. The positive effect of his support serves to enhance his own self-esteem in his new familial role. Support from the father has been shown to decrease the need for medication in labor (Parke 1986), to improve competence with breast- and bottle-feeding (Pedersen 1980), and to enhance maternal postpartum adjustment (Grossman et al. 1980). In addition, increased involvement of the father during pregnancy predicts his increased involvement with the child in the first 4 years of life (Barnard 1982).

The impact of involved fathers has often been overlooked. Historically, many cultures have tended to exclude the father, leaving the pregnancy and early childrearing to the mother. The influence of the father on his children is often mediated by the mother. Mothers can promote or dampen the paternal relationship with their children. Some mothers can be threatened by the fathers' involvement because of fears of the infant's emancipation. Others may promote letting the father into the triangle, thus improving the child's ability for attachment (Brazelton and Cramer 1990). Recent societal changes have allowed the father to be more extensively involved in the pregnancy and delivery. This may have a powerful impact on new paternal behavior and may change the nurturing capacity of men, as a group, in future generations.

Psychiatrists and other mental health professionals may have reason to address issues of fatherhood not only when care is sought or recommended for parenting difficulties, but also when they arise in the course of treatment undertaken for any reason. Obstetricians and gynecologists can also be encouraged to involve and counsel fathers along with mothers. The goal of the therapist in working with fathers is to help them understand their role and the source of the conflicts that have arisen. Fathers can be reassured that their function is as important as that of the mother. They need help to develop an appropriate mental representation of the child, which will enable them to make appropriate parenting decisions. The father's role in the decision to have a child and his involvement in the pregnancy and delivery can help reinforce his identity as an important, active participant in parenthood. This can prepare him for a more active role after the child is born. The rewards are seen in two ways: improving the relationship with the spouse and enjoyment of a personal role in the parenting process.

INFERTILITY

The diagnosis and treatment of infertility involves the "medicalization" of the most intimate aspects of a couple's relationship (see Chapter 10). The diagnosis of infertility may affect the mental, marital, and social adjustment of couples. Whether one or both partners are shown to have a problem, the other partner also has a strong interest in the investigation and treatment. Infertility is always a problem of the couple, and both partners should be involved from the onset.

Problems adjusting to infertility treatment may further exacerbate infertility itself by affecting the sexual relationship. Studies show that most couples report deleterious effects on their sexual relationship during infertility treatment (Dennerstein and Morse 1988; Mahlstedt 1985; Reading and Kerin 1989; Rosenthal 1985). Sexual intercourse, which previously occurred spontaneously in response to loving, erotic feelings, now occurs in response to clinical demand. Complaints that sex has become too cold and too purposeful are common. Both members of the couple are expected to perform. The male is expected to produce semen when required, to masturbate into a jar on demand. The woman is expected to ovulate and to become pregnant. These demands recur month after month in the course of attempts at artificial insemination, the only reassurance being the possibilities offered by subsequent attempts. The inability to conceive and bear a child after much emotional, physical, and financial investment may lead to feelings of failure in one or both members of the couple (Dennerstein and Morse 1988; Mahlstedt 1985; Rosenthal 1985).

Fifty percent of women and 15% of men treated for infertility report that infertility is the most upsetting experience of their lives (Freeman et al. 1985). Several studies have shown that female infertility patients have higher levels of anxiety and neuroticism than do their male partners or normally fertile men or women (Shaw et al. 1988). This may reflect the greater impact of infertility and its treatment on them. Women also showed evidence of less self-esteem than did their male partners (Dennerstein and Morse 1988). Men, however, showed a higher tendency than did women to offer misleadingly healthy responses on these scales (Dennerstein and Morse 1988). Men were significantly more hopeful regarding the success of the procedure (Mahlstedt 1985). The difficulty men face in expressing their true feelings often covers their concerns regarding their own virility. Men should be included in any therapy directed at lowering stress, even if the male partner appears to be more relaxed and less frustrated than the woman (Mahlstedt 1985; Reading and Kerin 1989; Rosenthal

1985; Wright et al. 1991). The man's understanding of what his spouse is feeling enables him to support her during this most difficult time.

Publicity regarding the success of in vitro fertilization (IVF) can detract attention from the high percentage of failures; recent figures are 80%–90% failure on a single attempt and a cumulative conception rate of approximately 40% after three treatment cycles (Damewood 1987; Reading and Kerin 1989; Shaw et al. 1988). There is evidence that couples seeking and undergoing IVF treatment underestimate the incidence of failure, which can set them up for disappointment when attempts at pregnancy are unsuccessful. By continuing to hope for a successful outcome of the next procedure, many couples avoid facing and addressing the personal meaning of childlessness. IVF is regarded as the final chance for treatment; when pregnancy does not occur, the couple is forced for the first time to confront their sterility as a pair.

In one study, 48% of men reported improvement in the marital relationship, but 17% of men reported negative effects on the marital relationship after unsuccessful attempts at IVF (Baram et al. 1988). Forty percent of men reported symptoms of depression after failure of IVF, and 30% of those were still feeling depressed after 18 months. Only a small number sought any treatment. This is a difficult time for couples, when, having endured costly, disruptive, stressful, and sometimes physically painful IVF cycles, they may have little to show for their efforts. As individuals, both can feel cheated and devastated. The couple is angry at themselves and at the IVF staff for not making a pregnancy occur.

For men, working through the issues after an unsuccessful infertility evaluation and treatment can be an isolating experience. Men are often secretive about the infertility problem, and no one is readily available to help them deal with their feelings. Health care practitioners need to be available to the man as well as the woman. Couples support groups can also be an important resource for those dealing with the finality of conception failure (Baram et al. 1988). It is important to encourage the male partner's attendance at support group meetings. Men have a tendency not to want to get involved in such activities in order to avoid the underlying feelings of anger and inadequacy.

Possible positive aspects of the infertility experience include improved communication and emotional closeness in the relationship. Most men state that their spouse is their primary source of support. This crisis, if successfully resolved, can lead to adaptation accompanied by an increase in the strength and security of the relationship. Some feel a sense of relief that they can finally go on with their lives and leave behind concerns with infertility.

BIRTH OF AN ABNORMAL CHILD

> It is as if human beings find it very difficult to believe that they are good enough to create within themselves something that is quite good. I doubt whether any mother really fully believes in her child at the beginning. Father comes in to this too, for he suffers just as much as mother does from doubt that he may not be able to create a healthy normal child. (Winnicott 1964)

The hope for a normal child is universal among parents. The birth of an abnormal child is a devastating blow. In response, the couple goes through stages of shock, disbelief, anger, and sadness; equilibrium; and reorganization (Drotar 1975) (see Chapter 8). Solnit and Stark (1961) discuss a therapeutic approach to parents who are overwhelmed with their infant's condition. These authors felt that the affected infant was a distortion of the parents' dreams and that the parents must mourn the loss of their fantasized, perfect infant. The parents' attempt to withdraw and mourn may be complicated by the demands of taking care of an ill child. This can be overwhelming at a time when they are emotionally and physically drained by grief. The caregiver must be patient in order to answer the bewildered parents' questions and, many times, to bear the parents' misplaced anger. If the child survives, the constant contact and heavy demands placed on the family can prolong the grief and mourning process (Solnit and Stark 1961).

Marital breakdown and disharmony are more common in families with a child with Down's syndrome than in control subjects (Gath 1977). Gath found that some fathers of children with Down's syndrome complained of feeling impotent and "less of a man." The delivery of a child with Down's syndrome, however, was also found to draw approximately half of the couples closer together. The effect on fathers is striking. They commonly are not ready for such a devastating event and react differently than do women, becoming more isolated and unwilling to discuss their feelings (Klaus and Kennell 1983). In one study, fathers who had a history of a psychiatric illness and who had children with Down's syndrome were noted to have a recurrence of psychiatric illness (Gath 1977). Although this is anecdotal evidence, it may be important to be aware of previous psychiatric difficulties in order to anticipate the needs of the father and mother of a child born with special needs.

Caregivers resonate with parents' pain under these circumstances. When parents of affected children were asked what aspects of care were helpful to them, most indicated that the answering of questions and the emotional support of the caregivers were very important. When asked what was least helpful, most were concerned about the way in which they were told about the child and that they were not told the news together (Klaus and Kennell 1983). The parents need a clear discussion of the known facts in layperson's terms. It is important not to overwhelm them with details or with complicated medical terms that may reinforce feelings of inadequacy. This is particularly true for the father who needs to maintain a sense of control at a time when he feels totally helpless.

Spending time alone with the father can be helpful, allowing him some private time to express his emotions without his having to feel that he needs to be strong for his spouse. In addition, support groups for parents who have lost children or who have severely impaired infants may be valuable. These groups can allow parents to identify with others in similar circumstances, and men can observe other men's expressions of feelings and learn about the ways in which they cope. Group therapy also provides an opportunity to regain feelings of competence by supporting other group members.

PREMENSTRUAL SYNDROME

Many women of reproductive age in the United States report mild premenstrual symptomatology that does not interfere with function. A smaller group (5%–10%) have severe premenstrual symptoms that disturb the individual and/or family (see Chapter 9). Premenstrual syndrome (PMS) has been said to affect relationships and to be associated with problems such as marital strife and divorce (Severino 1989). It should be remembered that many relationship issues may surface under the guise of PMS.

A self-help PMS group (PMS Access Newsletter 1985) published anecdotal responses of men, who expressed feelings of frustration, bitterness, and anger over the effects of this cyclic intrusion on their own, as well as their families', lives. A study by Cortese and Brown (1989), using Brown and Zimmer's Premenstrual Symptom Inventory, correlated women's perceptions of their premenstrual symptoms to their male partner's coping mechanisms, as indicated on the PMS Partner's Coping Inventory. Men were found to use a wide variety of coping mechanisms. The most common coping mechanisms used by men whose partners experienced more severe symptoms were "told myself that she can't help it," "lending support through educating (themselves) and giving reassurance to (their) partner," and "expressing anger toward (their) partner" (Cortese and Brown 1989). The coping mechanism particularly used by male partners of women with high levels of symptomatology was seeking knowledge about the symptoms and accompanying the woman to obtain professional help. This may suggest that problems in the relationship with more symptomatic women were significant enough to motivate the men to get outside help (Cortese and Brown 1989).

Psychotherapeutic interactions with the male partner of a woman with PMS may lead to improvement in the relationship of the family and couple. Encouraging the man to be aware of the cyclic nature of the syndrome and to abstain from sensitive issues during this period may be an effective coping strategy.

Most information on PMS is female oriented. Health care practitioners should focus on the couple, providing information for both partners. Individual sessions with the male partner are effective not only in providing information, but also in allowing the man to ventilate his concerns and perceptions. This provides an opportunity for men in such relationships to examine misconceptions and myths about PMS.

OTHER ISSUES

Women's gynecologic problems and treatments carry meanings for their male partners that may have an impact on the men's behaviors and attitudes toward the women in their lives. The implications of breast disease and mastectomy, hysterectomy, and gynecologic onco-logic procedures have important repercussions on the female patient (see Chapters 14 and 15). The male view of these events may include several emotions: anger toward the illness, his partner, and her care-givers; anxiety over the impact on their sexual relations; and feelings of fear or even repulsion. Misinformation about the illness and its treatment, as well as its etiology and sequelae, may exacerbate these negative feelings.

It is vital for the caregiver to talk to both members of the couple, discussing the implications of the gynecologic problem and the treat-ment possibilities. The more the male partner is included and in-formed regarding the situation, the more supportive he can be to his partner and the better mastery he will have of his own reactions. Ac-companying the patient to follow-up appointments should be encour-aged. Spending a few moments alone with the male partner may provide an opportunity for discussion of new problems, concerns, or misconceptions that have arisen. It is important to respect the confi-dentiality of the woman involved. Her wishes are paramount, and con-sulting her beforehand about what will be discussed with her partner is critical. If she has apprehensions, an explanation of the value of correct, relevant information for her partner may be helpful. Above all, however, her rights to confidentiality must be respected.

CONCLUSIONS

Many of the reproductive issues facing women have both direct and indirect impacts on the couple and on the men in their relationships. The man involved may have an opportunity to process some of his individual issues that surface around the reproductive concerns facing the couple. In addition, the involvement of both members of the cou-ple in discussions of problems encountered in pregnancy and related reproductive areas can often be a first step in improving feelings of intimacy and communication in their relationship.

REFERENCES

American Psychiatric Association: Diagnostic and Statistical Manual of Mental Disorders, 3rd Edition, Revised. Washington, DC, American Psychiatric Association, 1987

Assor A, Assor T: Emotional involvement in marriage during the last trimester of first pregnancy: a comparison of husbands and wives. J Psychol 119:243–252, 1985

Baram D, Tourtelot E, Muechler E, et al: Psychosocial adjustment following unsuccessful in vitro fertilization. Journal of Psychosomatic Obstetrics and Gynaecology 9:181–190, 1988

Barnard KE: Reported in Pedersen FA, Father influences viewed in a family context, in Role of Father in Child Development, 2nd Edition. Edited by Lamb ME. New York, Wiley, 1982

Brazelton TB, Cramer BG: The attachment of fathers to be, in The Earliest Relationship: Parents, Infants and the Dramas of Early Attachment. Edited by Brazelton TB, Cramer BG. Boston, MA, Addison-Wesley, 1990, pp 33–42

Chesler P: Women and Madness. Garden City, NY, Doubleday, 1972

Clinton JF: Physical and emotional responses of expectant fathers throughout pregnancy and the early post-partum period. Int J Nurs Stud 24:59–68, 1987

Cortese J, Brown MA: Coping responses of men whose partners experience premenstrual symptomatology. J Obstet Gynecol Neonatal Nurs, September/October 1989, pp 405–412

Damewood MD: Medical procedures and psychosexual evaluation for in vitro fertilization. Clinical Practice in Sexuality 3:14–21, 1987

Dennerstein L, Morse C: A review of psychological and social aspects of in vitro fertilization. Journal of Psychosomatic Obstetrics and Gynaecology 9:159–170, 1988

Drotar D: The adaptation of parents to the birth of an infant with congenital malformation: a hypothetical model. Pediatrics 56:710–717, 1975

Erikson EH: Eight stages of man, in Childhood and Society. Edited by Erikson EH. New York, WW Norton, 1950, pp 247–274

Freeman EW, Boxer AS, Rickels K, et al: Psychological evaluation and support in a program of in vitro fertilization and embryo transfer. Fertil Steril 43:48–53, 1985

Freud S: The Interpretation of Dreams (1905). Edited by Strachey J. New York, Discus Books, 1965, pp 430–438

Gath A: The impact of an abnormal child upon the parents. Br J Psychol 130:405–410, 1977

Gerzi S, Berman E: Emotional reactions of expectant fathers to their wives' first pregnancy. Br J Med Psychol 54:259–265, 1981

Grossman FK, Eichler LS, Winickoff SA: Pregnancy, Birth and Parenthood. San Francisco, CA, Jossey-Bass, 1980

Klaus MH, Kennell JH: Bonding: The Beginnings of Parent-Infant Attachment. St. Louis, MO, CV Mosby, 1983

Lerner HG: Origins of envy and devaluation of women, in Women in Therapy. Northvale, NJ, Aronson, 1988, pp 3–22

Mahlstedt PP: The psychological component of infertility. Fertil Steril 43:335–346, 1985

Osofsky H: Expectant and new fatherhood as a developmental crisis. Bull Menninger Clin 46:209–228, 1982

Parke R: Fathers, in In Support of Families. Edited by Yogman M, Brazelton TB. Cambridge, MA, Harvard University Press, 1986

Pedersen FA: The Father-Infant Relationship: Observational Studies in the Family Setting. New York, Praeger, 1980

PMS Access Newsletter: Men coping with PMS. Madison, WI, PMS Access, 1985

Potts L: Considering parenthood: group support for a critical life decision. Am J Orthopsychiatry 50:629–638, 1980

Quadagno DM, Dixon LA, Denny NW, et al: Post-partum moods in men and women. Am J Obstet Gynecol 154:1018–1023, 1986

Reading AE, Kerin J: Psychologic aspects of providing infertility services. J Reprod Med 34:861–871, 1989

Rosenthal MB: Grappling with the emotional aspects of infertility. Contemporary Ob/Gyn, July 1985, pp 97–103

Rubin SP: The over-35 reaction to pregnancy, in It's Not Too Late for a Baby. Edited by Rubin SP. Newark, NJ, Prentice-Hall, 1980

Severino SK: Premenstrual Syndrome: Clinician's Guide. New York, Guilford, 1989

Shaw P, Johnson M, Shaw R: Counselling needs, emotional and relationship problems in couples awaiting IVF. Journal of Psychosomatic Obstetrics and Gynaecology 9:171–180, 1988

Solnit AJ, Stark MH: Mourning the birth of a defective child. Psychoanal Study Child 16:523–527, 1961

Trad PV: Infant Previewing: Predicting and Sharing Interpersonal Outcome. New York, Springer-Verlag, 1990

Winnicott DW: The Child, the Family and the Outside World. London, UK, Tavistock, 1964

Wright J, Duchesne C, Sabocrin S, et al: Psychosocial distress and infertility: men and women respond differently. Fertil Steril 55:100–108, 1991

Zaslow M, Pedersen F, Kramer E, et al: Depressed Mood in New Fathers: Interview and Behavior Correlates. Boston, MA, Society for Research in Child Development, 1981

Chapter 20

ALCOHOL AND SUBSTANCE ABUSE IN THE PRACTICE OF OBSTETRICS AND GYNECOLOGY

Sheila B. Blume, M.D., C.A.C.
Marcia Russell, Ph.D.

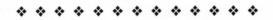

WOMEN, ALCOHOL, AND DRUGS

Historical and Social Factors

The abuse of alcohol and other psychoactive drugs predates recorded history. Although the types of drugs used and abused in different cultures have varied over time, nearly all societies that have permitted substance use have had separate rules for each sex. These rules have been based on deeply ingrained cultural stereotypes of the differential effects of these drugs on men and women.

Western thought, dating back as far as the ancient Romans and Israelites (Gomberg 1986; McKinlay 1959), has held that alcohol is a sexual stimulant that makes women promiscuous. Although careful studies of women in the United States have not substantiated this idea (Klassen and Wilsnack 1986), the stereotype is widely accepted and has led to a destructive stigma applied to all chemically dependent women. This stigma characterizes them as both generally and sexually immoral (i.e., as "fallen women") and in turn simultaneously enhances denial and leads to underrecognition of chemical dependence in middle-class and professional women (Moore et al. 1989). It further results in the social acceptance of physical and sexual victimization of chemically dependent women (Blume 1991). Rapists are considered less responsible for their acts if intoxicated at the time of the rape, whereas victims are held more to blame if intoxicated (Richardson and Campbell 1982). It is hardly surprising, therefore, that women suffering from addictive diseases are often the victims of violence, both at home and in society (Miller et al. 1989).

Social customs related to the use and abuse of substances affect women in a variety of ways:

❖ Drinking norms that dictate lower levels of intake by women protect them from developing alcoholism (Klee and Ames 1987).

❖ The evolution of social custom has produced a convergence of use patterns for some drugs among male and female teenagers. More girls are now initiating smoking than boys (Gritz 1987).

❖ The tendency of physicians to prescribe more psychoactive drugs for women than men (Cooperstock 1978) puts women at a higher risk for becoming dependent on prescription drugs and puts alcoholic women at increased risk for mixed addictions.

❖ Wives, daughters, and mothers of alcoholics or addicts often assume the social role of caretaker. In their efforts to cope with familial dysfunction, they may display maladaptive behavior characterized as "codependency" (Cermak 1986). Depression, somatic complaints, eating disorders, and alcohol or drug abuse are often seen in this group.

Epidemiology

Women's alcohol use has increased over the past half century. Although there have been no dramatic overall changes in the last few years, heavy drinking has continued to rise among younger cohorts. For the year 1990, Williams et al. (1989) estimated that 1.8 million women in the United States would be suffering from alcohol abuse and an additional 2.8 million from alcohol dependence, for a total of 4.6 million, or 5.1% of the adult female population. This compares to about 10.5 million alcoholic males, yielding a male-to-female ratio of about 2:1.

In the year 1988, approximately 5.8% of women in the United States admitted to some illicit drug use (including nonmedical use of prescription drugs) during the month prior to a household survey

(National Institute on Drug Abuse 1989). Women of childbearing age reported a higher prevalence: 14.1% for ages 18–25 and 9.6% for ages 26–34.

High-risk groups for alcohol and drug problems among women include inner-city and criminal justice populations, women in the military, and lesbian women (Wilsnack 1984). A family history of alcoholism increases the risk of alcohol abuse or dependence in women (Russell et al. 1990).

Studies of obstetric-gynecologic populations reveal higher prevalence rates than are found in the general public. For example, of 147 women visiting two private gynecologic practices for routine care, 12% met criteria for alcohol abuse or dependence. Of 95 women treated in the same locations for premenstrual syndrome, 21% were also alcoholic (Halliday et al. 1986). In a similar study of 1,967 gynecologic patients, 17% were heavy drinkers and 14% regularly used psychoactive drugs with the potential for nonmedical use (Russell and Coviello 1988). Among 631 obstetric patients, 18% reported one or more alcohol-related problems, which strongly predicted adverse pregnancy outcome (Russell and Skinner 1988). Positive urine toxicology screening tests have been reported in 13.1% of 335 women in private and 16.3% of 380 women in public obstetric practices (Chasnoff 1990) and in 29.5% of 200 women admitted in active labor to an inner-city hospital (Parente et al. 1990).

Psychological Aspects

Longitudinal studies of girls who later developed drinking problems have revealed feelings of low self-esteem and impaired ability to cope (Jones 1971) and drinking to relieve shyness, to get along better on dates, and to get "high" (Fillmore 1979). Additional risk factors have been identified in retrospective studies. In a large general-population sample of adult women, a history of sexual assault increased the risk for a lifetime diagnosis of alcohol abuse or dependence (3.5 times more likely) and drug abuse or dependence (4 times more likely) (Winfield et al. 1990). In addition, women who develop chemical dependency are more likely than men to satisfy diagnostic criteria for an additional psychiatric diagnosis, especially major depression (Helzer and Pryzbeck 1988; Hesselbrock et al. 1985). Alcoholic women are also at increased risk for suicide (Gomberg 1986). When alcoholism and major depression occur in the same woman, the depression predates the onset of alcoholism two-thirds of the time. Such "dual-diagnosis" patients have a favorable prognosis if they receive adequate treatment for both disorders (Rounsaville et al. 1987), whereas efforts to relieve chemical dependence by treating "underlying" disorders alone have usually been unsuccessful.

Physiological Factors

Women have been found to be more sensitive to alcohol than are men. When given equal doses of alcohol per pound of body weight under standard conditions, female subjects attain higher blood alcohol levels than do males. This is partly due to the lower average water content in the bodies of women, since alcohol is distributed in total body water. It may also be a result of more complete absorption of alcohol in women, which results from lower levels of the metabolic enzyme of alcohol, alcohol dehydrogenase, in gastric tissue (Frezza et al. 1990). Women also show more variable peak blood alcohol levels, which some, but not other, investigators have found to correlate with the menstrual cycle. Although there is little evidence that patterns of drug use vary with the menstrual cycle in normal women, those who suffer from premenstrual dysphoria tend to increase their use of alcohol and marijuana during the premenstruum (Mello 1986).

Sex differences in relative body water and fat content also lead to longer half-lives for lipid-soluble psychoactive drugs, such as diazepam and oxazepam, in women (Barry 1986). Aging further exaggerates this trend.

Effects of Alcohol and Drug Use on Sexuality and Reproduction

In examining the effects of psychoactive substance use on women's sexuality, the strong influence of socially conditioned expectations must be considered (Wilsnack 1984). Because alcohol is thought to be sexually stimulating, women report more subjective sexual arousal when they have consumed alcohol, even when physiological measurements show otherwise. In physiological experiments, alcohol has been shown objectively to have a dose-related depressant effect on sexual arousal (Wilson and Lawson 1976) and orgasm (Malatesta et al. 1982) in women. Alcoholic women report a wide variety of sexual dysfunctions, including premenstrual dysphoria, lack of sexual interest, anorgasmia, vaginismus, and dyspareunia. At the same time, these women believe that alcohol arouses them and fear that they will not enjoy sex if they are sober. Physicians can help these women by explaining alcohol's depressant effects and reassuring them that abstinence from alcohol and other drugs is likely to improve their sexual functioning in the long run. Another commonly held expectation is that cocaine and amphetamines function as enhancers of sexual functioning. In fact, chronic use of both drugs can cause impotence and ejaculatory failure in men, inhibition of orgasm in women, and loss of sexual desire in both sexes (Washton 1989).

Heroin dependence has been reported to depress sexual desire and suppress ovulation (Gaulden et al. 1964). Menstrual periods often return to normal within a few months after the institution of methadone maintenance treatment (Wallach et al. 1969). Methadone itself, however, depresses sexual activity in a dose-related fashion (Crowley and Simpson 1978). The abuse of sedative drugs and minor tranquilizers such as diazepam may also depress both sexual desire and orgasm in women.

Alcoholic women commonly experience amenorrhea, anovulatory cycles, luteal phase dysfunction, and early menopause (Mello et al. 1989). They may therefore seek help for infertility, unaware that their alcohol or sedative intake might play an etiological role. In addition, even at levels of social drinking, alcohol has also been shown to increase the risk of spontaneous abortion, especially in the midtrimester (Mello et al. 1989).

Adverse effects of alcohol and drug abuse on pregnancy and the developing fetus are produced by a complex interaction of pharmacological, life-style, and nutritional factors, including absent or insufficient prenatal care. Although some women use only one drug, multiple drug use, including heavy smoking, is common (Mello et al. 1989). Premature labor, abruptio placentae, stillbirth, and a wide variety of other obstetric complications have been reported to be associated with maternal abuse of alcohol and other chemicals (Levy and Koren 1990). Alcohol is also known to suppress uterine contractions and in the past was employed in the treatment of threatened preterm labor (Fadel and Hadi 1982).

Cocaine, because of its acute stimulant, vasoconstrictive, and cardiac arrhythmia-producing properties, has been linked to sudden death in pregnant women (Burkett et al. 1990), as well as to premature rupture of the membranes, preterm labor, and fetal distress (Mastrogiannis et al. 1990). Unfortunately, the association between acute ingestion of cocaine and premature labor has led to a mistaken belief among young women that cocaine can shorten their labor while making it less painful (Skolnick 1990). This misconception may actually lead to an increase in the use of cocaine in late pregnancy.

Cigarette smoking has been associated with an increased risk of spontaneous abortion, placenta previa, and abruptio placentae (Levy and Koren 1990). Studies of the influence of marijuana use on the course of pregnancy have been equivocal; some studies suggest an increased incidence of protracted labor and precipitate labor (Levy and Koren 1990).

Adverse effects of drugs of abuse on the fetus include both general and substance-specific influences. Table 20–1 summarizes these effects. In addition to those listed, an increased incidence of sudden infant death syndrome or neonatal apnea has been correlated with prenatal exposure to both cocaine and nicotine. Heroin dependence has been linked to a range of obstetric complications. On the other hand, women who are maintained on stable doses of methadone and are provided with adequate prenatal care and nutrition have an improved course of pregnancy and may produce offspring of normal size and weight (Blinick et al. 1973). Postnatal abstinence syndrome is common in such infants but can be managed (Hoegerman et al. 1990).

Evidence for long-term neurobehavioral abnormalities due to methadone exposure is equivocal (Rosen and Johnson 1985). Fetal alcohol syndrome (FAS), first described and named in 1973, consists of the following signs and symptoms (U.S. Department of Health and Human Services 1990):

Table 20–1. Commonly reported teratogenic effects of abused drugs

Specific fetal effects	Opiates	Alcohol	Other sedative-hypnotic drugs	Cocaine	Other stimulants	Hallu-cinogens	Marijuana	Nicotine
Structural nonspecific growth retardation	X	X	—	X	—	—	X	X
Specific dysmorphic effects	—	X	—	X	—	—	—	—
Behavioral	X	X	X	X	X	X	X	X
Neurobiochemical (abstinence syndrome)	X	X	X	—	—	—	—	—
Increased fetal and perinatal mortality	X	X	—	X	—	—	—	X
Percentage of women reporting use in pregnancy (varies with population)	5	>50	<5	≤20	<5	<5	5–34	>50

Note. — = effect not reported.
Source. Reprinted from Hoegerman G, Wilson CA, Thurmond E, et al.: "Drug-Exposed Neonates." *Western Journal of Medicine* 152:559–564, 1990. Used with permission.

❖ Prenatal and postnatal growth retardation
❖ Central nervous system dysfunction (including any combination of reduced head circumference; mental retardation; hyperactivity; and disordered learning, coordination, or balance)
❖ A characteristic facial dysmorphism, with shortened palpebral fissures, epicanthic folds, and a shortened, depressed nose bridge
❖ Elongated, flattened upper lip and displaced, deformed ears
❖ Additional birth defects ranging from mild (birthmarks, single palmar crease) to severe (cardiac, joint, eye, and ear abnormalities)

The term *fetal alcohol effects* (FAE) refers to abnormalities that are presumed or suspected to be related to maternal drinking during pregnancy and that do not meet the criteria for FAS. Although it has been established through both human and animal studies that heavy drinking throughout most of pregnancy produces both FAS and FAE, the relative risks of various amounts and patterns of drinking are still in question. Experiments in animals indicate that alcohol consumed in a binge pattern may produce more severe damage than an equal quantity consumed over a longer period.

Although no absolutely safe level of alcohol intake during pregnancy has been established, negative effects of "light," "moderate," or "social" drinking have been subtle and more difficult to document than the effects of heavier drinking (Blume 1986a; Russell 1991). Nevertheless, most authorities recommend abstinence, following the advice of the U.S. Surgeon General, who issued the following statement in 1981:

> The Surgeon General advises women who are pregnant (or considering pregnancy) not to drink alcoholic beverages and to be aware of the alcoholic content of foods and drugs.

Most drugs of abuse pass freely into breast milk and can cause harm to the nursing infant. Even small quantities of alcohol consumed during lactation may cause measurable differences in motor development (Little et al. 1989). Alcohol use has also been associated with a risk of breast cancer in women in a dose-response relationship (Longnecker et al. 1988).

Other Physical Complications of Alcohol and Drug Use

Alcoholism has been found to progress more rapidly in women than in men. This is also true for the physical complications of alcoholism, including fatty liver, hypertension, obesity, anemia, malnutrition, peptic ulcer, and cirrhosis of the liver (Ashley et al. 1977; Gavaler 1982). These conditions may in turn cause further obstetric and gynecologic morbidity (Blume 1986b).

Another important set of complications of alcohol and drug dependence are sexually transmitted diseases. The proportion of women among all newly reported cases of acquired immunodeficiency syndrome (AIDS) has grown steadily over the past decade. Seventy-nine percent of affected women are between the ages of 13 and 39 (Campbell 1990). Half of these women have been users of intravenous drugs, and 15% have been nonusing sexual partners of male intravenous drug users (Cohen et al. 1989). In New York City at present, approximately 60% of intravenous drug users are positive for antibodies to human immunodeficiency virus (HIV) (Des Jarlais et al. 1989). Studies of HIV-positive women in a methadone maintenance program showed no differences in fertility when compared with HIV-negative control subjects, and very few differences in the course of pregnancy were found between the two groups (Selwyn et al. 1989). About one-third of infants born to HIV-positive women will be HIV positive themselves at 18 months of age (Blanche et al. 1989).

In addition, there was a sharp rise in the incidence of both primary and secondary syphilis, especially among women, during the 1980s (Rolfs and Nakashima 1990). Seropositivity for syphilis in women has been linked to cocaine use (Minkoff et al. 1990), as well as to the use of other drugs.

IDENTIFICATION AND TREATMENT OF PSYCHOACTIVE SUBSTANCE ABUSE IN OBSTETRIC-GYNECOLOGIC PRACTICE

Screening

Among the available methods to identify those obstetric-gynecologic patients who are at risk for alcohol and other drug problems is the inclusion in the history-taking of specific questions, such as those in the CAGE (Ewing 1984), TWEAK (Russell et al. 1991), or T-ACE questionnaires (Sokol et al. 1989). A self-administered questionnaire (Figure 20–1) can be conveniently administered in the patient waiting room and reviewed by the clinician with the patient (Russell 1982). Laboratory approaches include drug testing of blood or urine and may involve drug testing of the newborn infant. Routine blood tests have also been helpful in the identification of alcoholism. Mean corpuscular volume and/or γ-glutamyltransferase were elevated in two-thirds of a group of female alcoholic outpatients who were free of physical complications (Hollstedt and Dahlgren 1987). Positive scores on the same tests were sensitive to levels of drinking and predictive of alcohol-related birth defects in obstetric patients who were problem drinkers (Ylikorkala et al. 1987).

Positive screening results should be followed in all cases by a careful diagnosis in which accepted criteria are used. A positive urine test should not be used as a substitute for a clinical assessment.

Treatment Considerations

The most important factors in approaching the chemically dependent woman identified in obstetric-gynecologic practice are a nonjudgmental, helping attitude; a thorough knowledge of available treatment resources in the community; and the involvement of family members or significant others in carrying out the referral to treatment for chemical dependency. Education or warnings about the need for abstinence are not sufficient for alcohol- or drug-dependent pregnant women. Although some are able to abstain during pregnancy without treatment, most relapse after delivery, to the detriment of their health, family life, and future pregnancies. These women need rehabilitative treatment, sometimes preceded by detoxification, to recover. Sample protocols are available to assist in detoxification of the pregnant woman who is dependent on alcohol or sedatives. Opiate-dependent pregnant women may be either detoxified or shifted to a methadone maintenance regimen (Hoegerman et al. 1990). Self-help fellowships such as Alcoholics Anonymous, Narcotics Anonymous, and Women for Sobriety are widely available and play an essential role in long-term recovery.

Both self-help (e.g., Al-Anon Family Groups, Nar-Anon, Adult Children of Alcoholics groups) and professional services are indicated for those obstetric-gynecologic patients whose lives have been adversely affected by the chemical dependence of a family member. At times a structured intervention can be arranged in which family and friends confront the alcohol- or drug-dependent person with the assistance of a trained professional (Johnson Institute 1983). Structured intervention should be considered as an approach if the chemically dependent obstetric-gynecologic patient is initially unwilling to accept the need for alcohol or drug treatment concomitant with her obstetric-gynecologic care.

Barriers to Treatment

Women are seriously underrepresented in alcoholism treatment in the United States. Although they constitute approximately one-third of alcoholic individuals, only one-fourth to one-fifth of patients in treatment are female. Likewise, there is a serious shortage of treatment for other drug dependence, especially for pregnant patients. A recent study (General Accounting Office 1990) reports that approximately 280,000 pregnant women needed drug abuse treatment in 1989, but less than 11% of this number received it.

Many women who are in need of care are single parents, unemployed, or underemployed, making them less likely to have adequate insurance coverage. Furthermore, the lack of available child care often prevents them from entering inpatient or residential programs. Although a few programs admit both mothers and children, such facilities are rare.

An additional barrier to treatment is the fear of losing child custody. Women who must rely on a public agency for child care in order to enter treatment are often reluctant to do so. Pregnant patients also fear criminal prosecution for "prenatal child abuse" or for the delivery of controlled substances to a minor (via the umbilical cord). Publicized cases of prosecution and incarceration of pregnant or newly delivered women have further eroded the fragile trust of chemically dependent women in the health care system and will lead to more births to mothers lacking prenatal care. In some jurisdictions, the re-

Please check answers below.

	Very helpful	Not helpful	Never tried

1. When you are depressed or nervous, do you find any of the following helpful to feel better or to relax?

   a. Smoking cigarettes ___ ___ ___

   b. Working harder than usual at home or job ___ ___ ___

   c. Taking a tranquilizer ___ ___ ___

   d. Taking some other kind of pill or medication ___ ___ ___

   e. Having a drink ___ ___ ___

   f. Talking it over with friends or relatives ___ ___ ___

2. Think of the times you have been most depressed; at those times, did you:

	Yes	No

   a. Lose or gain weight? ___ ___

   b. Lose interest in things that usually interest you? ___ ___

   c. Have spells when you couldn't seem to stop crying? ___ ___

   d. Suffer from insomnia? ___ ___

3. Have you ever gone to a doctor, psychologist, social worker, counselor, or clergy person for help with an emotional problem? ___ ___

4. How many cigarettes a day do you smoke? Check one.

   ___ More than 2 packs   ___ 1–2 packs   ___ Less than 1 pack   ___ None

5. How often do you have a drink of wine, beer, or other beverage containing alcohol?

   ___ 3 or more times a day   ___ Twice a day   ___ Almost every day
   ___ Once or twice a week   ___ Once or twice a month
   ___ Less than once a month   ___ Never

Figure 20–1. Health questionnaire.

6. a. If you drink wine, beer, or other beverages containing alcohol, how often do you have four or more drinks?

___ Almost always ___ Frequently ___ Sometimes ___ Never

   b. If you drink wine, beer, or other beverages containing alcohol, how often do you have one or two drinks?

___ Almost always ___ Frequently ___ Sometimes ___ Never

7. What prescribed medications do you take? _____

_____

_____

8. What other drugs or medications do you use? _____

_____

_____

	Yes	No
9. Does your drinking or taking other drugs sometimes lead to problems between you and your family, that is, spouse, children, parent, or other close relative?	___	___
10. During the past year, have close relatives or friends worried or complained about your drinking or taking other drugs?	___	___
11. Has a friend or family member ever told you about things you said or did while you were drinking or using other drugs that you do not remember?	___	___
12. Within the past year, have you started to drink alcohol and found it difficult to stop before becoming intoxicated?	___	___
13. Has your father or mother ever had problems with alcohol or other drugs?	___	___

Figure 20–1. Health questionnaire *(continued)*.

moval of newborn infants from their mothers solely on the basis of a positive drug test, without any effort at assessment, diagnosis, intervention, or treatment, has created a reluctance among both professionals and patients to make use of this important diagnostic tool. The ensuing policy debate has led to proposed legislation in several states to protect the rights of women and encourage chemical dependency treatment, rather than prosecution.

Educating Obstetrician-Gynecologists About Psychoactive Substance Abuse

Programs aimed at the prevention of chemical dependency in women and chemical-related birth defects in children have taken two related approaches: public and professional education. Both aim at acquainting young people and adults with the teratogenicity of alcohol and other drugs and with the concept of chemical dependencies as treatable diseases. Both also depend on enhancing the health care professional's recognition of these diseases in women and successful referral of these patients to treatment.

Evaluations of efforts at professional education have shown that obstetrician-gynecologists will read and respond to a state-sponsored fetal alcohol syndrome information packet (Russell et al. 1983) or a community education program (Little et al. 1983). To sustain appropriate screening and referral patterns in obstetric practice, however, ongoing educational efforts are necessary (Weiner et al. 1983). Primary care workers and health educators must also be involved, especially in high-risk populations such as Native Americans and Alaska Natives, but preliminary evidence indicates that such prevention programs can be effective (May and Hymbaugh 1989).

Psychiatrists have an important role in these prevention activities. The training of all obstetrician-gynecologists should include methods of identifying, motivating, and referring women with chemical dependencies. This training can be provided by psychiatrists with skills and experience in this area. Other opportunities arise around consultation and in continuing-education programs for physicians and other health professionals. Psychiatrists can also help improve procedures for screening and intervention in obstetric-gynecologic practice.

The goals of prevention through social change include education to remove the inaccurate social stigma attached to chemically dependent women. At the same time, they stress the promotion of supportive networks that preserve women's social protection from the expectation that they drink or take drugs "like men." Finally, they provide psychosocial support for women undergoing stressful transitions, such as separation, divorce, and bereavement, to help them cope with these changes without developing dependence on chemicals of abuse. Psychiatrists can participate by helping to organize such support systems and by acting as consultants to community-based prevention programs. Finally, all concerned citizens can advocate enlightened public policies that offer appropriate and accessible help to women in need, in place of punitive and stigmatizing measures.

REFERENCES

Ashley MJ, Olin JS, leRiche WH, et al: Morbidity in alcoholics: evidence for accelerated development of physical disease in women. Arch Intern Med 137:883–887, 1977

Barry PP: Gender as a factor in treating the elderly, in Women and Drugs: A New Era for Research (NIDA Research Monograph No 65). Edited by Ray BA, Braude MC. Washington, DC, U.S. Department of Health and Human Services, 1986, pp 65–69

Blanche S, Rouzious C, Moscato ML, et al: A prospective study of infants born to women seropositive for HIV type 1. N Engl J Med 32:1643–1648, 1989

Blinick G, Jerez E, Wallach RC: Methadone maintenance, pregnancy, and progeny. JAMA 225:477–479, 1973

Blume SB: Is social drinking during pregnancy harmless? there is reason to think not. Advances in Alcohol and Substances Abuse 5:209–219, 1986a

Blume SB: Women and alcohol: a review. JAMA 256:1467–1470, 1986b

Blume SB: Sexuality and stigma: the alcoholic woman. Alcohol Health and Research World 15:139–146, 1991

Burkett G, Bandstra ES, Cohen J, et al: Cocaine-related maternal death. Am J Obstet Gynecol 163:40–41, 1990

Campbell CA: Women and AIDS. Soc Sci Med 30:407–415, 1990

Cermak TL: Diagnosing and Treating Codependence. Minneapolis, MN, Johnson Institute, 1986

Chasnoff IJ: The prevalence of illicit drug or alcohol use during pregnancy and discrepancies in mandatory reporting in Pinellas Co. Florida. N Engl J Med 322:1202–1206, 1990

Cohen JB, Hauer LB, Wofsy CB: Women and IV drugs. Journal of Drug Issues 19:39–56, 1989

Cooperstock R: Sex differences in psychotropic drug use. Soc Sci Med 12:179–186, 1978

Crowley TJ, Simpson R: Methadone dose and human sexual behavior. Int J Addict 13:285–295, 1978

Des Jarlais DC, Friedman SR, Novick DM, et al: HIV-1 infection among intravenous drug users in Manhattan, New York City, from 1977 through 1987. JAMA 261:1008–1012, 1989

Ewing JA: Detecting alcoholism: the CAGE questionnaire. JAMA 252:1905–1907, 1984

Fadel HE, Hadi HA: Alcohol effects on the reproductive function, in Encyclopedic Handbook of Alcoholism. Edited by Pattison EM, Kaufman E. New York, Gardner Press, 1982, pp 293–300

Fillmore KM, Bacon SD, Hyman M: The 27-year longitudinal panel study of drinking by students in college: report 1979 to National Institute of Alcoholism and Alcohol Abuse (DHHS Publ No ADM-281-76-0015). Washington, DC, U.S. Government Printing Office, 1979

Frezza M, DiPadova C, Pozzato G, et al: High blood alcohol levels in women. N Engl J Med 322:95–99, 1990

Gaulden EC, Littlefield DC, Putoff OE, et al: Menstrual abnormalities associated with heroin addiction. Am J Obstet Gynecol 90:155–160, 1964

Gavaler JS: Sex-related differences in ethanol-induced liver disease: artifactual or real? Alcohol Clin Exp Res 6:186–196, 1982

General Accounting Office: Drug-exposed infants: a generation at risk (Publ No GAO/HRD 90-138). Washington, DC, General Accounting Office, June 1990

Gomberg ESL: Women: alcohol and other drugs, in Perspectives on Drug Use in the United States. Edited by Segal B. New York, Haworth Press, 1986, pp 75–110

Gritz ER: Which women smoke and why? in Not Far Enough: Women vs Smoking (DHHS Publ No 87-2942). Washington, DC, National Institutes of Health, 1987, pp 15–19

Halliday A, Bush B, Cleary P, et al: Alcohol abuse in women seeking gynecologic care. Obstet Gynecol 68:322–326, 1986

Helzer JE, Pryzbeck TR: The co-occurrence of alcoholism with other psychiatric disorders in the general population and its impact on treatment. J Stud Alcohol 49:219–224, 1988

Hesselbrock MJ, Meyer RE, Keener JJ: Psychopathology in hospitalized alcoholics. Arch Gen Psychiatry 49:1050–1055, 1985

Hoegerman G, Wilson CA, Thurmond E, et al: Drug-exposed neonates. West J Med 152:559–564, 1990

Hollstedt C, Dahlgren L: Peripheral markers in the female "hidden alcoholic." Acta Psychiatr Scand 75:591–596, 1987

Johnson Institute: Intervention, a Professional's Guide. Minneapolis, MN, Johnson Institute, 1983

Jones MC: Personality antecedents and correlates of drinking patterns in women. J Consult Clin Psychol 36:61–69, 1971

Klassen AD, Wilsnack SC: Sexual experiences and drinking among women in a US national survey. Arch Sex Behav 15:363–392, 1986

Klee L, Ames G: Reevaluating risk factors for women's drinking: a study of blue-collar wives. Am J Prev Med 3:31–41, 1987

Levy M, Koren G: Obstetric and neonatal effects of drug abuse. Emerg Med Clin North Am 8:633–652, 1990

Little RE, Streissguth AP, Guzinski GM, et al: Change in obstetrician advice following a two-year community educational program on alcohol use and pregnancy. Am J Obstet Gynecol 146:23–28, 1983

Little RE, Anderson KW, Ervin CH, et al: Maternal alcohol use during breast-feeding and infant mental and motor development at one year. N Engl J Med 321:425–430, 1989

Longnecker MP, Berlin JA, Orza MJ, et al: A meta-analysis of alcohol consumption in relation to risk of breast cancer. JAMA 260:652–656, 1988

Malatesta VJ, Pollack RH, Crotty TD, et al: Acute alcohol intoxication and female orgasmic response. Journal of Sex Research 18:1–17, 1982

Mastrogiannis DS, Decavalas GO, Verma U, et al: Perinatal outcome after recent cocaine usage. Obstet Gynecol 76:8–11, 1990

May PA, Hymbaugh KJ: A macro-level FAS prevention program for native Americans and Alaskan natives: description and evaluation. J Stud Alcohol 50:508–518, 1989

McKinlay AP: The Roman attitude toward women's drinking, in Drinking and Intoxication. Edited by McCarthy RG. New Haven, CT, College and University Press, 1959, pp 58–61

Mello NK: Drug use patterns and premenstrual dysphoria, in Women and Drugs: A New Era for Research (NIDA Research Monograph No 65). Edited by Ray BA, Braude MC. Washington, DC, U.S. Department of Health and Human Services, 1986, pp 31–48

Mello NK, Mendelson JH, Teoh SK: Neuroendocrine consequences of alcohol abuse in women. Ann N Y Acad Sci 562:211–240, 1989

Miller BA, Downs WR, Gondoli DM: Spousal violence among alcoholic women as compared to a random household sample of women. J Stud Alcohol 50:533–540, 1989

Minkoff HL, McCalla S, Delke I, et al: The relationship of cocaine use to syphilis and HIV infections among inner city parturient women. Am J Obstet Gynecol 163:521–526, 1990

Moore RD, Bone LR, Geller G, et al: Prevalence, detection and treatment of alcoholism in hospitalized patients. JAMA 261:403–408, 1989

National Institute on Drug Abuse: National household survey on drug abuse: population estimates, 1988 (DHHS Publ No ADM-89-1636). Washington, DC, U.S. Government Printing Office, 1989

Parente JT, Gaines B, Lockridge R, et al: Substance abuse during pregnancy. N Y State J Med 90:336–337, 1990

Richardson D, Campbell J: The effect of alcohol on attributions of blame for rape. Personality and Social Psychology Bulletin 8:468–476, 1982

Rolfs RT, Nakashima AK: Epidemiology of primary and secondary syphilis in the United States, 1981 through 1989. JAMA 264:1432–1437, 1990

Rosen TS, Johnson HL: Long-term effects of prenatal methadone maintenance, in Consequences of Maternal Drug Abuse (NIDA Research Monograph No 59). Edited by Pinkert TM. Washington, DC, U.S. Department of Health and Human Services, 1985, pp 73–83

Rounsaville BJ, Dolinsky ZS, Babor TF, et al: Psychopathology as a predictor of treatment outcome in alcoholics. Arch Gen Psychiatry 44:505–513, 1987

Russell M: Screening for alcohol-related problems in ob/gyn patients, in Fetal Alcohol Syndrome, Vol 2. Edited by Abel EL. Boca Raton, FL, CRC Press, 1982, pp 1–19

Russell M: Clinical implications of recent research on the fetal alcohol syndrome. Bull N Y Acad Med 67:207–222, 1991

Russell M, Coviello D: Heavy drinking and regular psychoactive drug use among gynecological outpatients. Alcohol Clin Exp Res 12:400–406, 1988

Russell M, Skinner JB: Early measures of maternal alcohol misuse as predictors of adverse pregnancy outcomes. Alcohol Clin Exp Res 12:824–830, 1988

Russell M, Kang GE, Uhteg L: Evaluation of an educational program on FAS for health professionals. Journal of Alcohol and Drug Education 29:48–61, 1983

Russell M, Cooper ML, Frone MR: The influence of sociodemographic characteristics on familial alcohol problems: data from a community sample. Alcohol Clin Exp Res 14:221–226, 1990

Russell M, Martier SS, Sokol RJ, et al: Screening for pregnancy risk-drinking: tweaking the tests (abstract). Alcohol Clin Exp Res 15:268, 1991

Selwyn PA, Schoenbaum EE, Davenny K, et al: Prospective study of human immunodeficiency virus and pregnancy outcomes in intravenous drug users. JAMA 261:1289–1294, 1989

Skolnick A: Cocaine use in pregnancy: physicians urged to look for problem where they least expect it. JAMA 264:306–309, 1990

Sokol RJ, Martier SS, Ager JW: The T-ACE questions: practical prenatal detection of risk-drinking. Am J Obstet Gynecol 160:863–870, 1989

U.S. Department of Health and Human Services: Fetal alcohol syndrome and other effects of alcohol on pregnancy outcome, in Seventh Special Report to the U.S. Congress on Alcohol and Health (DHHS Publ No ADM-90-1656). Washington, DC, U.S. Government Printing Office, 1990, pp 139–161

U.S. Surgeon General: Surgeon General's advisory on alcohol and pregnancy. FDA Drug Bulletin 11:1, 1981

Wallach RC, Jerez E, Blinick G: Pregnancy and menstrual function in narcotics addicts treated with methadone. Am J Obstet Gynecol 105:1226–1229, 1969

Washton AM: Cocaine Addiction. New York, WW Norton, 1989

Weiner L, Rosett HL, Edelin KC: Behavioral evaluation of fetal alcohol education for physicians. Alcohol Clin Exp Res 6:230–233, 1983

Williams GD, Grant BF, Harford TC, et al: Population projections using DSM-III criteria, alcohol abuse and dependence, 1990–2000. Alcohol Health and Research World 13:366–370, 1989

Wilsnack SC: Drinking, sexuality and sexual dysfunction in women, in Alcohol Problems in Women. Edited by Wilsnack SC, Beckman LJ. New York, Guilford, 1984, pp 189–227

Wilson GT, Lawson DM: Effects of alcohol on sexual arousal in women. J Abnorm Psychol 85:489–497, 1976

Winfield I, George LK, Swartz M, et al: Sexual assault and psychiatric disorders among a community sample of women. Am J Psychiatry 147:335–341, 1990

Ylikorkala O, Stenman U, Halmesmaki E: Gammaglutamyl transferase and mean cell volume reveal maternal alcohol abuse and fetal alcohol effects. Am J Obstet Gynecol 157:344–348, 1987

Chapter 21

Eating Disorders and Reproduction

Donna E. Stewart, M.D., D.Psych., F.R.C.P.C.
Gail Erlick Robinson, M.D., F.R.C.P.C.

❖ ❖ ❖ ❖ ❖ ❖ ❖ ❖ ❖ ❖ ❖ ❖ ❖ ❖

Social pressures for thinness in women have greatly escalated during the 20th century as a result of remarkable shifts in attitudes concerning women's attractiveness. After centuries of admiration for curvaceous women, thinness is now idealized. One paradoxical aspect of this quest for thinness is the fact that, as nutrition has improved, the average weight of women in industrialized societies has increased by 5 pounds (Polivy et al. 1986). These factors have led to a greatly increased pressure to diet.

Various theories have been proposed to explain the new emphasis on thinness. One factor may be the tendency of modern society to idealize youthfulness (Shainess 1979). Prepubescent girls acting as fashion models promote the idea that the ideal shape is that of a child. Excessive thinness eliminates the curves that are suggestive of adulthood. Moreover, throughout history, upper-class women have served as role models for fashion. In contradistinction to the past, being overweight no longer denotes wealth. Rather, in today's industrialized society, it is lower-class women with inadequate diets and insufficient exercise who are the most likely to be overweight (Polivy et al. 1986).

The devotion to thinness that began in upper classes has now spread throughout society. Medical science has also contributed to this fashion for thinness by linking obesity with heart disease, arthritis, and early mortality (Bray 1976). Evidence for the health dangers of thinness have received far less attention (Sorlie et al. 1980). Preoccupation with weight may also reflect the new pressures on women to

411

compete with men, and eliminating the feminine figure may be an attempt to reinforce the move away from traditional female stereotypes (Orbach 1978). Because dieting may be regarded as a sign of internal control, slim women are thereby viewed as disciplined and in control (Garner et al. 1983).

The pressures for thinness have resulted in a general increase in body consciousness that is much more marked for women than men. Surveys of high school students indicate that girls usually want to weigh less than their current weight (Jakobouits et al. 1977). National surveys of adults conclude that a woman's self-esteem often relates to her feeling pretty and slim (Berscheid et al. 1973). Surveys of college-age women have found dieting and disordered eating to be widespread (Herman and Polivy 1980).

Polivy et al. (1986) have concluded that our society's attitudes and behaviors connected with food, eating, and body weight are not unlike those of the anorexic patient. There is an intense preoccupation with food, gourmet cuisine, and cooking; at the same time, there are multiple articles in the popular press on weight reduction and fad diets. A great deal of attention is paid to exercising and fitness, and there is a strong belief that the pursuit of thinness is both normal and admirable. The extreme consequences of these social pressures and their resultant behavior is found in the clinical syndromes of anorexia nervosa and bulimia nervosa.

Many women with eating disorders are secretive about them, and problems in diagnosis are compounded by the fact that some women with eating disorders appear to be of normal weight by actuarial or population mean standards. Careful examination of their longitudinal weight histories, however, may reveal premorbid obesity that led to highly restrictive dieting coupled with bulimic behaviors. Relative starvation and nutritional chaos may thus be obscured. Eating disorders result in a mortality of approximately 5% and lead to significant morbidity secondary to weight loss, vomiting, electrolyte disturbances, gastrointestinal problems, osteoporosis, psychiatric sequelae, and reproductive complications (Garfinkel 1985). Although the medical effects have been described for many years, the reproductive aspects of eating disorders have been inadequately studied (Stewart and Robinson 1989).

It is known that many patients with eating disorders develop amenorrhea, and recently more attention has been paid to infertility in these women (Abraham et al. 1990; Allison et al. 1988; Stewart et al. 1990). As more effective treatment of eating disorders and infertility evolves, more of these women eventually become pregnant. Little is known about the course of their pregnancies or the health of their infants. Many psychological conflicts, such as body image, autonomy, sexuality, dependency, and relationships to parents, that are common in patients with eating disorders are highlighted during normal pregnancy. It is therefore possible that pregnancy is an especially stressful time for women with eating disorders (Stewart et al. 1987). This chapter examines what is currently known about the effects of eating disorders on menstruation, fertility, pregnancy, the fetus and newborn, and the infant and feeding.

DEFINITIONS

Anorexia nervosa is a psychiatric disorder characterized by 1) refusal to maintain body weight over the minimal normal weight for one's age and height—for example, weight loss leading to maintenance of a body weight that is 15% below that expected—or failure to achieve expected weight gain during a period of growth; 2) intense fear of gaining weight or of becoming fat even though underweight; 3) disturbance in the way in which one's body weight, size, or shape is experienced, for example, claiming to feel fat even when emaciated; and 4) in females, the absence of at least three consecutive menstrual cycles when otherwise expected to occur (American Psychiatric Association 1987). This self-imposed starvation triggered by the relentless pursuit of thinness and fear of fatness occurs in serious form in about 1% of adolescent and young adult women (Garfinkel and Garner 1982).

A related disorder, *bulimia nervosa,* is characterized by 1) recurrent episodes of binge eating of large amounts of food in a discrete period of time; 2) feeling a lack of control over eating behavior during eating binges; 3) regular use of self-induced vomiting, laxatives, or diuretics; strict dieting or fasting; or vigorous exercise in order to prevent weight gain; 4) a minimum average of two binge eating episodes a week for at least 3 months; and 5) persistent overconcern with body shape and weight (American Psychiatric Association 1987). Bulimia nervosa may occur within the context of anorexia nervosa or as a separate syndrome with little weight loss. Its prevalence in serious form is 1.7% among adolescent and young adult women (Ben-Tovim 1988).

A common, milder variant of these disorders is *eating disorder not otherwise specified*, which does not meet strict criteria for a specific eating disorder (American Psychiatric Association 1987). It occurs in a further 5% of the female population (Button and Whitehouse 1981; King 1986).

EFFECTS ON MENSTRUATION

It has long been known that women with anorexia nervosa may suffer from primary or secondary amenorrhea (Gull 1874). Indeed, one of the criteria for the diagnosis of anorexia nervosa includes absence of periods for three cycles. More recently, Pirke et al. (1985) have shown that 50% of patients with bulimia nervosa also suffer from amenorrhea. It is therefore prudent for clinicians to enquire about eating and dieting behaviors in women who report absent or irregular menstrual cycles.

Starkey and Lee (1969) looked at menstruation in 58 patients with a previous diagnosis of anorexia nervosa and found that all patients had established menstrual patterns prior to the onset of the disorder, but most became amenorrheic concurrent with the onset of the eating disorder. Most reported an improved weight gain with treatment, but in the group who did not gain weight, none experienced the return of menses. Nillius (1978) reported that 34% of 287 women with amenorrhea seen in his practice had amenorrhea caused by self-induced weight loss, but no mention was made of the presence of clinical eating disorders. A study by Fries (1974) found a high proportion of women with eating disorders among 30 Scandinavian women with secondary amenorrhea caused by self-induced weight loss.

Copeland and Herzog (1987) and Devlin et al. (1989) have described the endocrinologic findings associated with menstrual cycle abnormalities in women with anorexia nervosa and bulimia nervosa. In general, these women tended to have fewer secretory spikes of luteinizing hormone (LH) and a trend toward lower mean 24-hour LH levels than did control subjects. Stimulation with gonadotropin-releasing hormone produced elevated LH responses in women with bulimia nervosa and blunted LH responses in those with anorexia. Estradiol levels were uniformly lower in women with anorexia nervosa, and stimulation with estradiol revealed diminished LH augmentative responses and a trend toward diminished follicle-stimulating hormone augmentative responses in patients with anorexia nervosa and bulimia nervosa compared with control subjects. Pirke et al. (1985, 1988) have shown that approximately 50% of women of normal weight who have bulimia nervosa have menstrual abnormalities with impaired follicular maturation caused by impaired gonadotropin secretion. They have also shown that in normal young women of normal body weight who diet for 6 weeks (800–1,000 kilocalories per day), a variety of changes in endocrinologic function develop, with disruption of menstrual cycles for 3–6 months after dieting in approximately 20% of these women.

Kreipe et al. (1989) have shown that women with eating disorders not otherwise specified also frequently have menstrual dysfunction. As this disorder occurs more often than criteria-confirmed anorexia or bulimia nervosa, the full extent of the contribution of eating disorders to the clinical symptom of disordered menstruation is still unknown but is likely to be substantial in developed countries.

EFFECTS ON FERTILITY

Of all couples having regular, unprotected intercourse in the childbearing years, 15%–18% are unable to conceive within 1 year (Menning 1980). Until recently, it has been assumed that among women with eating disorders, only those with anorexia nervosa accompanied by amenorrhea contributed to the overall rates of infertility. Recent studies, however, have shown that unexplained infertility may sometimes be due to an undisclosed eating disorder or severe weight control. At the other end of the spectrum, compulsive eating with severe weight gain may also interfere with fertility.

Bates et al. (1982) found that 47 women with unexplained infertility or menstrual dysfunction who were referred to a reproductive endocrinology clinic had practiced weight control by caloric restriction in order to maintain a fashionable body habitus. All were below ideal body weight when compared with normative tables for height and weight. When 36 of the women followed a dietary regimen designed to increase their weight to predicted ideal body weight, 73% conceived spontaneously and 90% with secondary amenorrhea resumed menstruation. It is of interest that 97% of these "infertile" women and their husbands had been previously evaluated for infertility by a variety of diagnostic gynecologic studies without any reason being discovered. The authors concluded that the practice of weight control may be the cause of unexplained infertility and menstrual dysfunction in otherwise healthy women.

Nillius (1978) found that, in his infertility patients with amenorrhea, a number of costly and complicated gynecologic and endocrinologic investigations, and sometimes hormonal induction of ovulation, were carried out without an inadequate dietary intake ever coming to light. Allison et al. (1988) found an increased prevalence of abnormal eating attitudes in a small sample of infertility clinic patients. Stewart et al. (1990) reported a 17% prevalence of eating disorders in 66 consecutive patients attending a reproductive biology unit for infertility. The patients were prospectively screened with the Eating Attitudes Test—26 item (Garner et al. 1982), and women with positive screening tests were then interviewed to confirm or refute the diagnosis of an eating disorder. Of these women, 7.6% had anorexia nervosa or bulimia nervosa, and 9.1% had an eating disorder not otherwise specified. Among infertile women with amenorrhea or oligomenorrhea, 58% had eating disorders. It is of interest that none of these patients had previously disclosed their eating disorder to their gynecologist.

Abraham et al. (1990) raised the question of whether ovulation should be induced in women suffering or recovering from an eating disorder, in view of their poorer prognosis in pregnancy. She found that 13 of 14 consecutive women in whom ovulation had been induced met the criteria for an eating disorder at some time in the past, whereas 5 women currently fulfilled these criteria.

Several investigators have recommended that infertility specialists routinely ask questions about a woman's eating and dieting behavior, history of eating disorders, exercising habits, and past and present body weight before proceeding with infertility investigations (Abraham et al. 1990; Stewart and MacDonald 1987; Stewart et al. 1990). Patients often fail to volunteer information about eating disorders to their gynecologists, and they sometimes appear to be of normal weight. An awareness of the frequency of eating disorders in infertility patients, however, followed by careful clinical inquiry, should correctly identify most cases. It has become common for infertility clinics to provide psychiatric services for couples who are distressed by the diagnosis, investigation, and management of infertility problems (Stewart et al. 1992). Psychiatrists working with infertility patients can provide useful resources in the early identification and treatment of patients with a concurrent eating disorder or disordered eating that fails to meet the full diagnostic criteria for an eating disorder.

EFFECTS ON PREGNANCY

Hyperemesis Gravidarum

Hyperemesis gravidarum is intractable vomiting of pregnancy requiring hospitalization and accompanied by dehydration, electrolyte imbalance, ketonuria, and weight loss. In a study of hyperemesis gravidarum patients who were referred for psychiatric consultation (Stewart and MacDonald 1987), it was found that a number of these women had suffered from an eating disorder before conception but had initially failed to disclose this fact. A comparison of these patients with those who had hyperemesis gravidarum without a history of eating disorders found that those with eating disorders responded less favorably to treatment and spent twice as many days in the hospital during pregnancy. It is of interest that 50% of the hyperemesis patients with eating disorders had presented to an infertility clinic for induction of ovulation. Although hyperemesis gravidarum may be caused by a variety of psychological, social, physical, and physiologic problems, it is wise for obstetricians and consulting psychiatrists to remember that an eating disorder may also play an important role in some women. Further studies are required to investigate the true prevalence of eating disorders in women with hyperemesis gravidarum.

Food aversions, cravings, and pica are common occurrences in pregnancy. Their associations, if any, to eating disorders are unknown. These phenomena may accompany hyperemesis gravidarum but often present in the absence of vomiting. Food aversions and cravings are usually considered normal in pregnancy.

Low Maternal Weight Gain

Low maternal weight before pregnancy and poor weight gain during pregnancy correlate significantly with an increase in intrauterine growth retardation, low birth weight, congenital anomalies, and perinatal mortality (Abrams and Laros 1986). Although many of the data were collected during famines or in concentration camps, eating disorders are also a cause of low prepregnancy weight and failure to gain weight in pregnancy due to inadequate nutrition. Stewart et al. (1987) described 15 women who had previously suffered from anorexia nervosa or bulimia nervosa and who later conceived 23 pregnancies. Compared with women whose eating disorders were in remission, women who had an active eating disorder throughout pregnancy gained less weight and had more pregnancy complications. Lacey and Smith (1987) examined the impact of pregnancy in a report on eating behavior in 20 patients who had untreated bulimia nervosa and who were of normal weight. Although those authors found that the frequency of bulimic behavior generally diminished as pregnancy advanced, symptoms tended to return in the puerperium, and in nearly half of their sample, eating patterns were more disturbed after delivery than before conception.

Careful nutritional, weight, and psychosocial histories should be obtained in women who fail to gain weight adequately in pregnancy. Early psychiatric referral is indicated in women with psychiatric diagnoses or eating disorders.

EFFECTS ON THE FETUS AND NEWBORN

Several investigators (Brinch et al. 1988; Lacey and Smith 1987; Stewart et al. 1987; Strimling 1984; Treasure and Russell 1988) have described fetal problems associated with a maternal eating disorder. These difficulties may include intrauterine growth retardation, prematurity, low birth weight, low Apgar scores, increased risk of congenital anomalies, and higher perinatal mortality. The consequences of intrauterine growth retardation from any cause may be considerable in causing fetal antenatal or intrapartum asphyxia, resulting in fetal death or an increase in fetal distress and damage (Van der Spuy 1985). Once delivered, these small infants are at increased risk for hypothermia, hypoglycemia, and infection and have increased perinatal mortality (Van der Spuy 1985). Stewart et al. (1987) found that babies born to women with active eating disorders during their pregnancies were smaller and had lower 5-minute Apgar scores than did babies of mothers whose eating disorders were in remission. Lacey and Smith (1987) described higher incidences of fetal abnormalities, including cleft lip and palate; multiple gestation; obstetric complications, including breech presentation; and surgical intervention in 20 untreated bulimic women of normal weight. Brinch et al. (1988) followed 50 women with histories of eating disorders and found double the rate of premature births in their offspring and six times the expected rate of perinatal mortality. Treasure and Russell (1988) described the outcome of 7 pregnancies in women with anorexia nervosa who conceived despite low weight. The abdominal circumference of all 7 babies was well below the third percentile at birth. These studies all suffer from small sample sizes, and further work is required to replicate their findings in larger, controlled studies.

Feingold et al. (1988) reported a single case of bulimia nervosa in which the diagnosis of eating disorder was recognized in early pregnancy. By implementation of multidisciplinary management, including perinatology, nutrition, and psychiatry, the woman was able to gain adequate weight in pregnancy and delivered a healthy baby. Further study with effective case detection and larger sample sizes is necessary to determine whether this finding can be generalized.

EFFECTS ON THE INFANT AND FEEDING

Low-birth-weight infants who survive the early weeks of life may have long-term developmental consequences with continued delays in physical and neurological development and impaired intellectual ability, particularly when associated with low intrauterine growth before 26 weeks of gestation (Van der Spuy 1985). No work has yet been reported on the long-term follow-up of low-birth-weight infants born to mothers with eating disorders. It is hoped that, in view of the prevalence of eating disorders in young women, this work will soon be undertaken.

An additional problem in some mothers with eating disorders results from the worry that their infants will become obese, a concern leading to early nutritional deprivation or caloric restriction. Lacey and Smith (1987) found that 15% of bulimic mothers reported restricting calories in their child before 1 year of age. Stewart et al. (1987) found a decreased rate of breast-feeding in women with active eating disorders and more difficulties with postpartum adjustment. Brinch et al. (1988) reported a 17% rate of failure to thrive in the first year of life in the infants of mothers with eating disorders. Similarly, Treasure and Russell (1988) reported that children of four patients attending their eating disorders clinic had been investigated for poor growth attributed to inadequate feeding. They also reported that five of six mothers with anorexia nervosa had difficulty in breast-feeding and introduced bottle-feeds in the first few months of life. Stein and Fairburn (1989), Fahy and Treasure (1989), and Van Wezel-Meijler and Wit (1989) also found poor nutrition in infants of women with eating disorders. They also had concerns about the mother-child relationship and the infant's development.

Pediatricians (Pugliese et al. 1987) have also reported failure to thrive in infants whose parents had been restricting calories in their children because of fears that they might become overweight, although it is not clear that these parents actually suffered from eating disorders (as opposed to overconcern about obesity). Further investigations are required to establish the role of maternal eating disorders in nutritionally deprived children in wealthy, developed countries.

CONCLUSIONS

Currently available information suggests that a history of eating disorders or weight-reducing behavior should be part of the routine assessment of patients with amenorrhea, oligomenorrhea, and infertility, as well as in prenatal patients with hyperemesis gravidarum, those who fail to gain weight adequately in pregnancy, and those have babies who are small for gestational date. Those women in whom eating disorders are discovered before conception should be counseled to delay pregnancy until the eating disorder is adequately treated and truly in remission. If the woman has already conceived, the earliest possible diagnosis of an eating disorder should be made so that proper psychiatric treatment, dietary advice, and weight monitoring can be implemented to reduce the risk of maternal and fetal complications. The infants of mothers with eating disorders should also be carefully observed for failure to thrive so that early corrective measures can be implemented. Similarly, the parents of infants who fail to thrive should be assessed for eating disorders, overconcern about obesity, or abnormal eating behaviors. The field of reproductive effects of eating disorders offers many rich opportunities for psychiatrists to collaborate with obstetricians and gynecologists, nutritionists, nurses, and perinatologists in primary and secondary prevention programs directed toward both mother and infant.

REFERENCES

Abraham S, Mira M, Llewellyn-Jones D: Should ovulation be induced in women recovering from an eating disorder or who are compulsive exercisers? Fertil Steril 52:566–568, 1990

Abrams BF, Laros RK: Pregnancy weight, weight gain and birth weight. Am J Obstet Gynecol 154:503–509, 1986

Allison S, Kalucy R, Gilchrist P, et al: Weight preoccupation among infertile women. International Journal of Eating Disorders 7:743–748, 1988

American Psychiatric Association: Diagnostic and Statistical Manual of Mental Disorders, 3rd Edition, Revised. Washington, DC, American Psychiatric Association, 1987

Bates GW, Bates SR, Whitworth NS: Reproductive failure in women who practice weight control. Fertil Steril 37:373–378, 1982

Ben-Tovim DI: DSM-III, draft DSM-III-R and the diagnosis and prevalence of bulimia in Australia. Am J Psychiatry 145:1000–1002, 1988

Berscheid E, Walster E, Bohrnstedt GW: The happy American body: a survey report. Psychology Today, November 1973, pp 119–131

Bray G: The Obese Patient. Toronto, Canada, WB Saunders, 1976

Brinch M, Isager T, Tolstrup K: Anorexia nervosa and motherhood: reproductional pattern and mothering behaviour of 50 women. Acta Psychiatr Scand 77:98–104, 1988

Button EJ, Whitehouse A: Subclinical anorexia nervosa. Psychol Med 11:509–516, 1981

Copeland PM, Herzog DB: Menstrual abnormalities, in The Psychobiology of Bulimia. Edited by Hudson JI, Pipe HG. Washington, DC, American Psychiatric Press, 1987, pp 31–54

Devlin MJ, Walsh BT, Katz JL, et al: Hypothalamic-pituitary-gonadal function in anorexia nervosa and bulimia. Psychiatry Res 28:11–24, 1989

Fahy T, Treasure J: Children of the mothers with bulimia nervosa (letter). BMJ 299:1031, 1989

Feingold M, Kaminer Y, Lyons K, et al: Bulimia nervosa in pregnancy. Obstet Gynecol 71:1025–1027, 1988

Fries H: Secondary amenorrhea, self-induced weight reduction and anorexia nervosa. Acta Psychiatr Scand 248 (suppl):1–69, 1974

Garfinkel PE: Anorexia nervosa and bulimia. Ontario Medical Review, November 1985, pp 657–662

Garfinkel PE, Garner D (eds): Anorexia Nervosa: A Multidimensional Perspective. New York, Brunner/Mazel, 1982, pp 307–326

Garner DM, Olmsted MP, Bohr Y, et al: The Eating Attitudes Test: psychometric features and clinical correlates. Psychol Med 12:871–878, 1982

Garner DM, Garfinkel PE, Olmsted M: An overview of socio-cultural factors in the development of anorexia nervosa, in Anorexia Nervosa: Recent Developments. Edited by Darby PL, Garfinkel PE, Garner DM, et al. New York, Alan R Liss, 1983, pp 105–122

Gull WW: Anorexia nervosa. Trans Med Soc Lond 7:22–28, 1874

Herman CP, Polivy J: Restrained eating, in Obesity. Edited by Stunkard A. Philadelphia, PA, WB Saunders, 1980, pp 208–239

Jakobouits C, Halstead P, Kelley L, et al: Eating habits and nutritional intakes of college women over a thirty year period. J Am Diet Assoc 71:405–411, 1977

King MB: Eating disorders in general practice. BMJ 293:1412–1414, 1986

Kreipe RE, Strauss J, Hodgman CH, et al: Menstrual cycle abnormalities and subclinical eating disorders: a preliminary report. Psychosom Med 51:1–86, 1989

Lacey JH, Smith G: Bulimia nervosa: the impact of pregnancy on mother and baby. Br J Psychiatry 150:777–781, 1987

Menning BE: The emotional needs of infertile couples. Fertil Steril 34:313–319, 1980

Nillius SJ: Psycho-pathology of weight-related amenorrhea, in Advances in Gynaecological Endocrinology. Edited by Jacobs HS. London, UK, Royal College of Obstetricians and Gynaecologists, 1978, pp 118–130

Orbach S: Fat Is a Feminist Issue—The Anti-Diet Guide to Permanent Weight Loss. New York, Paddington Press, 1978

Pirke KM, Ulrich S, Lemmel W, et al: The influence of dieting on the menstrual cycle of healthy young women. J Clin Endocrinol Metab 60:1174–1179, 1985

Pirke KM, Dogs M, Fichter MM, et al: Gonadotrophins, oestradiol, and progesterone during the menstrual cycle in bulimia nervosa. Clin Endocrinol 29:265–270, 1988

Polivy J, Garner DM, Garfinkel PE: Causes and consequences of the current preference for thin female physiques, in Physical Appearance, Stigma and Social Behavior. Edited by Herman CP, Zanna MP, Higgins ET. Hillsdale, NJ, Lawrence Erlbaum, 1986, pp 89–112

Pugliese MT, Weyman-Daum M, Moses M, et al: Parental health beliefs as a cause of nonorganic failure to thrive. Pediatrics 80:175–182, 1987

Shainess N: The swing of the pendulum—from anorexia to obesity. Am J Psychoanal 39:225–234, 1979

Sorlie P, Gordon T, Kannel WB: Body build and mortality: the Framingham study. JAMA 243:1828–1831, 1980

Starkey TA, Lee RA: Menstruation and fertility in anorexia nervosa. Am J Obstet Gynecol 105:374–379, 1969

Stein A, Fairburn CG: Children of mothers with bulimia nervosa. BMJ 299:777–778, 1989

Stewart DE, MacDonald OL: Hyperemesis gravidarum and eating disorders in pregnancy, in Eating Disorders and Disordered Eating. Edited by Abraham S, Llewellyn-Jones D. Sydney, Australia, Ashwood House, 1987, pp 52–55

Stewart DE, Robinson GE: Pregnancy and eating disorders, in The Free Woman. Edited by Van Hall E. Carnforth, UK, Parthenon, 1989, pp 812–817

Stewart DE, Raskin J, Garfinkel PE, et al: Anorexia nervosa, bulimia, and pregnancy. Am J Obstet Gynecol 157:1194–1198, 1987

Stewart DE, Robinson GE, Goldbloom DS, et al: Infertility and eating disorders. Am J Obstet Gynecol 163:1196–1199, 1990

Stewart DE, Boydell KM, Redmond C, et al: A prospective study of the effectiveness of brief professionally led support groups for infertility patients. Int J Psychiatry Med 22:173–182, 1992

Strimling BS: Infant of a pregnancy complicated by anorexia nervosa. Am J Dis Child 138:68–69, 1984

Treasure JL, Russell GFM: Intrauterine growth and neonatal weight gain in babies of women with anorexia nervosa. BMJ 296:1038, 1988

Van der Spuy Z: Nutrition and reproduction. Clin Obstet Gynecol 12:579–604, 1985

Van Wezel-Meijler G, Wit JM: The off-spring of mothers with anorexia nervosa: a high-risk group for undernutrition and stunting? Eur J Pediatr 149:130–135, 1989

Chapter 22

BREAST DISORDERS AND BREAST CANCER

Barbara L. Andersen, Ph.D.
Susan Doyle-Mirzadeh, M.A.

❖ ❖ ❖ ❖ ❖ ❖ ❖ ❖ ❖ ❖ ❖ ❖ ❖ ❖

Although the diagnosis of cancer is a devastating experience, most women cope successfully. In fact, many report renewed vigor in their approach to life, stronger interpersonal relationships, and a "survivor" adaptation (Taylor 1983). These outcomes do not, however, describe the process of adjustment, which may include feelings of an emotional crisis at diagnosis, fears of cancer treatment and the changes it may bring, and a dread of life changes or adjustments. For decades the understanding of the psychological processes and outcomes for cancer patients was largely clinical, consisting of detailed case studies of patients and clinical descriptions of difficult treatment experiences (Sutherland et al. 1952). The message from these reports was that the psychological trajectory for women treated for breast cancer was guarded, at best.

More recently, controlled research on the behavioral and psychological aspects of cancer has described the specific difficulties that cancer patients may face, some proposed etiologic mechanisms for these processes, and the tested psychological interventions to enhance coping (Andersen 1989). In much of this research, women with breast cancer have been the study participants, although those with disease at other sites have also received recent study (Andersen et al. 1989a, 1989b; Cella and Tross 1986).

This chapter provides a scholarly overview of the psychological processes of adjustment to breast cancer, from symptom appearance to cure or death from disease. Also included are brief discussions of

intervention strategies for the consulting psychiatrist. As a preface, benign breast disorders are briefly reviewed, as many of these conditions
produce symptoms or signs closely resembling those of breast cancer.

BENIGN BREAST DISORDERS

Benign breast disorders are common (Hacker and Jochimsen 1986).
Fibrocystic disease, the most frequent condition, is clinically apparent
in about 50% of women. This disease is characterized by hyperplastic
changes that may involve any or all of the breast tissues. Changes may
be hormonally mediated and due to a relative or absolute decline in
progesterone or to an increase in estrogen. When hyperplastic changes
are also accompanied by cellular atypia, there is an increased risk for
malignancy. The clinical picture is usually one of multiple bilateral lesions that may become painful and/or tender, particularly premenstrually. The disease is often diagnosed and problematic during the
young adult years, with symptomatology ending at menopause (unless,
of course, exogenous estrogens are taken). Treatment decisions are
moderated by the age of the woman, symptom severity, and the relative
risk for breast malignancy. Particularly troublesome cysts are aspirated
to relieve pain (and to determine the absence of malignancy), but in
severe circumstances subcutaneous mastectomies may be considered.

   There are several other types of benign breast growths. Fibro-
adenomas are the most common benign tumors of the breast. Clinically, these neoplasms are circumscribed, solitary, and freely movable;
they are found most commonly in women less than 30 years of age.
These tumors require excision for definitive diagnosis and cure.
Other benign growths include intraductal papillomas, mammary duct
ectasias, and galactoceles. In diagnosing these conditions, mammography or cytologic examination of the fluids is required.

BREAST CANCER

Epidemiology, Clinical
Features, and Description of Disease

Breast cancer accounts for 32% of all cancers in women (Boring et al.
1992); no other cancer site among women or men approaches this

percentage. Incidence rates are higher for white females than for black females. For example, the 1978–1981 national breast cancer rate for white females was 85.6 per 100,000, whereas for black females it was 71.9 (Horm et al. 1984). Relative survival rates have fluctuated over the years but have remained basically unchanged. Survival rates have remained consistently lower for black women. For example, the 5-year survival rates for all stages among white females was 76% for the period 1974–1986, whereas it was 63% for black women (Boring et al. 1992).

Several variables have been identified as risk factors for breast cancer (Bean 1986). The demographic factors that have been studied include age (age increases risk), race (blacks have a lower incidence than whites, as mentioned previously), ethnicity (Jewish women have higher rates than non-Jewish women), and socioeconomic status (women in the highest socioeconomic status group have a risk almost twice as great as those in the lowest). Family history is important; the risk of breast cancer in women who have had a mother or a sister diagnosed with breast cancer is almost three times higher than in women without such a family history. A history of benign breast disease is usually correlated with the subsequent appearance of breast cancer. Reproductive variables are important. Women who have no pregnancy or who have their first child after the age of 30 have a risk almost three times higher than those giving birth for the first time at age 20 or younger. Various hypotheses for a hormonal factor have arisen from findings of increased risk among nulliparous women, women with late first birth, and women with late menopause. Finally, the role of diet in breast cancer is controversial, although it has led to recommendations such as reduction of fat intake to 25% of total calories or lower.

Despite the emphasis on mammography as a screening device, carcinoma of the breast is usually first discovered as a lump (usually in the upper outer quadrant of the breast) by the woman or her physician (Hacker and Jochimsen 1986). The mass is usually painless and freely mobile, but with progressive growth the tumor may become fixed to the chest wall. A less common sign is a serous or bloody discharge from the nipple. Extension to the skin may cause retraction and dimpling, and ductal involvement may cause nipple retraction. Blockage of skin lymphatics may cause lymphedema and thickening of the skin, a change referred to as "peu d'orange." Inflammatory signs may also appear, with warmth and redness of the overlying skin and swelling of the surrounding breast tissues.

A definitive diagnosis of breast cancer requires either tissue cytology (open breast biopsy) or fluid (fine-needle aspiration). The advantage of the latter is that it can be performed on an outpatient basis and, if positive, allows for a full discussion of treatment options preoperatively. Histology studies indicate a wide variety of malignant tumor types. Approximately 90% of cases arise in the ducts, and the remainder originate in the lobules. About 70% of all breast cancers are infiltrating duct carcinomas. Less common types include medullary, invasive lobular, mucinous, tubular, and papillary; in many tumors, several patterns exist.

Breast cancer spreads by local infiltration, moving directly into the surrounding breast tissue and eventually involving the overlying skin or the underlying muscle. When it occurs, lymphatic spread is mainly to the axillary nodes, with 40%–50% of patients having progressed to nodal involvement by the time of diagnosis. The most important prognostic factors for women with breast cancer are the presence of spread to the villa and the level of spread relative to the pectoralis minor muscle. Lymphatic spread can also occur via the internal mammary node chain; supraclavicular nodes are involved only after axillary involvement. Hematogenous spread occurs mainly to the lungs and liver, but other sites include the bone, pleura, adrenals, ovaries, and brain.

Approximately a century ago, in 1894, the primary treatment for breast cancer—radical mastectomy—was described. The procedure consisted of en bloc dissection of the entire breast, the pectoralis major and minor muscles, and the axilla. By 1970, however, controversy surrounding the surgical management of breast cancer was apparent, and a prospective, randomized clinical trial was begun by the National Surgical Adjuvant Breast Project (NSABP) (Harris et al. 1984). Over 1,700 women with clinically negative axillary nodes were entered in this study and received either radical mastectomy, a total (simple) mastectomy followed by local or regional radiation, or a total mastectomy alone. No differences in survival times were found in node-negative and surgically determined node-positive women, indicating that the less radical surgery could significantly reduce morbidity (e.g., leave the pectoralis major intact and provide superior functional and cosmetic results) without compromising mortality. Breast reconstruction, performed at the time of mastectomy or later, was also possible with this approach.

Radiation therapy is used postoperatively for women with positive axillary nodes. Although it significantly reduces local and regional relapse, its effect on survival remains controversial. There is increased use of radiation as initial therapy for small primary tumors (≤ 2 cm diameter).

Because breast cancer is often a systemic disease, adjuvant chemotherapy or hormonal therapy is required. Although many drugs can exert some control over the spread of disease, the four most commonly used drugs are cyclophosphamide, methotrexate, 5-fluorouracil, and doxorubicin (adriamycin). As single agents, each of these drugs is capable of inducing responses in 25%–45% of patients, although combinations of drugs (the most popular being cyclophosphamide, methotrexate, and 5-fluorouracil) are more effective. As noted above, the presence and extent of nodal disease are the most important prognostic factors for survival. For example, in the NSABP studies, women with negative lymph nodes had an actuarial 5-year survival of 83%, compared to 73% for patients with 1–3 positive nodes, 45% for those with 4 or more positive nodes, and 28% for those with more than 13 positive nodes (Fisher et al. 1983). In patients with metastatic disease, symptoms may be palliated with combination chemotherapy. Partial responses are obtained in 50%–75% of patients, but complete clinical responses are seen infrequently (5%–10%). Finally, hormonal therapy is often used, and the response is correlated with the incidence of estrogen receptors (ER) and progesterone receptors (PR). For example, the response rate to progesterone treatment in ER-positive tumors is 50%–60%, whereas it is less than 10% in ER-negative tumors.

Prevention

Unlike many medical problems, the development of malignancy and the appearance of symptoms are usually protracted, and a complex and changing symptom picture can be typical of patients with breast cancer. The psychological and behavioral aspects of people's commonsense understanding of illnesses (Leventhal et al. 1980) and symptom interpretation (Cacioppo et al. 1986) have been offered as theoretical frameworks for understanding illness interpretations and patient delay. Recent studies indicate that patient delay (i.e., the time from a patient's awareness of signs and symptoms to her appearance before a physician for consultation) is most often accounted for by the time that is necessary for the patient to decide that the symptoms indicate "illness" rather than a normal and nonserious health condition. An example of this type of patient delay is represented by the 45-year-old perimenopausal woman who eventually decides that her irregular vaginal bleeding may indicate something else, perhaps cancer, rather than menopause, as she originally assumed (Cacioppo et al. 1986). Interestingly, the delayed "serious" judgment also appears in the few studies of physician delay in making diagnoses (Howson 1950; Mommsen et al. 1983).

Diagnosis

The diagnosis of cancer, whether initial or recurrent, is the period of greatest acute stress for the cancer patient. This crisis is defined by the emotions of sadness (depression), fear (anxiety), confusion, and on some occasions, anger (Andersen et al. 1989b). It has been suggested that the cognitive coping responses prompted by the diagnosis include positive and confronting strategies, fatalistic responses, hopeless and helpless attitudes, and/or denial and avoidance (Burgess et al. 1988). Understanding these psychological processes is important for interpreting women's responses as they comprehend their diagnosis, complete a tumor evaluation, and begin treatment.

To examine the emotional responses at diagnosis, we assessed the moods of 65 women with cancer (clinical stage I or II gynecologic cancer) within 5–10 days of their learning of their diagnosis and prior to treatment (Andersen et al. 1989b). Their responses on a self-report mood questionnaire, the Profile of Mood States (McNair et al. 1971), were compared with those of women from two age-matched comparison groups—a group of women with recently diagnosed benign gynecologic disease and healthy women receiving routine gynecologic examinations. The cancer patients were also followed for approximately 4 years. Cancer recurred in a subset of the women during that time, and their moods were reassessed at this second diagnosis.

A significant elevation in depression was noted in the cancer patients only at the time of the initial diagnosis, and a further, significant increment in distress was noted at recurrence. In combination, these data indicate the unique and significant role of depressed affect for the cancer patient during diagnostic periods. In contrast, anxiety was a common affective experience for all women who had a medical diagnosis and were anticipating medical treatment, whether the disease was benign or malignant. However, there were no further elevations in anxiety at the time of recurrence. This pattern would suggest that anxiety may be prompted in part by treatment-related fears. Anger was present to a significant degree in the cancer patients only at the time of recurrence; the levels at the time of the initial diagnosis were not elevated and were as low as those for the healthy women or the women with benign disease. These data indicate that the initial diagnosis of cancer is characterized by significant depressed affect, whereas recurrence may be characterized by even greater depression and anger. Significant anxiety is also present during diagnostic periods.

In an early report of hospitalized cancer patients who were referred for psychiatric consultation, Levin et al. (1978) noted that most (56%) of these women had been diagnosed with depression. More recent surveys still cite depression as the most prevalent affective problem in women cancer patients, but estimates of unipolar diagnoses among unscreened patients are on the order of 5%–6% (Derogatis et al. 1983; Lansky et al. 1985). When major depression and adjustment disorder with depressed mood are considered, prevalence rates are higher (e.g., 16% in Derogatis et al. 1983) but still not of the magnitude noted in the previous decade's research. In general, higher rates of depression are found in patients undergoing active treatment than on follow-up or in those receiving palliative rather than curative treatment, those with pain or other disturbing symptoms, or those with histories of affective disorders. Among women without these characteristics, the base rate of major depression is likely to be on the order of 6%, a rate comparable to that of the general population.

As with patients with other serious illnesses, it is difficult to diagnose depression in cancer patients. First, a determination must be made about the vegetative symptoms, that is, poor appetite or actual weight loss, sleep disturbance (e.g., insomnia, hypersomnia), loss of energy or fatigue, and loss of sexual desire or interest. The diagnostician must determine whether such symptomatology represents depression, disease-related events, or a combination of factors. If, for example, the disease is disseminated or accompanied by pain, the case would be stronger for disease-initiated, rather than psychological, symptoms.

Another difficult issue in recognizing major depression in women with cancer is distinguishing between the psychological symptoms of depression (e.g., dysphoric mood, loss of interest or pleasure) and the normal psychological reactions to a life-threatening illness. This is particularly difficult because depression in cancer patients is reactive, that is, it occurs soon after the diagnosis, and the content of the depressive ruminations reflects the diagnostic event (Noyes and Kathol 1986). When depressive symptoms are present at the time of diagnosis, they tend to be intermittent and rarely persist once treatment has begun or is concluded. Emotional "rebound" following treatment is rapid, usually occurring by 3–4 months, if recovery proceeds smoothly (Andersen et al. 1989b). Finally, because cancer is a realistic health stressor, patients and physicians alike regard a depressive reaction to the diagnosis as "normal." As such, patients may not feel comfortable (or able) enough to complain about their moods or feelings, even when extreme. Similarly, physicians or nurses may not recognize severe depressive reactions because of their infrequency and the "normality" of less severe reactions. In combination, these circumstances conspire to contribute to underrecognition and undertreatment of major depression among cancer patients (Derogatis et al. 1979). The effects of depressive symptoms and medical conditions on adjustment and well-being are additive, however; individuals experiencing depression within the context of cancer report roughly twice the reduction in social functioning associated with either condition alone (Wells et al. 1989).

When depression does occur, some symptoms may be more or less characteristic for the cancer patient. In addition to dysphoric mood, other common symptoms may include loss of interest or pleasure, loss of energy, fatigue, and difficulty thinking or concentrating (e.g., feeling confused or bewildered). Other common feelings include inter-mittent anxiety, feelings of helplessness, and concern about the future (Lansky et al. 1985). Endicott (1984) has suggested that other possible but less common reactions include fearful or depressed appearance, social withdrawal or decreased talkativeness, brooding or pessimism, and mood that is not reactive (i.e., the patient cannot be cheered up, does not smile, and does not react to good news). Reactions such as these can be considered as symptoms and signs of major depression in medical patients. In contrast, psychological characteristics of de-pressed psychiatric patients that are uncommon for cancer patients include feelings of low self-esteem and guilt. Finally, it is rare for can-cer patients to be melancholic, psychotic, or suicidal (Bukberg et al. 1984; Saunders and Valente 1988).

Anxiety disorder is the second most frequently encountered psy-chiatric problem in cancer patients. Derogatis et al. (1979) have esti-mated the prevalence to be 7% among outpatient cancer patients currently undergoing treatment. In a study of 44 breast cancer pa-tients interviewed at the time of diagnosis, Hughes (1981) estimated that 25% of the patients in the sample had severe anxiety reactions. Anxiety-related problems are typically manifested by the symptoms of generalized anxiety: classic fear, worry, and rumination. Other symp-toms include motor tension (e.g., shakiness, muscle tension, restless-ness, easy fatigability), autonomic hyperactivity (e.g., abdominal distress, frequent urination), and/or indications of vigilance and scanning (e.g., difficulty concentrating, trouble falling or staying asleep, feeling on edge). Much of the content of the anxiety-provok-ing thoughts is focused on medical examinations and cancer treat-ments (e.g., fear of pain or disfigurement) and the short- and long-term disruption they may produce. Other targets of anxiety in-clude the life disruption and change that may occur because the indi-vidual has cancer; the most common spheres of worry include family, money, work, and illness (e.g., "Who will care for the children when I am in the hospital?" "What if our insurance does not cover the bills?" "Will I be able to go back to work?" "What if I never get well?").

The emotion of anger has occupied a special role in theorizing, with hypotheses that it is relevant to the etiology and/or progression of cancer (Morris et al. 1981). As discussed here, we have not found any evidence of elevated anger at initial diagnosis, although there may be higher levels reported at the time of cancer recurrence. Clinical reports of the foci for anger at recurrence include frustration with the failure of presumably curative treatments.

Treatment

A component of the emotional distress occurring at diagnosis is the anticipation of difficult treatment(s). The current therapies of surgery, radiotherapy and radioactive substances, chemotherapy, hormonal therapy, immunotherapy, and combination regimens are preceded by physical examinations, biopsy, and/or laboratory studies. These treatments are significant stressors, and supporting data consistently portray more distress (particularly fear and anxiety), slower rates of emotional recovery, and perhaps additional behavioral difficulties (e.g., conditioned anxiety reactions) than are found in relatively healthy women undergoing medical treatment (e.g., hysterectomy, cholecystectomy) for benign conditions.

There have been few investigations of the psychological reactions to cancer surgery. For breast cancer patients, part of the fear surrounding surgery is responding to the feelings of loss of all or part of a breast. In addition, however, women are fearful of surgery per se, and there are numerous descriptive and intervention studies of the reactions of healthy women undergoing surgery for benign conditions, such as uterine fibroids (Anderson and Masur 1983). The latter studies are consistent in their portrayal of high levels of self-reported preoperative anxiety that are predictive of lowered postoperative anxiety. Further, postoperative anxiety is predictive of recovery: those with lower levels of postoperative anxiety recover more quickly (e.g., get out of bed sooner, complain less) than do those with higher levels of anxiety. What may distinguish cancer surgery patients are higher overall levels of distress and slower emotional rebound. Gottesman and Lewis (1982), for example, found greater and more lasting feelings of crisis and helplessness among cancer patients than in patients undergoing surgery for benign conditions for as long as 2 months following discharge.

Considering the latter data, findings on the patterns of interaction between physicians and cancer patients on morning surgical rounds are disturbing. Gathering behavioral data on the content and frequency of interactions, Blanchard et al. (1987) found attending physicians on a cancer unit to be less likely to engage in supportive behaviors and to address patients' needs than were physicians treating general medical patients. The heavier volume and more seriously ill patients common to cancer units may be reasons for this unfortunate relationship. Related survey findings indicate that oncology nurses may find their job significantly more stressful than other assignments (e.g., cardiac, intensive care, or operating room nursing) (Stewart et al. 1982). Taken together, these data suggest that the interactions of oncologists and oncology nurses with cancer inpatients may be even more important in influencing patients' adjustment to treatment than is commonly acknowledged.

For an empirical understanding of fears of radiation, the surgical anxiety studies described here have been used as a paradigm. Here, again, high levels of anticipatory anxiety are found, and if interventions to reduce distress are not conducted (Rainey 1985), heightened posttreatment anxiety is also found (Andersen and Tewfik 1985; Andersen et al. 1984) and may be maintained for as long as 3 months posttherapy (King et al. 1985). When the acute side effects of treatment resolve, however, there is no higher incidence of emotional difficulties for radiotherapy patients than for surgery patients (Hughson et al. 1987).

Of all cancer treatments, the behavioral and psychological aspects are best understood for chemotherapy, particularly the side effects of nausea and vomiting. Regarding the latter, a classical conditioning conceptualization has been offered to explain anticipatory nausea and vomiting. That is, the administration of chemotherapy (an unconditioned stimulus) produces posttreatment nausea and/or vomiting (the unconditioned response). Each chemotherapy infusion, however, is also paired with environmental stimuli (conditioned stimuli), such as visual (sight of the nurse), olfactory (the smell of rubbing alcohol), and gustatory (recently eaten food or drink) stimuli. With repeated "pairings" (i.e., the administration of chemotherapy in the same environmental context) and sufficiently severe posttreatment nausea and vomiting, conditioned stimuli alone may eventually elicit the same or a related response (i.e., nausea and vomiting—the conditioned response). Thus, following at least one cycle of chemotherapy, patients may report nausea and/or vomiting in response to chemotherapy administration (usually on the first day) of the second or subsequent cycles.

Research has progressed from prevalence estimates and single-subject and large-sample descriptive investigations to controlled investigations focused on eliminating or reducing disruptive side effects through hypnosis, progressive muscle relaxation with guided imagery, systematic desensitization, attentional diversion or redirection, and biofeedback (Carey and Burnish 1987). Research has also targeted individual differences among patients (i.e., high pretreatment anxiety or general distress, severity of posttreatment vomiting in the early cycles, age) and situations (i.e., more emetogenic regimens, higher doses, or greater amounts of chemotherapy) that place individuals at risk for developing anticipatory reactions.

With continued psychological research, improvement in anti-emetic drugs, and efforts to reduce drug toxicity, many of the gastrointestinal effects discussed above may be reduced, if not eliminated. There are, however, other problematic psychological and behavioral side effects of chemotherapy that remain. Appetite and weight loss may be significant clinical problems for women with disseminated disease. Learned aversions to food as a result of side effects from chemotherapy appear to be robust, with rapid acquisition (usually after a single course) and maintenance even after long delays between presentations of the conditioned stimulus (the taste of food) and the onset of the unconditioned stimulus (aversive internal sensations of nausea and vomiting following chemotherapy) (Bernstein 1986). This important psychological research has pointed the way, for example, to interventions employing novel tastes to "block" conditioning to familiar diet items, reducing food intake prior to drug administration, and ingesting diets high in carbohydrates rather than protein.

Immediate Posttreatment Recovery

Despite the difficulties of cancer treatment, the crisis levels of emotional distress that occur at diagnosis lessen during treatment initiation, continuance, and early recovery (i.e., 2–12 months posttreatment) (Andersen et al. 1989b; Bloom 1987; Devlen et al. 1987a, 1987b). Bloom (1987) reported the results of a controlled, prospective, longitudinal study of women with stage I or II breast cancer that had been treated with modified radical mastectomy. Comparison was made with women undergoing biopsy for benign disease, women having cholecystectomy for gall bladder disease, and healthy women. All women were seen within 3 months of surgery and again at 6, 9, and 12 months posttreatment. Women with breast cancer showed greater psychological distress related to social and interpersonal relationships. Further, women with stage II disease had more distress, as well as more negative attitudes toward self and the future, concern with physical symptoms, anxiety, strain, and interpersonal difficulties. They did not, however, show any greater evidence of psychopathology warranting psychiatric intervention during the first posttreatment year. Similar patterns of positive long-term adjustment have been found in retrospective research (Cella and Tross 1986) and in longitudinal studies of patients with gynecologic disease (Andersen et al. 1989b) and Hodgkin's disease and non-Hodgkin's lymphoma (Devlen et al. 1987a, 1987b).

Following these generally positive findings, investigators have tested moderators for adjustment. For example, early (e.g., 4 months posttreatment) physical impairment from treatment has been found to be an important predictor of poorer mental health functioning at the end of the first recovery year (Vinokur et al. 1989). Furthermore, younger age (e.g., women less than 60 years at diagnosis) can exacerbate this effect (Vinokur et al. 1990).

There have been several investigations of psychological counseling provided to breast cancer patients during the early months of recovery. Interventions are typically provided in one of two formats: individual or group therapy. Although studies have varied in their methodologic sophistication, they have generally demonstrated more positive outcomes for intervention patients. A visitation program in the Netherlands was reported by van den Borne et al. (1987). It appeared that regular contacts between patients decreased negative affect and feelings of uncertainty and increased self-esteem.

Telch and Telch (1986) compared supportive group therapy with a coping skills intervention offered to male and female cancer patients. Participants were randomly assigned to either of the interventions or to a no-treatment control group. Analyses revealed the coping intervention that had provided relaxation and stress management, communication and assertion skills, problem solving, emotional management, and activity planning as consistently superior. The final assessment at 6 weeks posttreatment indicated that the patients receiving the coping intervention reported improvement across all outcome variables, including mood, self-efficacy, reduction in the number of problems, and activity management.

Long-Term Recovery and Survival

For the "cured" cancer patient (a term typically referring to individuals surviving for at least 5 years), it has been suggested that there are two broad classes of stressors (Cella and Tross 1986). The first class of stressors includes residual sequelae, including lingering emotional distress from the cancer experience and the threat to life. This might be manifested when patients dread follow-up physical examinations or ruminate about the recurrence of disease. The second class of stressors includes continuing sequelae, such as coping with the changes to one's premorbid life and adjustment requiring new behaviors and emotions.

The earliest writings (from the 1950s to the 1980s) suggested that the psychological trajectory was troubled with somatic problems, psychological distress (Bard and Sutherland 1952; Maguire et al. 1978), impaired relationships (Dyk and Sutherland 1956; Wortman and Dunkel-Schetter 1979), preoccupation with death (Gullo et al. 1974), and/or general life disruption, such as reduced employment or career opportunities (Schonfield 1972). Many of these pioneering reports (primarily of breast cancer patients) were clinical in focus and, in general, controls were not in place for disease variables that are now recognized as moderators of adjustment. By the end of this same period, cancer had become more of a public issue and more survivable, and clinical trials were able to examine treatment toxicity following the establishment of effectiveness. Although it is unfortunate that the age-adjusted death rate for breast cancer has changed little since the 1950s (American Cancer Society 1992), dramatic changes in standard therapy have taken place, with a shift to less radical surgical treatments. The latter change has dramatically improved the quality of life for patients with breast cancer and accounts, in part, for the positive findings emerging in studies of long-term adjustment.

Data on the interpersonal relationships of cancer patients suggest that, in general, satisfaction predominates. Studies of women treated for breast cancer indicate that most relationships remain intact and satisfactory and, on occasion, become stronger (Lichtman and Taylor 1986; Tempelaar et al. 1989). The most important relationships are those within the family, so most studies have focused on them. When problems do occur, they include estrangement and distress that were originally hypothesized for most of the patients (Wortman and Dunkel-Schetter 1979). A common scenario may be for the woman to be inclined to discuss her feelings and experiences in attempts to cope with or understand the cancer stressor, but for her partner to be more inclined to advise her to "put the experience behind her" and not want to listen (Lichtman and Taylor 1986). It is clear that the distress of the patient's kin may approach that of the patient herself (B. R. Cassileth et al. 1985). Another common stressor for women with breast cancer is the subsequent risk of disease for her female children.

For many patients with breast cancer, it is clear that the one life area that is at risk for disruption is sexual functioning, although the incidence of these problems has dramatically declined with the development of less radical surgical therapies. Following is a brief summary of the major outcomes specific to type and choice of treatment, the two most influential variables in determining outcome for women treated for local or regional breast disease.

Controlled longitudinal studies indicate that 30%–40% of women treated with modified radical mastectomy report significant sexual problems (e.g., loss of desire, reductions in arousal) from 1–2 years posttreatment, compared to 10% of women with benign disease receiving diagnostic biopsy (Maguire et al. 1978; Morris et al. 1977). Studies from clinical trials have compared modified radical mastectomy with lumpectomy and radiotherapy. With few exceptions, studies have reported a clear benefit of the less-disfiguring form of treatment (Steinberg et al. 1985). For the lumpectomy patients, such differences include less alteration in body image and greater comfort with nudity and discussing sexuality with one's partner, no or few changes in frequency of intercourse, and a lower incidence of sexual dysfunction. Even if sexual disruption occurs, however, it need not portend disturbance of other life areas, such as marital adjustment, as indicated in studies comparing breast cancer patients with healthy women (Andersen and Jochimsen 1985). Finally, women with disseminated or recurrent disease confront a variety of other sexual difficulties, such as those arising from combination chemotherapy and surgery regimens that adversely affect the woman's interest in and ability to engage in sexual activity.

Recurrence and Death

The recurrence of cancer is devastating. As noted above, the magnitude of distress is even greater than that found with the initial diagnosis, and studies contrasting cancer patients with no evidence of disease with those receiving palliative treatment (B. R. Cassileth et al. 1985) report the greatest distress for those with disseminated disease. Difficult decisions, such as those between beginning a regimen that offers side effects and little chance for cure and receiving no treatment, are made within a context of extreme emotional distress and physical debilitation (P. A. Cassileth and Cassileth 1983a, 1983b).

A frequent and less controllable complication of disseminated disease is pain (Ahles et al. 1984). The major cause of cancer pain, accounting for roughly 70% of the cases, is due to direct tumor involvement (e.g., metastatic bone disease, nerve compression). Another 20%–30% of cases are due to therapy (e.g., postoperative pain, radiation-induced pain), and the remaining cases are individuals with pain problems unrelated to their cancer (Foley 1985). The most difficult case is chronic pain associated with disease progression, and combinations of antitumor therapy, anesthetic blocks, and behavioral approaches to pain control are considered. Behavioral research has focused on assessment strategies (Daut et al. 1983; Keefe et al. 1985) and pain reduction interventions; hypnosis has been used effectively with breast cancer patients (Spiegel and Bloom 1983). When palliative therapy is of little use and/or brings further debilitation, psychological interventions may provide pain control and, secondarily, prevent or treat pain sequelae, such as sleep disturbances, reduced appetite, irritability, and other behavioral difficulties.

Reducing Psychological Distress
Throughout the Cancer Experience:
Roles for the Psychiatrist

Suggestions have been made regarding the management of emotional distress in the cancer patient (Massie and Holland 1990). An often-overlooked strategy is the continuing emotional support of the patient's oncologist; psychiatrists are also in a unique position to assist their physician colleagues with such supportive efforts. Supplementary psychiatric consultation may be considered when severe affective symptoms last more than a week, when they worsen, or when they interfere with the patient's ability to function or cooperate with treatment. Brief, crisis-oriented therapy may be particularly useful at the time of diagnosis of cancer, whether initial or recurrent, and may assist the woman to regain a sense of self in this difficult circumstance, to correct misconceptions regarding the diagnosis or treatment, and to integrate the illness experience into prior life experiences. Other therapeutic efforts may be to include family members in the intervention sessions or to suggest participation in patient support groups.

Surveys of current psychotropic medications indicate that hypnotics (43% of all prescriptions), antipsychotics (28%), anxiolytics (27%), and antidepressants (3%) are typically chosen for psychological and physical management of symptoms (e.g., hypnotics and antipsychotics are often prescribed for nausea and vomiting rather than affective distress) (Stiefel et al. 1990). Specifically, the tricyclic antidepressants can be safely and effectively prescribed for depression (Massie and Holland 1990).

In addition to psychological interventions to assist coping with difficult treatments or the recovery process, data also indicate that important gains can be achieved during the terminal stages of illness (Linn et al. 1982). Group support interventions have been important, as they can serve a variety of purposes that individual therapy cannot offer (Taylor et al. 1986). Group members can serve as role models for each other in their coping efforts and in confronting the possibility of decline and death, and they can provide altruistic support to one another.

Spiegel et al. (1981) have provided two important reports on the emotional and survival benefits of such an intervention. In a randomized, prospective study, women with metastatic breast cancer were assigned to group therapy or to no-treatment conditions (Spiegel et al. 1981). The study assessments occurred at the beginning of the group and 4, 8, and 12 months later. The groups continued to meet for 2 additional years. Outcome data indicated that the women participating in the support groups reported lower emotional distress and fewer maladaptive coping responses, such as overeating, smoking, or drinking. A later report provided data on 10-year survival differences between the groups (Spiegel et al. 1989). At that time, only 3 of the 86 patients were alive, and death records were obtained on all other participants. Survival from time of randomization and onset of intervention was a mean of 36.6 months in the intervention group and 18.9 months in the control group, a significant difference. Survival plots indicated that divergence in survival began at 20 months after entry, or 8 months after the formal intervention study ended. Hypotheses for this important effect include the additional provision of social support from the therapy sessions, or enhanced self-care (e.g., better treatment compliance, improved diet, hypnosis for pain control, more exercise), among others. Future studies will examine the reliability and the mechanisms for these remarkable findings.

REFERENCES

Ahles TA, Rucksdeschel JC, Blanchard EG: Cancer related pain, I: prevalence in an outpatient setting as a function of stage of disease and type of cancer. J Psychosom Res 28:115–119, 1984

American Cancer Society: Cancer Facts and Figures—1992. Atlanta, GA, American Cancer Society, 1992

Andersen BL: Health psychology's contribution to addressing the cancer problem: update on accomplishments. Health Psychol 8:683–703, 1989

Andersen BL, Jochimsen PR: Sexual adjustment among breast cancer, gynecologic cancer and healthy women. J Consult Clin Psychol 53:25–32, 1985

Andersen BL, Tewfik HH: Psychological reactions to radiation therapy: reconsideration of the adaptive aspects of anxiety. J Pers Soc Psychol 48:1024–1032, 1985

Andersen BL, Karlsson JA, Anderson B, et al: Anxiety and cancer treatment: response to stressful radiotherapy. Health Psychol 3:535–551, 1984

Andersen BL, Anderson B, deProsse C: Controlled prospective longitudinal study of women with cancer, I: sexual functioning outcomes. J Consult Clin Psychol 57:683–691, 1989a

Andersen BL, Anderson B, deProsse C: Controlled prospective longitudinal study of women with cancer, II: psychological outcomes. J Consult Clin Psychol 57:692–697, 1989b

Anderson KO, Masur FT: Psychological preparation for invasive medical and dental procedures. J Behav Med 6:1–40, 1983

Bard M, Sutherland AM: Adaptation to radical mastectomy. Cancer 8:656–671, 1952

Bean JA: Epidemiologic review of cancer in women, in Women With Cancer: Psychological Perspectives. Edited by Andersen BL. New York, Springer-Verlag, 1986, pp 59–92

Bernstein IL: Etiology of anorexia in cancer. Cancer 58:1881–1886, 1986

Blanchard CC, Ruckdeschel JC, Labrecque MS, et al: The impact of a designated cancer unit on house staff behaviors toward patients. Cancer 60:2348–2354, 1987

Bloom JR: Psychological aspects of breast cancer study group: psychological response to mastectomy. Cancer 59:189–196, 1987

Boring CC, Squires TS, Tong T: Cancer statistics, 1992. Ca—A Cancer Journal for Clinicians 42:19–38, 1992

Bukberg J, Penman D, Holland JC: Depression in hospitalized cancer patients. Psychosom Med 46:199–212, 1984

Burgess C, Morris T, Pettingale KW: Psychological response to cancer diagnosis, II: evidence for coping styles (coping styles and cancer diagnosis). J Psychosom Res 32:263–272, 1988

Cacioppo JT, Andersen BL, Turnquist DC, et al: Psychophysiological comparison processes: interpreting cancer symptoms, in Women With Cancer: Psychological Perspectives. Edited by Andersen BL. New York, Springer-Verlag, 1986, pp 141–171

Carey MP, Burnish TG: Etiology and treatment of the psychological side effects associated with cancer chemotherapy. Psychol Bull 104:307–325, 1987

Cassileth BR, Lusk EJ, Strouse TB, et al: A psychological analysis of cancer patients and their next-of-kin. Cancer 55:72–76, 1985

Cassileth PA, Cassileth BR: Clinical care of the terminal cancer patient: Part I. Medical Times, March 1983a, pp 57s–66s

Cassileth PA, Cassileth BR: Clinical care of the terminal cancer patient: Part II. Medical Times, April 1983b, pp 9s–22s

Cella DF, Tross S: Psychological adjustment to survival from Hodgkin's disease. J Consult Clin Psychol 54:616–622, 1986

Daut RL, Cleeland CS, Flanery RC: Development of the Wisconsin Brief Pain Questionnaire to assess pain in cancer and other diseases. Pain 17:197–210, 1983

Derogatis LR, Feldstein M, Morrow G, et al: A survey of psychotropic drug prescriptions in an oncology population. Cancer 44:1919–1929, 1979

Derogatis LR, Morrow GR, Fetting J, et al: The prevalence of psychiatric disorders among cancer patients. JAMA 249:751–757, 1983

Devlen J, Maguire P, Phillips P, et al: Psychological problems associated with diagnosis and treatment of lymphomas, I: retrospective study. BMJ 295:953–954, 1987a

Devlen J, Maguire P, Phillips P, et al: Psychological problems associated with diagnosis and treatment of lymphomas, II: prospective study. BMJ 295:955–957, 1987b

Dyk RB, Sutherland AM: Adaptation of the spouse and other family members to the colostomy patient. Cancer 9:123–138, 1956

Endicott J: Measurement of depression in patients with cancer. Cancer 53:2243–2248, 1984

Fisher B, Bauer M, Wickerham DL, et al: Relation of number of positive axillary nodes to the prognosis of patients with primary breast cancer. Cancer 52:1551–1557, 1983

Foley KM: The treatment of cancer pain. N Engl J Med 313:84–95, 1985

Gottesman D, Lewis M: Differences in crisis reactions among cancer and surgery patients. J Consult Clin Psychol 50:381–388, 1982

Gullo V, Cherico J, Shadick R: Suggested stages and response styles in life threatening illness: a focus on the cancer patient, in Anticipatory Grief. Edited by Schoenberg C, Carr E, Kutscher F, et al. New York, Columbia University Press, 1974, pp 54–63

Hacker NF, Jochimsen PR: Common malignancies among women: sites and treatment, in Women With Cancer: Psychological Perspectives. Edited by Andersen BL. New York, Springer-Verlag, 1986, pp 3–58

Harris JR, Beadle GF, Hellman S: Clinical studies on the use of radiation therapy as primary treatment of early breast cancer. Cancer 53:705–711, 1984

Horm JW, Asire AJ, Young JL Jr, et al: SEER program: cancer incidence and mortality in the United States, 1973–1981 (DHHS Publ No NIH-85-1837). Washington, DC, U.S. Government Printing Office, 1984

Howson JT: The procedures and results of the Philadelphia Committee for the Study of Pelvic Cancer. Wis Med J, March 1950, pp 215–219

Hughes J: Emotional reactions to the diagnosis and treatment of early breast cancer. J Psychosom Res 26:277–283, 1981

Hughson AVM, Cooper AF, McArdle CS, et al: Psychosocial effects of radiotherapy after mastectomy. BMJ 294:1515–1518, 1987

Keefe FJ, Brantley A, Manuel S, et al: Behavioral assessment of head and neck cancer pain. Pain 23:327–336, 1985

King KB, Nail LM, Kreamer K, et al: Patients' descriptions of the experience of receiving radiation therapy. Oncol Nurs Forum 12:55–61, 1985

Lansky SB, List MA, Herrmann CA, et al: Absence of major depressive disorders in female cancer patients. J Clin Oncol 3:1553–1560, 1985

Leventhal H, Meyer D, Nerenz D: The common sense representation of illness danger, in Contributions to Medical Psychology, Vol 2. Edited by Rachman S. Oxford, UK, Pergamon, 1980, pp 7–30

Levin PM, Silberfarb PM, Lipowski ZJ: Mental disorders in cancer patients: a study of 100 psychiatric referrals. Cancer 42:1385–1391, 1978

Lichtman RR, Taylor SE: Close relationships and the female cancer patient, in Women With Cancer: Psychological Perspectives. Edited by Andersen BL. New York, Springer-Verlag, 1986, pp 233–256

Linn MW, Linn BS, Harris R: Effects of counseling for late stage cancer patients. Cancer 49:1048–1055, 1982

Maguire GP, Lee EG, Bevington DJ, et al: Psychiatric problems in the first year after mastectomy. BMJ 1:963–965, 1978

Massie MJ, Holland JC: Depression and the cancer patient. J Clin Psychiatry 51 (suppl):12–17, 1990

McNair DM, Lorr M, Droppleman IF: Profile of Mood States. San Diego, CA, Educational Testing Service, 1971

Mommsen S, Aagaard J, Sell A: Presenting symptoms, treatment delay and survival in bladder cancer. Scand J Urol Nephrol 17:163–167, 1983

Morris T, Greer HS, White P: Psychological and social adjustment to mastectomy: a two-year follow-up study. Cancer 40:2381–2387, 1977

Morris T, Greer S, Pettingale KW, et al: Patterns of expression of anger and their psychological correlates in women with breast cancer. J Psychosom Res 25:111–117, 1981

Noyes R, Kathol RG: Depression and cancer. Psychiatric Developments 2:77–100, 1986

Rainey LC: Effects of preparatory patient education for radiation oncology patients. Cancer 56:1056–1061, 1985

Saunders JM, Valente SM: Cancer and suicide. Oncol Nurs Forum 15:575–581, 1988

Schonfield J: Psychological factors related to delayed return to an earlier lifestyle in successfully treated cancer patients. J Psychosom Res 16:41–46, 1972

Spiegel D, Bloom JR: Group therapy and hypnosis reduce metastatic breast carcinoma pain. Psychosom Med 45:333–339, 1983

Spiegel D, Bloom JR, Yalom I: Group support for patients with metastatic cancer. Arch Gen Psychiatry 38:527–533, 1981

Spiegel D, Bloom JR, Kraemer HC, et al: Effect of psychosocial treatment on survival of patients with metastatic breast cancer. Lancet 2:888–891, 1989

Steinberg MD, Juliano MA, Wise I: Psychological outcome of lumpectomy versus mastectomy in the treatment of breast cancer. Am J Psychiatry 142:34–39, 1985

Stewart BE, Meyerowitz BE, Jackson IE, et al: Psychological stress associated with outpatient oncology nursing. Cancer Nurs, October 1982, pp 383–387

Stiefel FC, Kornblith AB, Holland JC: Changes in the prescription patterns of psychotropic drugs for cancer patients during a 10 year period. Cancer 65:1048–1053, 1990

Sutherland AM, Orbach CF, Dyk RB, et al: The psychological impact of cancer and cancer surgery, I: adaptation to the dry colostomy. Cancer 5:857–872, 1952

Taylor SE: Adjustment to threatening events: a theory of cognitive adaptation. Am Psychol 38:1161–1173, 1983

Taylor SE, Falke RI, Shoptow SJ, et al: Social support, support groups, and the cancer patient. J Consult Clin Psychol 54:608–615, 1986

Telch CF, Telch MJ: Group coping skills instruction and supportive group therapy for cancer patients: a comparison of strategies. J Consult Clin Psychol 54:802–808, 1986

Tempelaar R, DeHaes JCJM, DeRuiter JH, et al: The social experiences of cancer patients under treatment: a comparative study. Soc Sci Med 29:635–642, 1989

van den Borne HW, Pruyn JFA, van den Heuvel WJA: Effects of contacts between cancer patients on their psychosocial problems. Patient Education and Counseling 9:33–51, 1987

Vinokur AD, Threatt BA, Caplan RD, et al: Physical and psychosocial functioning and adjustment to breast cancer: long-term follow-up of a screening population. Cancer 63:394–405, 1989

Vinokur AD, Threatt BA, Vinokur-Kaplan D, et al: The process of recovery from breast cancer for younger and older patients: changes during the first year. Cancer 65:1242–1254, 1990

Wells KB, Steward A, Hays RD, et al: The functioning and well-being of depressed patients: results from the medical outcomes study. JAMA 262:914–919, 1989

Wortman CB, Dunkel-Schetter C: Interpersonal relationships and cancer: a theoretical analysis. Journal of Social Issues 35:120–155, 1979

Chapter 23

SEXUAL ASSAULT, DOMESTIC VIOLENCE, AND INCEST

Deborah S. Rose, M.D.

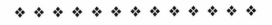

IDENTIFICATION IN THE OBSTETRIC-GYNECOLOGIC AND EMERGENCY SETTING

For victims of sexual assault, domestic violence, and incest, the port of entry into the health care system is frequently the obstetrician-gynecologist (Herman 1981; Renshaw 1989). Among the presenting issues are pregnancy, therapeutic abortion, and rape. Physical injuries need to be documented and treated. In these crises, the victim needs psychiatric evaluation. The family is also in need; it may include witnesses to the assault, the assailant, and family members who learn of the victimization after the fact.

As chronic sequelae of victimization develop, a wider range of psychological and physical symptoms develop. The emergency room is a common site for the first or only contact victims make with the health care system (Briere and Zaidi 1989).

Four factors operate to make obstetric and gynecologic problems often the first and only ones for which the victim will seek help. First, victims have a high rate and extensive range of gynecologic somatic symptoms, resulting from the interaction of actual physical injury, somatic memories of the assault, and somatization (Krystal 1978b, 1984; Loewenstein 1990; Morrison 1989; Rose 1986b, 1991). Physical injury and the threat of death are common in all forms of rape. In rape by a stranger, the assailant often uses unnecessary violence to force com-

447

pliance (Rose 1991). Furthermore, contrary to common belief, rape by a spouse or an acquaintance is perceived by the victim as more likely to lead to injury or death than is rape by a stranger (Kilpatrick et al. 1988).

Second, although physical assault and sexual assault are severe psychological stressors that usually cause posttraumatic stress disorder (PTSD), the psychological sequelae of PTSD are often too threatening to the victim and significant others to allow them to be acknowledged. The victim may be able to tolerate noticing only physical symptoms and often tries to go on with her life as if nothing has happened (Rose 1986b, 1991).

Third, problems with self-care are a frequent consequence of trauma (Krystal 1978a; Rose 1991), which are manifested as erratic care for emergencies only. The use of the emergency room in this manner is a symbolic reenactment of the psychological emergency that victimization creates and is a clue to an undisclosed history of victimization.

Last, in cases of domestic violence and incest, the only health care that the tyrannical, paranoid assailant may be able to allow is prenatal care or induced abortion. If the victim tries to seek health care beyond these measures, she is in danger of being assaulted emotionally and also often physically (Gise and Paddison 1988; Hilberman 1980; L. E. Walker 1979).

Awareness of the common presenting symptoms in this population of frightened, reluctant patients is essential, but impediments to awareness are common in the victim and health care system (Renshaw 1989). The victim is often unaware of the etiology of the symptoms because of the psychological damage from PTSD. A similar need to defend against the threat of trauma limits awareness in all providers of care (Blank 1985; Goodwin 1985a; Haley 1978; Kluft 1990a; Rose 1991). The standard history and physical examination that are taught in medical training routinely omit inquiry for a history of exposure to violence and violation (Briere and Zaidi 1989; Jacobson and Richardson 1987). The health care provider is thus left unequipped and ignorant, a psychological state that increases the need to defend against inquiring about victimization. This meshes all too well with the victim's defenses.

FREQUENCY OF SHORT- AND LONG-TERM PSYCHIATRIC COMPLICATIONS

A wide range of immediate and long-term sequelae of victimization have been observed. Most research on these complications is retrospective and lacks standardization. Studies often omit control groups and may overlook bias based on the sex of the observer (Bassuk and Apsler 1983). Even with these limitations, the studies clearly demonstrate that victimization is a major etiologic factor in a wide range of severe psychiatric disorders (Finklehor 1984; Green 1988a, 1988b, 1988c; Schetky 1990).

Studies of Nonclinical Populations

In studies of nonclinical populations, correlations between a history of victimization and psychiatric complications are repeatedly observed. In a prospective, long-term study of rape victims, beginning at 6–21 days after the rape, Kilpatrick et al. (1979, 1985) found that the victim's level of distress during this time was a reliable predictor of the level of distress at a 3-month follow-up visit. The level of distress present at 3 months after the rape continued unchanged during the next 4 years. All victims had enduring symptoms seen in PTSD. No evidence was found to support the concept of delayed PTSD.

Similarly, in a controlled study of a National Institute of Mental Health Epidemiologic Catchment Area, Winfield et al. (1990) noted that five lifetime DSM-III-R disorders (American Psychiatric Association 1987) were significantly correlated with a history of sexual assault: major depression, alcohol or drug abuse and dependence, PTSD, and obsessive-compulsive disorder. On the basis of data from two national telephone interview studies that focused mainly on domestic violence that had occurred in the prior year, Gelles and Straus (1988) observed that the experience of severe domestic violence (i.e., violence that has the potential to produce an injury) is highly correlated with significant psychiatric morbidity when compared with nonviolent homes. Women from these homes were found to have high rates of depression, despair, hopelessness, feelings of worthlessness and inadequacy, and fearfulness. The women also had many more days in bed and more ill health, somatic symptoms, substance abuse and dependency, suicidal ideation, and suicide attempts. The abused women were more likely to act out their aggression verbally and physically against non-family members, and 50% abused their children, a rate equal to that of their male partners. Children from homes with severe violence had significantly higher rates of difficulties than those from other homes.

In a study of retrospective, self-reported, long-term effects of child-hood incestuous abuse, in which a population of women selected from the community was compared with one from a psychiatric outpatient sample, Herman et al. (1986) found that 92% of the women from the community-based sample reported having been upset at the time the abuse occurred, with over 50% having been very upset. In comparison, over 50% thought of themselves as having recovered well, with one-half of those noting no long-lasting effects. The remainder of the women noted significant, lasting impact, with difficulties affecting feelings about themselves, men, and sex and problems with mistrust, anxiety, and intimate relationships, including sexual ones. The impact of the incest was positively correlated with the amount of force or violence used, the degree of physical violation, the nature of the familial relationship, and the age difference between the victim and the perpetrator. A nonsignificant positive association was observed between the age at onset of incest and lasting impact. The retrospective self-reporting and the exclusion of women who were too impaired to function in the community at large, however, may have skewed the results.

Studies of Clinical and Special Populations

A wide range of retrospective studies of psychiatric inpatient and out-patient populations and special populations, such as rapists and pros-titutes, have consistently shown an overrepresentation of victims. These populations also include some of the most difficult-to-treat di-agnoses (Beck and van der Kolk 1987; Borins and Forsythe 1985; Briere and Zaidi 1989; Brown and Anderson 1991; Burgess et al. 1987, 1988; Carmen et al. 1984; Emslie and Rosenfeld 1983; Herman 1986; Herman et al. 1989; Jacobson and Richardson 1987; Morrison 1989; Rosenfeld 1979; van der Kolk 1987a; E. Walker et al. 1988).

Carmen et al. (1984) noted that patients with a history of abuse had significantly longer hospitalizations and also differed noticeably in their handling of aggression. Women were much more likely to direct aggression inward in an acutely self-destructive manner, whereas the majority of abused men directed it outward in abuse toward others, with conduct disorders and involvement with the criminal justice system. The experiences of abuse resulted in aggression and hatred directed against the self. Victims were left with extreme problems of trust, self-image, and aggression, all of which profoundly affected the capacity of the victim to enter into therapy.

In a study by Brown and Anderson (1991) of 1,040 consecutive inpatient admissions in a U.S. Air Force tertiary-care hospital, 18% of patients reported a history of abuse. A history of physical abuse, but not of sexual abuse, correlated with current and past alcohol and drug abuse. The rate of drug abuse in females with a history of both physical and sexual abuse was nearly twice as high as in those with either physical or sexual abuse alone. Suicidality was significantly higher in all patients with a history of abuse. The rate of Axis II diagnoses, particularly borderline personality disorder, was significantly higher in all categories of patients with a history of abuse. Abuse was predominantly intrafamilial.

Rape victims who had received crisis intervention and counseling services through agencies were evaluated for symptoms of PTSD with self-report instruments. The scores of rape victims were significantly higher than nonpatient normal scores and were about the same as, or were not significantly higher than, those of women attending a psychiatric stress clinic. The amount of time that had elapsed since the rape was not correlated with severity of symptomatology (Burge 1988).

A study by Kemp et al. (1991) of battered women in shelters found that 84% met criteria for PTSD. Self-report data revealed that the presence and degree of PTSD were correlated with subjective distress regarding the battery experience and with extent of the abuse. L. E. Walker (1979, p. 55) noted a cyclical pattern in battering relationships consisting of three phases: the "tension building phase, the acute battering incident, and the calm, loving respite." Victims and batterers, as well as some researchers, have misinterpreted the "calm, loving," repentant, appeasing phase as love. Actually, it is a combination of the use of projective identification, denial, and dissociation in which the batterer projects onto the victim a variety of internal object and self images and relates to those projections, not the victim, just as is done in the other two phases. The victim uses similar defenses.

Goodwin (1985b) stated that most incest victims who seek therapy meet the criteria for PTSD, although this can be difficult to detect because of the severity of the symptoms, the victim's difficulty in being aware of the symptoms, the need to conceal the symptoms and the history of abuse, and the victim's young age. In studies of child victims of sexual abuse, most of the children met the criteria for PTSD, and many more exhibited significant symptoms of PTSD. These symptoms include reexperiencing and reenacting behaviors; avoidant behaviors; symptoms of autonomic hyperarousal; identification with the aggressor; fears of the mundane and specific trauma-related fears; developmental delays in speech, motility, and personal and social development; and learning disabilities secondary to the typical defenses employed (Burgess et al. 1987; Fish-Murray et al. 1987; Goodwin 1990; Green 1988a, 1988b; Kiser et al. 1988; MacVicar 1979; McLeer et al. 1988; Ornitz and Pynoos 1989; Terr 1979, 1991). Child witnesses to violence, such as murder, rape, severe domestic violence, and suicide of parents, are also at high risk for PTSD; these suffering, young witnesses are routinely overlooked (Pynoos and Eth 1985, 1986). Adults with such histories may show any or all of these symptoms throughout their posttraumatic development and into adulthood (Coons 1990; Goodwin 1985b; Putnam et al. 1986; Terr 1979, 1991).

Victims with PTSD are at increased risk for major depressive disorders; substance abuse, including nicotine and caffeine; panic disorder; suicide and homicide; phobias; sleep disturbances; and possibly shortened life span secondary to immune system impairment (Frank and Anderson 1987; van der Kolk 1987a, 1987b). Learning disorders are common. The hyperarousal that occurs in response to reminders of the traumatic stressor disrupts learning, and defenses typically used against remembering the trauma lead to cognitive malfunctioning (Fine 1990; Fish-Murray et al. 1987; Green 1988a, 1988b, 1988c; Greenberg and van der Kolk 1987; Terr 1979, 1983a, 1983b, 1987; van der Kolk 1987a, 1989).

Other long-term sequelae are equally devastating. Multiple personality disorder is the most dramatic outcome of childhood victimization (Braun 1990; Kluft 1987; Putnam et al. 1986; Ross et al. 1990). Coons et al. (1989), studying a population of psychiatric patients drawn from four settings, observed that in patients with multiple personality disorder, 80% had a history of childhood sexual abuse, 45% of physical abuse, 35% of verbal abuse, and 25% of neglect. Other dissociative disorders had a similar pattern but usually were associated with lower frequencies of childhood abuse. The frequency of neglect was higher in patients with psychogenic amnesia or atypical dissociative disorder. In a study of 100 patients with multiple personality disorder, Putnam et al. (1986), using a detailed questionnaire, found a very high rate of significant trauma in almost all patients.

In populations of patients with borderline personality disorder, Herman and van der Kolk (1987), Briere and Zaidi (1989), Brown and Anderson (1991), and Stone (1990), among others, have found high rates of histories of physical abuse, sexual abuse, and witnessing serious domestic violence. Herman (1986) observed that, in a population of psychiatric outpatients, women with a history of abuse were four to five times as likely to be given a diagnosis of borderline personality disorder and were at least twice as likely to be given a diagnosis of substance abuse as those who had no history of victimization. Herman et al. (1989) conceptualize borderline personality disorder as, in part, representing an integration and elaboration into the personality organization of the memories of the abuse and its posttraumatic sequelae; these are reexperienced and reenacted over time in somatic sensations, visual and other sensory images (Brett and Ostroff 1985), affective states, dissociated aspects of the self (Putnam 1990), and behavioral reenactments (Blum 1986; Carmen and Rieker 1989; Cooper 1986; Furst 1986; Gillman 1986; Rose 1991; Terr 1991). The memory of the trauma may thus be disguised and lost, and current symptoms of PTSD may not be reported.

Other diagnoses in which the frequency of a history of victimization is high are multiple personality disorder (Ross et al. 1990), antisocial personality disorder, conduct disorders, hysterical psychosis, and hysterical personality disorder (Burgess et al. 1987, 1988). Conversion disorder and somatization disorders (Loewenstein 1990; Morrison 1989; Schei and Bakketeig 1989; E. Walker et al. 1988)—in particular, pelvic pain, regardless of the kind and degree of pelvic pathology (Borins and Forsythe 1985)—have been linked with a history of sexual and/or physical abuse. In addition, victims are at significant risk for self-mutilation, self-starvation, revictimization, and becoming abusive themselves or failing to protect themselves and their children from abuse (Carmen and Rieker 1989; Gelinas 1983; Gelles and Straus 1988; Goodwin 1990; Green 1978, 1988a; Jacobson and Richardson 1987; Rose 1991; Russell 1986; Schultz 1990; Spiegel 1989; Steele 1986; Terr 1991; van der Kolk 1987a, 1989).

One form that the revictimization takes is that of being sexually misused by health care providers; victims have an increased likelihood of this and are overrepresented in this population (Kluft 1989, 1990b). A significant number of chronically institutionalized female psychiatric patients may have misdiagnosed dissociative disorders rather than schizophrenia. Beck and van der Kolk (1987) observed that these patients, who had failed to respond to antipsychotic medications, had a history of childhood incest; these patients were also noted, in comparison with controls, to be younger and to have a higher rate of possible organicity, sexual delusions and preoccupation, depressive symptoms, substance abuse, more threatened or actual violent behavior, more engagement socially with the staff, and more major medical problems.

A large majority of prostitutes and participants in pornography have a history of childhood incest, as do many people with paraphilias (van der Kolk 1987a). Victimization may contribute to homosexual orientation as a defense (Finkelhor 1984). Criminal behavior, the transformation from being abused to becoming abusive, is another outcome, particularly in male victims (Burgess et al. 1987, 1988; Pollock et al. 1990; Risin and Koss 1987; van der Kolk 1989).

Physical sequelae may have serious psychological consequences. Severe physical damage, deformity, and death are real dangers, as are sexually transmitted diseases, particularly bacterial vaginosis, trichomoniasis, and chlamydial infection, and the possibility of acquiring acquired immunodeficiency syndrome (AIDS) (Jenny et al. 1990). Because of damage to self-care (Krystal 1978a; Rose 1991), routine preventive medical care and interventions during illness are often postponed.

HISTORY

Demographics

Myth, religious beliefs, art forms such as drama and fairy tales, and laws reflect the prevalence of sexual assault, domestic violence, and incest in far-flung cultures throughout the history of humanity (Dickstein 1988; Goodwin 1990; Hilberman 1980). The content of some creative works has been found to be a reenactment of actual psychic trauma and its sequelae (Shengold 1989; Terr 1987, 1989). Victimization spares no socioeconomic group, age, or sex, but certain populations are more at risk.

Factors that are correlated with an increased risk for rape are youth, urban residence, being married or previously married, and higher level of education. The incidence of child witnesses to the mother's rape is estimated to be 10% of all reported rapes (Pynoos and Eth 1985; Pynoos and Nader 1988). When rape is reported to the police, the alleged rapist is arrested in only half of these cases. Of these arrests, only 60% result in prosecution. Only half of cases that are prosecuted are strong enough to be brought to trial, and of these, only 16% result in conviction (Gise and Paddison 1988).

No single factor explains the demography of domestic violence (Gelles and Straus 1988). The occurrence of domestic violence is correlated with an increased rate of life stresses, a history of having experienced abuse in childhood, and particularly, a history of having witnessed marital violence in childhood. Although lower-income and minority populations are overrepresented among families reported for child abuse and neglect, this is only partly related to their increased likelihood of being violent; another key factor is a well-documented bias in favor of the more well-to-do. Although alcohol use in association with violent behavior is reported by almost half of couples who commit acts of marital or parental violence, alcohol use is not causal, and moderate consumption is most commonly found in violent families.

The "typical" family in which violence between partners occurs does exist (Gelles and Straus 1988; Hilberman 1980). The man in this family is 18–24 years old, has been married for less than 10 years, and works part-time or not at all. He is very concerned about economic security and feels inadequate. He is dissatisfied with the standard of living he and his wife have; he works at a level below his educational background or below that of his wife's occupational or educational level. The woman has low self-esteem and inhibited aggression. She is dependent and feels helpless and hopeless. Both partners commonly come from homes in which neglect, physical and sexual abuse, emotional deprivation, and lack of protection prevail. The woman flees from her family of origin and her often seductive or overtly incestuous family into marriage. Frequently she is pregnant at the time of marriage.

Age is the best predictor of the risk of being beaten, the greatest likelihood occurring between the ages of 18 and 24 years. Abuse, however, may begin at any time in the relationship. Pregnancy does not increase the risk that battering will begin, but in relationships already characterized by violence, the nature and frequency of the violence often change. The man shifts the attacks to assaults against the fetus, in the form of blows to the woman's abdomen and breasts, rape, and increased demands for intercourse (L. E. Walker 1979).

Incest occurs in families with many predisposing factors that can be understood as sequelae of PTSD (Green 1988b, 1988c; Herman 1981). In the fathers and other perpetrators (Daie et al. 1989; Green 1988c), these include a background of childhood sexual and/or physical abuse; emotional deprivation; tyrannical, paranoid attitudes; alcohol abuse; unstable employment; social and physical isolation; and lower socioeconomic status. In the mothers, common findings include a similar history of abuse, passivity, and dependency; an increased likelihood of future victimization; absence and/or unavailability due to depression or illness; and a higher rate of pregnancy and sexual aversion. For daughters, being the oldest or the only daughter increases the likelihood of victimization.

Incestuous activity characteristically begins when the child is 8–12 years old and may start with genital fondling or oral-genital sex, later proceeding to intercourse when the victim reaches puberty, but it may begin in infancy (Chasnoff et al. 1986). Accompanying the victimization is alienation from the mother, who is unavailable before the incest, fails to protect, and may herself abuse the child (Gelinas 1983; Green 1988a, 1988b, 1988c; Herman 1981, 1988; Schultz 1990).

Freud and the Seduction Hypothesis Controversy

Charcot (Ellenberger 1970), Janet (van der Kolk and van der Hart 1989), and Freud (1896a, 1896b) linked symptoms they observed in their patients to traumatic experiences. Freud's early theories focused on incestuous experiences as etiologic in many of the patients he treated. He later shifted to the role of conflict and defense in normal psychosexual development to explain the states he observed in his patients. Although all of the information that led to this profound change in focus may never be available, it is well known that the normative response of the victim, the victimizer, significant others, and societal institutions is to defend against recognizing traumatic occurrences because of the profound threat they pose for all people (Blank 1985; Goodwin 1985a; Haley 1978; Rose 1991). In turning to the intrapsychic factors in psychopathology, Freud provided essential tools for understanding the impact of trauma on psychological functioning and for treating the psychological sequelae of trauma. A careful scrutiny of his later works indicates that Freud did not relinquish his belief in the occurrence and impact of trauma (Levine 1990).

CULTURAL AND CROSS-CULTURAL ISSUES

Among the variables that are important in understanding cultural and cross-cultural issues in violence are cultural beliefs about female and male sex roles, the role of children, and sexuality and violence. The impact of political and historical events on the culture may be of great significance, as are religious beliefs. Within the Anglo-American culture, the belief that family violence is acceptable prevails (Gelles and Straus 1988). Were a stranger to hit or to hurl epithets at anyone not in his family, the victim and bystanders would be shocked and consider it an assault. Help would be forthcoming. In families, however, even in public, assaults rarely are identified as such, and intervention is rare. Knowledge of these factors is crucial for the identification of victims of violence; for understanding the intrapsychic, interpersonal, and societal meanings of the victimization; and for conducting treatment (Hamilton 1989; Kinzie et al. 1990; Kroll et al. 1989; Mollica and Son 1989; Mollica et al. 1990; Parson 1985).

The therapist who is unprepared for working in cross-cultural settings may feel threatened and inadequate, defending against this by making erroneous interpretations. The following are some guidelines for interviewing in cross-cultural situations.

First, make no assumptions about the meanings of the victim's discomfort in seeking help; instead, ask the victim. Meaning may be culture bound and/or personal. For example, in Appalachian and Native American cultures, self-reliance is highly valued; offers of help from others are seen as a sign of disrespect and also may be viewed with suspicion. Second, seek consultation from someone who is knowledgeable about the culture. Third, be alert to limitations and differences in the contents of languages that may impede the victim's ability to verbalize. Ask the victim to explain the problem that is limiting communication and what would help. For example, the victim may not have any words in English to describe the act committed and the body parts violated and may find speaking of these in the native language offensive. Fourth, address the sex and culture of the therapist. For example, a Southeast Asian woman may find a therapist of her cultural group to be dangerous because of a fear that, owing to the therapist's contact with the victim's culture, her history of rape may get back to the community and result in her being divorced, disowned, battered, or even murdered. Individuals of some cultures may prefer an English-speaking therapist, despite the victim's limited English, because members of their own culture are believed to have inferior training or lower status. Fifth, be alert to one's own prejudices and that of the victim. Sixth, note that certain populations, such as Pacific Asians, Central and South Americans, and Africans, have a very high rate of victimization because of the political problems of their countries of origin (Mid-Peninsula Rape Crisis Center, undated).

ETIOLOGY

Rape, domestic violence, and incest and their sequelae have multiple interacting etiologies. None is sufficient by itself to explain these outcomes. Evidence is accruing, however, that psychic trauma resulting in PTSD is a crucial etiologic agent that may serve to explain and organize a wide range of biologic, intrapsychic, interpersonal, and cultural data from studies of victims, victimizers, significant others, and societal institutions (Brett and Ostroff 1985; Burgess and Holmstrom 1979; Burgess et al. 1987; Coons et al. 1989; Gelinas 1983; Hilberman 1980; Horowitz 1976; Terr 1979, 1991; van der Kolk 1987a; Walker 1991). Kardiner and Spiegel (1947) were the first to describe fully the outcome of psychic trauma as a "physioneurosis," that is, a disorder with both psychological and physiological components and unique pathophysiology.

Biological Etiology

Research on subjects with PTSD has demonstrated the impact of psychic trauma on central noradrenergic activity, the endogenous opioid system, the hypothalamic-pituitary-adrenal axis, and the sleep cycle (Friedman 1988, 1991; van der Kolk 1987a, 1987b, 1989; van der Kolk and Greenberg 1987). The model of learned helplessness secondary to inescapable shock may be directly applicable as a model for PTSD. Alternatively, prolonged excess stimulation of the central nervous system (CNS) from traumatic exposure may result in chronic cortical synaptic and neuronal changes in subjects with PTSD (Kolb 1987; Ornitz and Pynoos 1989; van der Kolk and Greenberg 1987). The neurobiological model, kindling (in which repeated subthreshold stimulation of an area of the brain results in response in the brain), may be a mechanism by which limbic nuclei may become altered in response to the chronic noradrenergic arousal in subjects with PTSD (van der Kolk and Greenberg 1987).

Excessive reactivity of the sympathetic nervous system is one consequence of alterations in CNS noradrenergic activity. Excessive adrenergic activity may also suppress endogenous opioid activity. Exogenous opiates tranquilize, exert an antidepressant effect, and decrease aggression, anxiety, paranoia, and feelings of inadequacy. Subjects with PTSD experience hyperalgesia, which may be a factor in the chronic pain syndromes frequently seen in victims. Exposure to a stressor that is a reminder of the original stressor has been observed to induce a temporary analgesia that can be partially blocked by naloxone. This analgesia may be an important etiologic factor in the "addiction to trauma" seen in victims of abuse, war veterans, and other populations with PTSD. Opiate withdrawal symptoms can result when exposure to traumatic reminders ceases. Some victims of child abuse use self-mutilation, in part, to stop the withdrawal. Clonidine, a blocker of autonomic manifestations of opiate withdrawal, stops self-mutilation and other forms of self-destructive actions in some victims.

Central adrenergic hyperactivity may be the cause of decreased functioning of the hypothalamic-pituitary-adrenal axis, reflected in decreased levels of urinary cortisol. Sleep disturbances secondary to nightmares arising out of rapid eye movement (REM) or non-REM sleep have been clearly documented. But controversy surrounds the question of alteration of sleep architecture in subjects with PTSD. With such disruption of basic neurophysiologic functioning in many systems, substance abuse, which commonly coexists with PTSD, may have, in part, a biologic basis. Substances that are CNS depressants, such as alcohol, marijuana, and narcotics, down-regulate the central adrenergic activity and consequently ameliorate the endogenous opioid deficiency.

Intrapsychic Etiology

A model that integrates many psychodynamic theories (Rose 1991) is based on the assumption that a victim, by definition, has experienced an event that is outside the norm of those human experiences that can be expected to occur. The victim, regardless of prior experience, is thus psychologically unprepared to cope adequately. Consequently, the victim's intrapsychic world of basic beliefs, internalized object relations, defenses, familiar affects and mechanisms for regulating them, and accompanying neurophysiologic stability are experienced as having been rendered useless and as having failed and betrayed the victim. The victim's psychological life is felt to have been destroyed and lost, to be supplanted by a new inner world of intense primitive affects such as terror and murderous rage, dissociative defenses (Braun 1989; Spiegel 1984; Spiegel et al. 1988), and unfamiliar self and object images. Associated with this is an outpouring of neurotransmitters and subsequent alterations in their regulation and metabolism, adding to the victim's altered self-experience. The experience of loss, failure, betrayal, and psychological death—"soul murder" (Shengold 1989)—evokes murderous rage in the victim (Rose 1991; Schultz 1990; Winnicott 1960), who attacks and devalues the intrapsychic world. These changes cause the victim to lose the capacity for empathy and to dread empathy from others. The victim projects both the loss of the capacity to empathize and the dread of empathy (Burgess et al. 1987; Rose 1991). Clinically, the projections present in two forms: the victim's belief that no one, particularly the mother and maternal representatives in society, can understand the victim unless that person has had a very similar experience; and the victim's extreme reticence in revealing anything other than repetitive, very limited information about the assault (Rose 1991).

The use of dissociative defenses during the traumatic event protects ego functioning and creates the illusion that the victim has escaped from the abuser. These defenses persist after the assault because of the psychological damage that has occurred; the defenses then impair psychic integrity and sense of identity (Putnam 1990; Rose 1991; Spiegel et al. 1988). They also cause alterations in consciousness and memory functioning (Clary et al. 1984; Rose 1991). When the dissociative defenses fail, the victim experiences intrusive thoughts, nightmares (Rose 1991; van der Kolk 1987a), and flashbacks, as well as physical symptoms of hyperarousal (Rose 1991; van der Kolk 1989). The victim then uses avoidance of any stimuli that remind her of the assault to protect against future intrusive phenomena (Brett and Ostroff 1985; Nader et al. 1990; Rose 1991; Terr 1979, 1991), thus circumscribing her life further. Projective identification (Catherall 1991; Clary et al. 1984; Rose 1991) and reenactment are also employed by the victim (Burgess et al. 1987, 1988; Carmen and Rieker 1989; MacVicar 1979; Rose 1986b, 1991; van der Kolk 1989; van der Kolk and Kadish 1987). Unfortunately, these strengthen the belief that other people are threatening and dangerous. Significant others may comply with the projection or may participate in the reenactment (Green 1988b, 1988c; Kluft 1990a, 1990b; Krugman 1987; Moss et al. 1990; Rose 1991). The typical conflicts developed and the defenses used by subjects with PTSD may result in the victim's becoming the victimizer (Burgess et al. 1987, 1988; Green 1988; Krugman 1987; Rose 1991).

Substance abuse, including alcohol, drugs, cigarettes, and caffeine, may be used in an attempt to remedy the sequelae of hyperarousal and constriction resulting from PTSD; it may also be used as a means to create an externally induced dissociative state, when dissociative defenses are inadequate to prevent return of the traumatic state. Both the victim and the victimizer may also blame the substance abuse as a defense against recognizing the real origin of the violence (Burgess et al. 1987; Rose 1991; Terr 1991).

If the victims of or witnesses to rape, domestic violence, or incest are seen very soon after the first assault, the vast majority of them will have easily detectable symptoms of acute PTSD. Without intervention, chronic PTSD, "posttraumatic decline" (Titchener 1986, p. 5), is the usual outcome. In chronic PTSD, although the symptoms resulting from intrusive phenomena and hyperarousal may still be detectable, the predominant findings reflect the constriction that has occurred, intertwined with preexisting personality, normal development, and the responses of significant others (Eth and Pynoos 1985; Herman et al. 1989; MacVicar 1979; Pynoos and Nader 1988; Rose 1991; Schultz 1990; Terr 1979, 1981, 1991).

Interpersonal Etiology

The interpersonal world of the victim and victimizer reflects and enacts the typical defenses against the threat that psychic trauma poses to all human beings (Bard et al. 1986; Kluft 1990a; Rose 1986b, 1991). Blaming the victim for the violence is common. In families in which domestic violence and child abuse occur, the other family members usually have their own histories of victimization and thus the defenses, dissociative states, cognitive distortions, beliefs, internalized object relations, and conflicts similar to those of the victim. These reinforce the pathological changes that can occur in any victim of violence, causing alterations in cognition that then disconfirm the reality of the abuse.

Rieker and Carmen (1986) note the transition from victim to patient. The defenses typically used by the victim of child abuse or domestic violence interact with those of the family members. Remarkable distortions and disconfirmations of abuse, such as believing that the abuse is a display of love, result from these ongoing interactions among the victim, victimizer, family, and societal institutions. In these families, the conflict over aggression and extensive use of primitive defenses distort object relations and impair the development of physical and psychological boundaries, separateness, individuation, autonomy, and intimacy (Green 1988a; Hilberman 1980; Schultz 1990).

The family members are impaired in their ability to protect themselves and one another. The family atmosphere is one of terror, secrecy, mistrust, extensive control, and paranoia. The family and its individual members become increasingly isolated from the community. Their resulting psychological, cognitive, and intellectual impairment limits their academic achievement, career opportunities, and skills to support themselves. The children may be able to separate only in adolescence, when they are under the threat of severe physical harm or pregnancy, often fleeing into relationships that repeat this vicious cycle (Green 1988a; Krugman 1987; Madonna et al. 1991; Russell 1986).

Revictimization is a common occurrence. It presents in many forms: the victim with a history of two or more rapes; the marriage of a victim of child abuse or a witness to domestic violence to an abusive spouse; the prostitute who is a victim of incest; and the incest victim, in psychotherapy, who is sexually abused by the therapist. The psychodynamics of PTSD predispose to revictimization. The defenses employed to prevent reexperiencing the traumatic helplessness and intrapsychic changes prevent the use of fear and anger as signal affects to inform and alert the victim to danger. Turning passive to active compels the victim to seek out dangerous situations (Green 1988a; MacVicar 1979; Rose 1991; Terr 1979, 1991; van der Kolk 1989); the "addiction to trauma" also contributes to this. The impact of trauma results in the victim's becoming dependent, turning aggression against the self, with idealization of others and devaluing of the self. This, in concert with severe conflicts over aggression, renders the victim unable to be separate and to use her observing ego. The victim's desperate need for relief from self-hatred and feeling unlovable make her unable to protect herself from, or compel her to seek, inappropriate and abusive objects (Chasnoff et al. 1986; Kluft 1989, 1990b; Yates 1982).

Sociocultural Factors

Sociocultural attitudes are important contributing factors for victims of rape, domestic violence, and incest (Bard et al. 1986; Blank 1985; Goodwin 1985a; Rose 1991). The sequelae of PTSD are played out within society's attitudes and institutions. Thus, laws that are punitive toward the victim have been commonplace, as has minimalizing the extent and impact of these forms of violence. Rape continues to be the only violent crime in which the victim's testimony is insufficient for conviction (Gise and Paddison 1988). Until recently, rape victims who pressed charges commonly found their veracity and private lives on trial at the alleged rapist's trial. Victims of domestic violence were told to patch up their relationship, if the police even responded to their call for help. This attitude coexisted with the knowledge that police are in grave danger from the abuser when responding to calls for help from the victim of domestic violence. Incest was considered to be extremely rare; the victim was viewed as seducing the adult; only psychotic adults were thought to be perpetrators.

CURRENT REALITIES

Incidence

Only 20 years ago rape, domestic violence, and incest were thought to be rare experiences that happened only to highly deviant females who unconsciously or consciously wished for and solicited the assault (Bard and Sangrey 1979; Burgess and Holmstrom 1974, 1979; Horowitz 1976; Kempe et al. 1962; Meiselman 1978; Rosenfeld 1979; L. E. Walker 1979). A reluctant society and its health care providers began to confront these terrifying and staggering realities. If only a small fraction of victims develop PTSD and its comorbid disorders, a major epidemic of a disabling psychological and physiological disorder that is transgenerationally transmitted has now been detected (Krugman 1987).

Rape is defined legally as "carnal knowledge of a person by force and against the person's will" (Gise and Paddison 1988, p. 630). Estimates of the prevalence of completed rape have ranged from 6% to 16%. Rape by strangers has been estimated to be underreported by as much as a 10:1 ratio, with date and marital rape even more underreported (Bowie et al. 1990; Gise and Paddison 1988; Pynoos and Nader 1988; Stewart et al. 1987). Kilpatrick et al. (1988) found that, among female rape victims, rape by a stranger occurred in 21%, date rape in 17%, rape by other non-strangers in 39%, and marital rape in 24%. Date and marital rape were more likely to result in physical injury.

Domestic violence includes the physical abuse of a spouse and children, sexual abuse, emotional abuse, and neglect, as well as witnessing abuse. The home, thought of in our culture as a refuge, is actually the most dangerous place to be. Although the frequency and types of assaults are alike for men and women, men inflict more injury because of their greater physical strength. Researchers disagree over whether women's physical attacks on men are predominantly in self-defense or are the initial attack at least 50% of the time. The incidence of domestic violence is dismaying (Gelles and Straus 1988; Hilberman 1980; McNeely and Robinson-Simpson 1987; L. E. Walker 1979):

❖ Physical abuse by a spouse is estimated to occur to 4 million women and men per year, with an equal occurrence to women and men.

❖ Marital rape has been reported to occur in 3%–14% of marriages.

❖ Three percent of parents report that they punch, kick, or bite their child each year. More than 4% report that they have beaten their child. Women abuse children at an equal or slightly higher rate than men. Some researchers suggest that this is a result of women's having more contact with and responsibility for the care of children.

❖ Children are almost always witnesses to all forms of abuse.

❖ Adults have revealed that 20%–30% approved of hitting the spouse.

❖ Violence in courtship occurs in 22%–67% of dating relationships.

❖ Over 85% of adults approve of strong discipline for children.

❖ Sibling violence, ranging from slaps and pushes to the use of weapons, occurs in 80% of homes each year.

❖ Between 20% and 50% of all murders in this country occur within the family.

❖ Forty percent of all female homicide victims are killed by their husbands, and 10% of male victims are killed by their wives, most often in self-defense. Equal numbers of men and women kill their spouses.

The rate of sexual victimization of women in childhood has been consistently found to be 16%–38%, with 6.5%–12% reporting intrafamilial abuse. Men as perpetrators account for 92% of sexual abuse of girls and 84% of abuse of boys. Women alone account for 6% of sexual abuse of girls and 14% of abuse of boys. Most often the abusive woman is the mother. Burgess et al. (1988) consider this figure for women to be low and attribute underreporting to the cultural stereotype of boys being initiated into adult sexuality by older women.

Legal Ramifications

In the legal definition of rape, penetration, however slight, is "carnal knowledge." The law provides protection and redress for victims through both criminal and civil processes. It is necessary to learn the legal options for the victim in both the state in which she was assaulted and the one in which she resides. Areas of the law with which the psychiatrist treating a victim must become familiar include the victim's filing a police report, collection of evidence, the steps in criminal prosecution (Spiegel 1986), victims' rights, ways to provide police and physical protection, restraining orders, financial support and maintenance, divorce and child visitation, compensation via civil suits, and statutes of limitation (Schetky and Benedek 1989; L. E. Walker 1988; Young 1988b).

This information may be available through rape crisis centers, programs for victims of domestic violence, the district attorney, family law specialists, and personal injury attorneys. Each step taken by the victim in the legal process may activate severe psychological conflict over this appropriate, socially sanctioned expression of self-assertion and/or autonomy, particularly when this includes retaliating by pressing a criminal or civil suit or filing for divorce. These conflicts underlie many of the failures to report victimization and also the phenomenon of the battered woman's returning to the abusive man several times before being able to make a final separation. These phenomena have contributed to society's belief that these forms of victimization are rare and not to be taken seriously and that women want to be mistreated and are masochistic.

Although the criminal and civil justice systems are more informed than they once were about the consequences of victimization, the victim remains very vulnerable to experiencing retraumatization in her contacts with them. Also, not infrequently, law enforcement officers, the judicial system, and attorneys fail to carry through on their responsibilities (Schetky and Benedek 1989).

In cases of domestic violence and incest, much of the mental health community has traditionally preferred an intervention in which the family and abuser seek treatment, with the family remaining intact (Gelles and Straus 1988; Giarretto 1989; Phelan 1987). It is now thought by many experts, however, that divorce is almost inevitable. Both of these groups think that arrest of the abuser is essential for any further kind of intervention to become possible (Dickstein 1988; Gelles and Straus 1988; Goodwin and Talwar 1989).

Social Attitudes

The Women's Movement and the Victims of Crime Movement (Young 1988a) have made accurate information about victimization available to the public and to legal and health professionals. Consequently, social attitudes toward rape, domestic violence, and incest are undergoing a change. Blaming the victim and ignoring or minimizing the damage from victimization are less prevalent now. In many areas of the country, there are agencies that provide services for the victim and significant others, laws have changed at both the federal and state levels, and funding is guaranteed for financial compensation of monetary losses by victims and witnesses under the Victims of Crime Program.

Reporting

Rape victims have complete control over reporting rape. Statutes of limitation vary by state. Immediate reporting is much more likely to result in arrest and conviction, because evidence can be gathered and the victim's credulity is less in question. In domestic violence, the victim, the spouse abuser, and the police have the power to report (Walker 1988).

In cases of child abuse, all health care providers, teachers, and others who provide care for children are required to report child abuse in all states. More recently, legislation has been enacted requiring mandatory reporting to a national data bank of all abusers who have current contact with children. This is a highly controversial issue. On one hand, many psychiatrists and other providers of services to victims fear that informing the victim of this requirement will deter victims from seeking help or will cause them to flee. On the other hand, others believe that reporting, when handled properly, can be salutary and that the major impediment is countertransference (Rose 1986a).

EMERGENCY MANAGEMENT

At the time of reporting a crime of assault or abuse, the victim and, in the case of domestic violence, the children and batterer are often in grave physical and psychological danger (Gise and Paddison 1988; Hilberman 1980; Rose 1986a, 1986b, 1991; L. E. Walker 1979). Once safety is secured, other interventions can be explored and provided.

Victims need many kinds of emergency and long-term assistance. These range from a safe and supportive place to stay and help in negotiating medical, legal, and criminal justice issues to education of significant others, employers, health care providers, and the criminal justice system and referral for psychotherapy. Financial aid provided by state and federal Victims of Crime programs permits restitution for uninsured medical costs, psychotherapy costs, and lost wages. The victim is usually unfamiliar with these areas and ill equipped to cope with them (Young 1988b).

The staff and volunteers of rape crisis centers, battered women's shelters, Victims of Crime programs, agencies responsible for emergency interventions for child incest victims, and support programs for adults abused as children may be able to provide this necessary range of services. By their doing so, the psychiatrist is more easily able to maintain the usual boundaries and neutrality. When these services are absent, the psychiatrist needs to assist the victims. Simultaneously, the psychiatrist must inquire about the meanings these interventions hold for the victim.

A psychiatric emergency occurs not only when the victim has just recently been assaulted or is first disclosing it (Sauzier 1989; Schatzow and Herman 1989), but also when the victim begins to have access to previously dissociated material. Whether in the emergency room or the consultation room, the evaluation consists of an assessment of PTSD, the pre-assault personality structure and level of functioning, availability of support, and interventions needed. When this segment of the emergency evaluation is conducted properly, psychotherapy for the victim and significant others has begun. Following this, the psychiatrist needs to give the victim and significant others, if present, an explanation of the impact of the trauma on the victim and on significant others, addressing presenting symptoms and defenses. Then follows the recommendation for psychotherapy, including a statement that, in the psychiatrist's experience, the victim can expect to recover and an explanation of how psychotherapy works to effect recovery.

THERAPEUTIC INTERVENTIONS

Diagnosis

Usually no single diagnosis describes all the sequelae of victimization. PTSD is readily diagnosed when the victim can report the traumatic experience and when acute symptomatology is present. Within a short time, the characteristic defenses and characterologic changes often obscure the history of trauma and acute symptoms of PTSD (Kluft 1990a; Rose 1991). Terr (1991) has suggested that, from childhood trauma, four characteristics persist for years, irrespective of the patient's diagnosis. These are 1) repeated reexperiencing of memories of the trauma in visual or other sensory modalities, 2) reenactments in play and behavior, 3) fears linked to the trauma, and 4) altered beliefs about the self, others, and life course. If the victims are not treated shortly after the trauma, all children except those experiencing the mildest of traumas are destined to have the impact of the trauma last for years.

Later, comorbid mental disorders begin to appear. Victims are then likely to have a wide range of diagnoses applied. Diagnostic errors commonly include panic disorder, anorexia nervosa, somatization disorder, conversion reaction, conduct disorder, and antisocial personality disorder (Pollock et al. 1990); major depression, substance abuse, borderline personality disorder (Catherall 1991; Clary et al. 1984; Horevitz and Braun 1984); and atypical psychosis, hysterical psychosis, and multiple personality disorder or other dissociative disorders (Putnam 1990; Ross et al. 1990; Schetky 1988).

The crucial history of victimization may not be obtained. It may take many years of therapeutic work before the history of victimization becomes accessible. Thus, categories such as "masochistic personality disorder" and "self-defeating personality disorder" carry the possibility of being misused. The study of PTSD and its etiologic factors, pathophysiology and psychopathology, symptomatology, comorbidity with other mental disorders, and long-term course, treatment, and outcome is in its infancy.

Difficulties in Recovering the History of Trauma

Recovery and working through of traumatic memories are difficult, even when the victim is highly motivated and is supported by significant others. Memories may be evanescent, distorted, and incomplete secondary to both the use of dissociative defenses and the impact of neurochemical changes on memory storage (Goodwin 1985a; Greenberg and van der Kolk 1987; Rieker and Carmen 1986; Rose 1991; van der Kolk 1987c). Remembering also brings with it the risk of being retraumatized. When the victim has been physically assaulted, many of the memories are stored in the form of sensory perceptions and actions, such as nonverbal communication, reenactment, and acting out; regression also contributes to this phenomenon (Carmen and Rieker 1989; Krystal 1978b, 1984; Rose 1986b, 1991). In spite of these obstacles to remembering, victims have been found to recover memories of trauma that can usually be validated (Herman and Schatzow 1987).

Treatment

A history of violence should alert the therapist to the likely need for psychotherapy, as should evidence of posttraumatic sequelae. The few prospective studies of victim populations beginning shortly after the traumatic event indicate that no one escaped unscathed psychologically (Kilpatrick et al. 1985; Nader et al. 1990; Terr 1983b, 1991). The recognition of the experience of psychological helplessness is central to understanding the damage that has occurred. The purpose of the interventions is to enable the victim to gain understanding. The range of efficacious treatments includes psychodynamic psychotherapy (Catherall 1991; Gillman 1986; Horowitz 1976, 1986; Kluft 1989; Lindy 1986; Rose 1986b, 1991; Shengold 1989; Steele 1986); cognitive therapies and behavioral therapies (Courtois 1988; Frank et al. 1988; Lyons and Keane 1989; Pitman et al. 1991); hypnotherapy (Spiegel 1984, 1990); pharmacotherapy (Friedman 1988, 1991; Silver et al. 1990); and self-help organizations (Goodwin and Talwar 1989). Regardless of theoretical orientation or technique used, several principles of technique prevail (Bowie et al. 1990; Braun 1989; Carmen and Rieker 1989; Horowitz 1986; Jacobson and Richardson 1987; Kluft 1989; Lindy 1986; MacVicar 1979; Pynoos and Eth 1986; Rose 1986b, 1991; Rozynko and Dondershine 1991; Sonnenberg 1988):

- ❖ The therapist should inquire routinely, actively, and thoroughly about victimization and its resolution (Briere and Zaidi 1989; Courtois 1988; Stone 1989).
- ❖ The therapist needs to present himself or herself as an expert on the impact of victimization and PTSD. This is crucial, because the victim has lost the belief that others can understand and tolerate the victim's experience. The therapist must be able to understand and explain the impact of victimization to the victim and significant others and thus restore and increase the victim's self-knowledge and capacity to cope (Pynoos and Eth 1986; Rose 1991).
- ❖ The therapist, in recognition of the severe damage to psychic

structure that results from trauma, needs to provide a psychological "holding environment" (Winnicott 1960, p. 44) until the victim can perform these ego supportive functions for himself or herself (Rose 1991).

❖ The therapist should not focus on abreaction and catharsis to the exclusion of exploration and interpretation of defenses and conflicts, thus retraumatizing the victim and causing a negative therapeutic reaction or resulting in a "transference cure" with ongoing vulnerability (Coons et al. 1989; Herman et al. 1989; Lyons and Keane 1989; Pynoos and Eth 1986; Rose 1991; Spiegel 1989).

❖ The personal meanings of the traumatic experience must be explored (Gelinas 1983; Rose 1986b, 1991).

❖ The autonomy of the victim must be meticulously respected; victims have suffered gross violations of fundamental autonomy in the course of victimization and are very vulnerable to any impingement on their autonomy, such as pressures to report the victimization or to confront the victimizer, to tell others of the victimization, or to take medication. At the same time, through reenactment, the victim commonly elicits violations by the therapist. Common examples include the victim's being so reticent to discuss anything, especially the trauma, that the psychiatrist probes (intrudes); and the victim's being so enraged that the psychiatrist feels threatened and fearful and hospitalizes the victim (Catherall 1991; Rose 1991).

❖ The comorbid diagnoses need to be treated (Rose 1991; Silver et al. 1990). Not only do they cause the victim great suffering, but they are also defenses against reexperiencing the trauma. They need to be treated so that all aspects of the traumatic experience can be worked through.

Prognosis

Despite the severity and chronicity of damage resulting from victimization, the treatment of victims of violence can be successful and rewarding. Once the posttraumatic sequelae are identified and the process of working through begins, significant improvement in symptomatology, changes in characterologic defenses, and psychological integration and autonomy may occur. Correspondingly, if the post-traumatic etiology is missed, relentless therapeutic stalemates and negative therapeutic reactions are to be expected (Herman et al. 1989; Rose 1991). Victims are vulnerable to reactivation of the disorder in response to future important life events, as are any psychiatric patients. It is hoped that future studies will provide further information on the factors leading to successful interventions and outcome.

REFERENCES

American Psychiatric Association: Diagnostic and Statistical Manual of Mental Disorders, 3rd Edition, Revised. Washington, DC, American Psychiatric Association, 1987

Bard M, Sangrey D: The Crime Victims' Handbook. New York, Basic Books, 1979

Bard M, Arnone HC, Nemiroff D: Contextual influences on the post-traumatic stress adaptation of homicide survivor-victims, in Trauma and Its Wake, Vol 2: Traumatic Stress, Theory, Research, and Intervention. Edited by Figley CR. New York, Brunner/Mazel, 1986, pp 292–304

Bassuk E, Apsler R: Are there sex biases in rape counseling? Am J Psychiatry 140:305–308, 1983

Beck JC, van der Kolk B: Reports of childhood incest and current behavior of chronically hospitalized psychotic women. Am J Psychiatry 144:1474–1476, 1987

Blank AS Jr: Irrational reactions to post-traumatic stress disorder and Viet Nam veterans, in The Trauma of War: Stress and Recovery in Viet Nam Veterans. Edited by Sonnenberg SM, Blank AS Jr, Talbott JA. Washington, DC, American Psychiatric Press, 1985, pp 69–98

Blum HP: The concept of the reconstruction of trauma, in The Reconstruction of Trauma: Its Significance in Clinical Work. Edited by Rothstein A. Madison, CT, International Universities Press, 1986, pp 7–27

Borins EFM, Forsythe PJ: Past trauma and present functioning of patients attending a women's psychiatric clinic. Am J Psychiatry 142:460–463, 1985

Bowie SI, Silverman DC, Kalick SM, et al: Blitz rape and confidence rape: implications for clinical intervention. Am J Psychother 44:180–188, 1990

Braun BG: Psychotherapy of the survivor of incest with a dissociative disorder. Psychiatr Clin North Am 12:307–324, 1989

Braun BG: Dissociative disorders as sequelae to incest, in Incest-Related Syndromes of Adult Psychopathology. Edited by Kluft RP. Washington, DC, American Psychiatric Press, 1990, pp 227–245

Brett EA, Ostroff R: Imagery and posttraumatic stress disorder: an overview. Am J Psychiatry 142:417–424, 1985

Briere J, Zaidi LY: Sexual abuse histories and sequelae in female psychiatric emergency room patients. Am J Psychiatry 146:1602–1606, 1989

Brown GR, Anderson B: Psychiatric morbidity in adult inpatients with childhood histories of sexual and physical abuse. Am J Psychiatry 148:55–61, 1991

Burge SK: Post-traumatic stress disorder in victims of rape. Journal of Traumatic Stress 1:193–210, 1988

Burgess AW, Holmstrom LL: Rape trauma syndrome. Am J Psychiatry 131:981–986, 1974

Burgess AW, Holmstrom LL: Rape: Crisis and Recovery. Bowie, MD, Robert J Brady, 1979

Burgess AW, Hartman CR, McCormack A: Abused to abuser: antecedents of socially deviant behaviors. Am J Psychiatry 144:1431–1436, 1987

Burgess AW, Hazelwood RR, Rokous FE, et al: Serial rapists and their victims: reenactment and repetition. Ann N Y Acad Sci 528:277–295, 1988

Carmen EH, Rieker PP: A psychosocial model of the victim-to-patient process: implications for treatment. Psychiatr Clin North Am 12:431–443, 1989

Carmen EH, Rieker PP, Mills T: Victims of violence and psychiatric illness. Am J Psychiatry 141:378–383, 1984

Catherall DR: Aggression and projective identification in the treatment of victims. Psychotherapy 28:145–149, 1991

Chasnoff IJ, Burns WJ, Schnoll SH, et al: Maternal-neonatal incest. Am J Orthopsychiatry 56:577–580, 1986

Clary WF, Burstin KJ, Carpenter JS: Multiple personality and borderline personality disorder. Psychiatr Clin North Am 7:89–99, 1984

Coons PM, Bowman ES, Pellow TA, et al: Post-traumatic aspects of the treatment of victims of sexual abuse and incest. Psychiatr Clin North Am 12:325–335, 1989

Coons PM, Cole C, Pellow TA, et al: Symptoms of posttraumatic stress and dissociation in women victims of abuse, in Incest-Related Syndromes of Adult Psychopathology. Edited by Kluft RP. Washington, DC, American Psychiatric Press, 1990, pp 205–225

Cooper AM: Toward a limited definition of psychic trauma, in The Reconstruction of Trauma: Its Significance in Clinical Work. Edited by Rothstein A. Madison, CT, International Universities Press, 1986, pp 41–56

Courtois CA: Healing the Incest Wound: Adult Survivors in Therapy. New York, WW Norton, 1988

Daie N, Witztum E, Eleff M: Long-term effects of sibling incest. J Clin Psychiatry 50:428–431, 1989

Dickstein LJ: Spouse abuse and other domestic violence. Psychiatr Clin North Am 11:611–628, 1988

Ellenberger HF: The Discovery of the Unconscious: The History and Evolution of Dynamic Psychiatry. New York, Basic Books, 1970

Emslie GJ, Rosenfeld A: Incest reported by children and adolescents hospitalized for severe psychiatric problems. Am J Psychiatry 140:708–711, 1983

Eth S, Pynoos RS: Developmental perspective on psychic trauma in childhood, in Trauma and Its Wake: the Study and Treatment of Post-Traumatic Stress Disorder. Edited by Figley CR. New York, Brunner/Mazel, 1985, pp 36–52

Fine CG: The cognitive sequelae of incest, in Incest-Related Syndromes of Adult Psychopathology. Edited by Kluft RP. Washington, DC, American Psychiatric Press, 1990, pp 161–182

Finkelhor D: Child Sexual Abuse. New York, Free Press, 1984

Fish-Murray CC, Koby EV, van der Kolk BA: Evolving ideas: the effect of abuse on children's thought, in Psychological Trauma. Edited by van der Kolk BA. Washington, DC, American Psychiatric Press, 1987, pp 89–110

Frank E, Anderson BP: Psychiatric disorders in rape victims: past history and current symptomatology. Compr Psychiatry 28:77–82, 1987

Frank E, Anderson B, Stewart BD, et al: Immediate and delayed treatment of rape victims. Ann N Y Acad Sci 528:296–309, 1988

Freud S: Further remarks on the neuropsychoses of defense (1896a), in The Standard Edition of the Complete Psychological Works of Sigmund Freud, Vol 3. Translated and edited by Strachey J. London, Hogarth Press, 1962, pp 157–185

Freud S: The aetiology of hysteria (1896b), in The Standard Edition of the Complete Psychological Works of Sigmund Freud, Vol 3. Translated and edited by Strachey J. London, Hogarth Press, 1962, pp 191–221

Friedman MJ: Toward rational pharmacotherapy for posttraumatic stress disorder: an interim report. Am J Psychiatry 145:281–285, 1988

Friedman MJ: Biological approaches to the diagnosis and treatment of posttraumatic stress disorder. Journal of Traumatic Stress 4:67–92, 1991

Furst SS: Psychic trauma and its reconstruction with particular reference to postchildhood trauma, in The Reconstruction of Trauma: Its Significance in Clinical Work. Edited by Rothstein A. Madison, CT, International Universities Press, 1986, pp 29–39

Gelinas DJ: The persisting negative effects of incest. Psychiatry 46:312–332, 1983

Gelles RJ, Straus MA: Intimate Violence: The Causes and Consequences of Abuse in the American Family. New York, Touchstone, 1988

Giarretto H: Community-based treatment of the incest family. Psychiatr Clin North Am 12:351–361, 1989

Gillman RD: Physical trauma and actual seduction, in The Reconstruction of Trauma: Its Significance in Clinical Work. Edited by Rothstein A. Madison, CT, International Universities Press, 1986, pp 73–94

Gise LH, Paddison P: Rape, sexual abuse, and its victims. Psychiatr Clin North Am 11:629–648, 1988

Goodwin J: Credibility problems in multiple personality disorder patients and abused children, in Childhood Antecedents of Multiple Personality Disorder. Edited by Kluft RP. Washington, DC, American Psychiatric Press, 1985a, pp 1–19

Goodwin J: Post-traumatic symptoms in incest victims, in Post-Traumatic Stress Disorder in Children. Edited by Pynoos RS, Eth S. Washington, DC, American Psychiatric Press, 1985b, pp 155–168

Goodwin JM: Applying to adult incest victims what we have learned from victimized children, in Incest-Related Syndromes of Adult Psychopathology. Edited by Kluft RP. Washington, DC, American Psychiatric Press, 1990, pp 55–74

Goodwin JM, Talwar N: Group psychotherapy for victims of incest. Psychiatr Clin North Am 12:279–293, 1989

Green AH: Self-destructive behavior in battered children. Am J Psychiatry 135:579–582, 1978

Green AH: Child maltreatment and its victims: a comparison of physical and sexual abuse. Psychiatr Clin North Am 11:591–610, 1988a

Green AH: Overview of the literature on child sexual abuse, in Child Sexual Abuse: A Handbook for Health Care and Legal Professionals. Edited by Schetky DH, Green AH. New York, Brunner/Mazel, 1988b, pp 30–54

Green AH: Special issues in child sexual abuse, in Child Sexual Abuse: A Handbook for Health Care and Legal Professionals. Edited by Schetky DH, Green AH. New York, Brunner/Mazel, 1988c, pp 125–135

Greenberg MS, van der Kolk BA: Retrieval and integration of traumatic memories with the "painting cure," in Psychological Trauma. Edited by van der Kolk BA. Washington, DC, American Psychiatric Press, 1987, pp 191–215

Haley SA: Treatment implications of post-combat stress response syndromes for mental health professionals, in Stress Disorders Among Vietnam Veterans: Theory, Research and Treatment. Edited by Figley CR. New York, Brunner/Mazel, 1978, pp 254–267

Hamilton JA: Emotional consequences of victimization and discrimination in "special populations" of women. Psychiatr Clin North Am 12:35–51, 1989

Herman J: Father-Daughter Incest. Cambridge, MA, Harvard University Press, 1981

Herman JL: Histories of violence in an outpatient population: an exploratory study. Am J Orthopsychiatry 56:137–141, 1986

Herman JL: Father-daughter incest, in Post-Traumatic Therapy and Victims of Violence. Edited by Ochberg FM. New York, Brunner/Mazel, 1988, pp 175–195

Herman J, Schatzow E: Recovery and verification of memories of childhood trauma. Psychoanalytic Psychology 4:1–14, 1987

Herman JL, van der Kolk BA: Traumatic antecedents of borderline personality disorder, in Psychological Trauma. Edited by van der Kolk BA. Washington, DC, American Psychiatric Press, 1987, pp 111–126

Herman J, Russell D, Trocki K: Long-term effects of incestuous abuse in childhood. Am J Psychiatry 143:1293–1296, 1986

Herman JL, Perry JC, van der Kolk BA: Childhood trauma in borderline personality disorder. Am J Psychiatry 146:490–495, 1989

Hilberman E: Overview: the "wife-beater's wife" reconsidered. Am J Psychiatry 137:1336–1347, 1980

Horevitz RH, Braun BG: Are multiple personalities borderline? an analysis of 33 cases. Psychiatr Clin North Am 7:69–87, 1984

Horowitz M: Stress Response Syndromes. Northvale, NJ, Jason Aronson, 1976

Horowitz M: Stress Response Syndromes, 2nd Edition. Northvale, NJ, Jason Aronson, 1986

Jacobson A, Richardson B: Assault experiences of 100 psychiatric inpatients: evidence of the need for routine inquiry. Am J Psychiatry 144:908–913, 1987

Jenny C, Hooton TM, Bowers A, et al: Sexually transmitted diseases in victims of rape. N Engl J Med 322:713–716, 1990

Kardiner A, Spiegel H: War Stress and Neurotic Illness, 2nd Edition. New York, Hoeber, 1947

Kemp A, Rawlings EI, Green BL: Post-traumatic stress disorder (PTSD) in battered women: a shelter sample. Journal of Traumatic Stress 4:137–147, 1991

Kempe CH, Silverman FN, Steele BF, et al: The battered child syndrome. JAMA 181:17–24, 1962

Kilpatrick DG, Veronen LJ, Resick PA: The aftermath of rape: recent empirical findings. Am J Orthopsychiatry 49:658–669, 1979

Kilpatrick DG, Veronen LT, Best CL: Factors predicting psychological distress among rape victims, in Trauma and Its Wake: The Study and Treatment of Post-Traumatic Stress Disorder. New York, Brunner/Mazel, 1985, pp 113–141

Kilpatrick DG, Best CL, Saunders BE, et al: Rape in marriage and in dating relationships: how bad is it for mental health? Ann N Y Acad Sci 528:335–344, 1988

Kinzie JD, Boehnlein JK, Leung PK, et al: The prevalence of posttraumatic stress disorder and its clinical significance among Southeast Asian refugees. Am J Psychiatry 147:913–917, 1990

Kiser LJ, Ackerman BJ, Brown E, et al: Post-traumatic stress disorder in young children: a reaction to purported sexual abuse. J Am Acad Child Adolesc Psychiatry 27:645–649, 1988

Kluft RP: An update on multiple personality disorder. Hosp Community Psychiatry 38:363–373, 1987

Kluft RP: Treating the patient who has been sexually exploited by a previous therapist. Psychiatr Clin North Am 12:483–500, 1989

Kluft RP: On the apparent invisibility of incest: a personal reflection on things known and forgotten, in Incest-Related Syndromes of Adult Psychopathology. Edited by Kluft RP. Washington, DC, American Psychiatric Press, 1990a, pp 11–34

Kluft RP: Incest and subsequent revictimization: the case of therapist-patient sexual exploitation, with a description of the sitting duck syndrome, in Incest-Related Syndromes of Adult Psychopathology. Edited by Kluft RP. Washington, DC, American Psychiatric Press, 1990b, pp 263–287

Kolb LC: A neuropsychological hypothesis explaining posttraumatic stress disorders. Am J Psychiatry 144:989–995, 1987

Kroll J, Habenicht J, Mackenzie T, et al: Depression and posttraumatic stress disorder in Southeast Asian refugees. Am J Psychiatry 146:1592–1597, 1989

Krugman S: Trauma in the family: perspectives on the intergenerational transmission of violence, in Psychological Trauma. Edited by van der Kolk BA. Washington, DC, American Psychiatric Press, 1987, pp 127–151

Krystal H: Self representation and the capacity for self-care. The Annual of Psychoanalysis 6:209–264, 1978a

Krystal H: Trauma and affects. Psychoanal Study Child 33:81–116, 1978b

Krystal H: Psychoanalytic views on human emotional damages, in Post-Traumatic Stress Disorder: Psychological and Biological Sequelae. Edited by van der Kolk BA. Washington, DC, American Psychiatric Press, 1984, pp 1–28

Levine HB: Introduction, in Adult Analysis and Childhood Sexual Abuse. Edited by Levine HB. Hillsdale, NJ, Analytic Press, 1990, pp 3–19

Lindy JD: An outline for the psychoanalytic psychotherapy of post-traumatic stress disorder, in Trauma and Its Wake, Vol 2: Traumatic Stress Theory, Research, and Intervention. Edited by Figley CR. New York, Brunner/Mazel, 1986, pp 195–212

Loewenstein RJ: Somatoform disorders in victims of incest and child abuse, in Incest-Related Syndromes of Adult Psychopathology. Edited by Kluft RP. Washington, DC, American Psychiatric Press, 1990, pp 75–111

Lyons JA, Keane TM: Implosive therapy for the treatment of combat-related PTSD. Journal of Traumatic Stress 1:137–152, 1989

MacVicar K: Psychotherapeutic issues in the treatment of sexually abused girls. Journal of the American Academy of Child Psychiatry 18:342–353, 1979

Madonna PG, van Scoyk S, Jones DPH: Family interactions within incest and nonincest families. Am J Psychiatry 148:46–49, 1991

McLeer SV, Deblinger E, Atkins MS, et al: Post-traumatic stress disorder in sexually abused children. J Am Acad Child Adolesc Psychiatry 27:650–654, 1988

McNeely RL, Robinson-Simpson G: The truth about domestic violence: a falsely framed issue. Soc Work 32:485–490, 1987

Meiselman K: Incest: A Psychological Study of Causes and Effects With Treatment Recommendations. San Francisco, CA, Jossey-Bass, 1978

Mid-Peninsula Rape Crisis Center: Working With Women of Color. Palo Alto, CA, Mid-Peninsula Rape Crisis Center (undated)

Mollica RF, Son L: Cultural dimensions in the evaluation and treatment of sexual trauma: an overview. Psychiatr Clin North Am 12:363–379, 1989

Mollica RF, Wyshak G, Lavelle J, et al: Assessing symptom change in Southeast Asian refugee survivors of mass violence and torture. Am J Psychiatry 147:83–88, 1990

Morrison J: Childhood sexual histories of women with somatization disorder. Am J Psychiatry 146:239–241, 1989

Moss M, Frank E, Anderson B: The effects of marital status and partner support on rape trauma. Am J Orthopsychiatry 60:379–391, 1990

Nader K, Pynoos R, Fairbanks L, et al: Children's PTSD reactions one year after a sniper attack at their school. Am J Psychiatry 147:1526–1530, 1990

Ornitz EM, Pynoos RS: Startle modulation in children with posttraumatic stress disorder. Am J Psychiatry 146:866–870, 1989

Parson ER: Ethnicity and traumatic stress: the intersecting point in psychotherapy, in Trauma and Its Wake: the Study and Treatment of Post-Traumatic Stress Disorder. Edited by Figley CR. New York, Brunner/Mazel, 1985, pp 314–337

Phelan P: Incest: socialization within a treatment program. Am J Orthopsychiatry 57:84–92, 1987

Pitman RK, Altman B, Greenwald E, et al: Psychiatric complications during flooding therapy for posttraumatic stress disorder. J Clin Psychiatry 52:17–20, 1991

Pollock VE, Briere J, Schneider L, et al: Childhood antecedents of antisocial behavior: parental alcoholism and physical abusiveness. Am J Psychiatry 147:1290–1293, 1990

Putnam FW: Disturbances of "self" in victims of childhood sexual abuse, in Incest-Related Syndromes of Adult Psychopathology. Edited by Kluft RP. Washington, DC, American Psychiatric Press, 1990, pp 113–131

Putnam FW, Guroff JJ, Silberman EK, et al: The clinical phenomenology of multiple personality disorder: review of 100 recent cases. J Clin Psychiatry 47:285–293, 1986

Pynoos RS, Eth S: Children traumatized by witnessing acts of personal violence: homicide, rape, or suicide behavior, in Post-Traumatic Stress Disorder in Children. Edited by Eth S, Pynoos RS. Washington, DC, American Psychiatric Press, 1985, pp 17–43

Pynoos RS, Eth S: Witness to violence: the child interview. J Am Acad Child Adolesc Psychiatry 25:306–319, 1986

Pynoos RS, Nader K: Children who witness the sexual assaults of their mothers. J Am Acad Child Adolesc Psychiatry 27:567–572, 1988

Renshaw DC: Treatment of sexual exploitation: rape and incest. Psychiatr Clin North Am 12:257–277, 1989

Rieker PP, Carmen EH: The victim-to-patient process: the disconfirmation and transformation of abuse. Am J Orthopsychiatry 56:360–370, 1986

Risin LE, Koss MP: Sexual abuse of boys: prevalence and descriptive characteristics of childhood victimization. Journal of Interpersonal Violence 2:309–319, 1987

Rose DS: Reporting a patient for child abuse: countertransference in ongoing psychotherapy. Paper presented at Child Psychiatry Grand Rounds, Stanford University School of Medicine, Stanford, CA, April 1986a

Rose DS: "Worse than death": psychodynamics of rape victims and the need for psychotherapy. Am J Psychiatry 143:817–824, 1986b

Rose DS: A model for psychodynamic psychotherapy with the rape victim. Psychotherapy 28:85–95, 1991

Rosenfeld AA: Incidence of a history of incest among 18 female psychiatric patients. Am J Psychiatry 136:791–795, 1979

Ross CA, Miller SD, Reagor P, et al: Structured interview data on 102 cases of multiple personality disorder from four centers. Am J Psychiatry 147:596–601, 1990

Rozynko V, Dondershine HE: Trauma focus group therapy for Vietnam veterans with PTSD. Psychotherapy 28:157–161, 1991

Russell D: The Secret Trauma: Incest in the Lives of Girls and Women. New York, Basic Books, 1986

Sauzier M: Disclosure of child sexual abuse: for better or for worse. Psychiatr Clin North Am 12:455–469, 1989

Schatzow E, Herman JL: Breaking secrecy: adult survivors disclose to their families. Psychiatr Clin North Am 12:337–349, 1989

Schei B, Bakketeig LS: Gynaecological impact of sexual and physical abuse by spouse: a study of a random sample of Norwegian women. Br J Obstet Gynaecol 96:1379–1383, 1989

Schetky DH: Child sexual abuse in mythology, religion, and history, in Child Sexual Abuse: A Handbook for Health Care and Legal Professionals. Edited by Schetky DH, Green AH. New York, Brunner/Mazel, 1988, pp 13–29

Schetky DH: A review of the literature on the long-term effects of childhood sexual abuse, in Incest-Related Syndromes of Adult Psychopathology. Edited by Kluft RP. Washington, DC, American Psychiatric Press, 1990, pp 35–54

Schetky DH, Benedek EP: The sexual abuse victim in the courts. Psychiatr Clin North Am 12:471–481, 1989

Schultz R: Secrets of adolescence: incest and developmental fixations, in Incest-Related Syndromes of Adult Psychopathology. Edited by Kluft RP. Washington, DC, American Psychiatric Press, 1990, pp 133–159

Shengold L: Soul Murder. New Haven, CT, Yale University Press, 1989

Silver JM, Sandberg DP, Hales RE: New approaches in the pharmacotherapy of posttraumatic stress disorder. J Clin Psychiatry 51:33–38, 1990

Sonnenberg SM: Victims of violence and post-traumatic stress disorder. Psychiatr Clin North Am 11:581–590, 1988

Spiegel D: Multiple personality as a post-traumatic stress disorder. Psychiatr Clin North Am 7:101–110, 1984

Spiegel D: Dissociating damage. Am J Clin Hypn 29:123–131, 1986

Spiegel D: Hypnosis in the treatment of victims of sexual abuse. Psychiatr Clin North Am 12:295–305, 1989

Spiegel D: Trauma, dissociation, and hypnosis, in Incest-Related Syndromes of Adult Psychopathology. Edited by Kluft RP. Washington, DC, American Psychiatric Press, 1990, pp 247–261

Spiegel D, Hunt T, Dondershine HE: Dissociation and hypnotizability in posttraumatic stress disorder. Am J Psychiatry 145:301–305, 1988

Steele BF: Child abuse, in The Reconstruction of Trauma: Its Significance in Clinical Work. Edited by Rothstein A. Madison, CT, International Universities Press, 1986, pp 59–72

Stewart BD, Hughes C, Frank E, et al: The aftermath of rape: profiles of immediate and delayed treatment seekers. J Nerv Ment Dis 175:90–94, 1987

Stone MH: Individual psychotherapy with victims of incest. Psychiatr Clin North Am 12:237–255, 1989

Stone MH: Incest in the borderline patient, in Incest-Related Syndromes of Adult Psychopathology. Edited by Kluft RP. Washington, DC, American Psychiatric Press, 1990, pp 183–204

Terr LC: Children of Chowchilla: a study of psychic trauma. Psychoanal Study Child 34:547–623, 1979

Terr LC: Psychic trauma in children: observations following the Chowchilla school-bus kidnapping. Am J Psychiatry 138:14–19, 1981

Terr LC: Time sense following psychic trauma: a clinical study of ten adults and twenty children. Am J Orthopsychiatry 53:244–261, 1983a

Terr LC: Chowchilla revisited: the effects of psychic trauma four years after a school-bus kidnapping. Am J Psychiatry 140:1543–1550, 1983b

Terr LC: Childhood trauma and the creative product. Psychoanal Study Child 42:545–572, 1987

Terr LC: Terror writing by the formerly terrified. Psychoanal Study Child 44:369–390, 1989

Terr LC: Childhood traumas: an outline and overview. Am J Psychiatry 148:10–20, 1991

Titchener JL: Post-traumatic decline: a consequence of unresolved destructive drives, in Trauma and Its Wake, Vol 2: Traumatic Stress Theory, Research, and Intervention. Edited by Figley CR. New York, Brunner/Mazel, 1986, pp 5–19

van der Kolk BA: The psychological consequences of overwhelming life experiences, in Psychological Trauma. Edited by van der Kolk BA. Washington, DC, American Psychiatric Press, 1987a, pp 1–30

van der Kolk BA: The separation cry and the trauma response: developmental issues in the psychobiology of attachment and separation, in Psychological Trauma. Edited by van der Kolk BA. Washington, DC, American Psychiatric Press, 1987b, pp 31–62

van der Kolk BA: The role of the group in the origin and resolution of the trauma response, in Psychological Trauma. Edited by van der Kolk BA. Washington, DC, American Psychiatric Press, 1987c, pp 153–171

van der Kolk BA: The compulsion to repeat the trauma: re-enactment, revictimization, and masochism. Psychiatr Clin North Am 12:389–411, 1989

van der Kolk BA, Greenberg MS: The psychobiology of the trauma response: hyperarousal, constriction, and addiction to traumatic reexposure, in Psychological Trauma. Edited by van der Kolk BA. Washington, DC, American Psychiatric Press, 1987, pp 63–87

van der Kolk BA, Kadish W: Amnesia, dissociation, and the return of the repressed, in Psychological Trauma. Edited by van der Kolk BA. Washington, DC, American Psychiatric Press, 1987, pp 173–190

van der Kolk BA, van der Hart O: Pierre Janet and the breakdown of adaptation in psychological trauma. Am J Psychiatry 146:1530–1540, 1989

Walker E, Katon W, Harrop-Griffiths J, et al: Relationship of chronic pelvic pain to psychiatric diagnoses and childhood sexual abuse. Am J Psychiatry 145:75–80, 1988

Walker LE: The Battered Woman. New York, Perennial Library, 1979

Walker LE: The impact of forensic issues on women's rights. Ann N Y Acad Sci 528:361–372, 1988

Walker LE: Post-traumatic stress disorder in women: diagnosis and treatment of battered woman syndrome. Psychotherapy 28:21–29, 1991

Winfield I, George LK, Swartz M, et al: Sexual assault and psychiatric disorders among a community sample of women. Am J Psychiatry 147:335–341, 1990

Winnicott DW: The theory of the parent-infant relationship, in The Maturational Processes and the Facilitating Environment. New York, International Universities Press, 1960, pp 37–55

Yates A: Children eroticized by incest. Am J Psychiatry 139:482–485, 1982

Young MA: The crime victims' movement, in Post-Traumatic Therapy and Victims of Violence. Edited by Ochberg FM. New York, Brunner/Mazel, 1988a, pp 319–329

Young MA: Support services for victims, in Post-Traumatic Therapy and Victims of Violence. Edited by Ochberg FM. New York, Brunner/Mazel, 1988b, pp 330–351

Chapter 24

EMERGING ISSUES IN MEDICAL ETHICS

Carol C. Nadelson, M.D.

❖ ❖ ❖ ❖ ❖ ❖ ❖ ❖ ❖ ❖ ❖ ❖ ❖ ❖

Ethical principles are influenced by personal values and beliefs, and by societal context. They are not immutable. In medicine, as new technologies have developed and changes in health care delivery have resulted, historically held views about the responsibilities, obligations, and relationships between health care providers and patients have been challenged.

The increasing complexity and cost of new technology, coupled with limited resources to provide care for all those who need and want it, create new ethical dilemmas. These are related to the need for decision making that is based on competing priorities, without establishing policies regarding who should make decisions and what the guiding principles should be. Current codes of medical ethics appear to be inadequate to address today's emerging questions, because values and ethical systems vary widely and often conflict. Choices that enable one to preserve personal moral accountability in a pluralistic society are difficult to make.

Furthermore, the process of medical decision making, as well as the delivery of medical care, is increasingly directed by those whose ethical frameworks do not originate from health care training or practice. This affects the decisions themselves as well as their implementation. For example, a businessman running a private hospital does not expect to deliver care in the same way as a charitable institution. He is

A previous version of this chapter was published as Nadelson CC: "Emerging Issues in Medical Ethics." *British Medical Journal* 158 (supplement 10):9–16, 1991. Used with permission.

485

bound by the interests of his investors and not primarily by a concept of public good. Likewise, the computerization of medical records and requirements for disclosure of data on diagnosis and treatment in order to provide reimbursement make the transfer of confidential information routine. The concept of consent is altered by the financial pressure on individual patients to permit disclosure.

Medical ethics encompass an enormous range of issues. This chapter focuses on aspects of current and emerging concerns, particularly some that relate specifically to women. Recognizing that overt as well as subtle cultural differences exist, major references herein are to the United States.

CHANGING CODES OF MEDICAL ETHICS

Codes of medical ethics have existed since ancient times and have varied with culture and era. The Hippocratic oath was unique in emphasizing the cure of the patient as the single overriding responsibility of the physician. Subsequently, medical ethics has also been concerned with the dignity, honor, and reputation of the profession. Currently, most Western countries emphasize as guiding principles the autonomy or self-determination of patients, a concept of beneficence that implies doing "good" rather than merely doing no harm, a concept of justice related to access to resources, and the physician's responsibility to his or her individual patients.

Different priorities are placed on these principles in different societies. Patient autonomy may be limited by decreasing the availability of procedures. Denial of access may be based on socioeconomics, age, or prognosis; family and societal needs may outweigh the desires of the individual in certain situations, such as forbidding the performance of induced abortion despite the wishes of a woman (Newman and Brody 1988). Engelhardt (1986) emphasized the tension that exists in ethics, deriving from the difference between respecting the freedom of individuals and securing their best interests.

This tension points to one of the fundamental problems of medical ethics: the definition and scope of paternalism. Generally, in the ethical literature, paternalism refers to practices that restrict the liberty of individuals without their consent, with the justification for such actions given as either the prevention of some harm they will do to themselves or the production of some benefit for them that they would not otherwise secure (Beauchamp 1978). Thus, the debate centers upon whether paternalistic justifications can be morally acceptable and where the limits and boundaries might be.

Other principles of medical ethics that are further elucidated in Western countries include considerations of confidentiality and boundaries of therapeutic relationships. These areas encompass issues such as valid consent and refusal on the part of the patient; the responsibilities of the physician, including failure to appropriately inform a patient and deception in practice and research; and sexual interaction between physicians and patients.

Decisions about access to and rationing of care are often dealt with by omission rather than by clearly stated policies. For example, patients may not have access to certain types of care because the resources are not available in their community or because they cannot pay for them. In other situations, ambiguities surrounding conflicting ethical principles make it difficult to be definitive about policy. For example, considerations of patient confidentiality preclude disclosure of the diagnosis of acquired immunodeficiency syndrome (AIDS), yet not to disclose this diagnosis may endanger the health of family members and others in the community. The policy to keep confidential the results of patients' tests for human immunodeficiency virus (HIV) has recently been vigorously debated in the United States, because reports of health care workers transmitting the virus to patients have resulted in public pressure to test health care workers and disclose their test results (Altman 1990).

Pellegrino and Thomasma (1988) imply that shifting ethical paradigms and conflicting moral principles may be related to some of today's health care dilemmas. They discuss the effects of conflicting ethical principles of health care on business, contractual, preventive, covenantal, and beneficent models. From the business perspective, they suggest that medicine has been considered to be a commodity and that the ethical obligation of physician to patient has become that of businessperson to consumer. The contractual mode is an extension of this model, whereby a contract formalizes the relationship, protecting the patient from excessive paternalism or economic self-interest from the physician. The preventive, or public health, model obligates the health care provider to protect many "healths" and does not place as high a priority on the individual physician-patient relationship.

A different perspective is derived from the traditionally held covenantal model. It is grounded in the trust and obligation between the physician and the patient. Pellegrino and Thomasma (1988), in reemphasizing the importance of the principle of beneficence, suggest that the physician and patient are joined because of the needs of the patient. Both partners recognize the patient's dependence upon the physician and the physician's responsibility to make good and moral judgments on behalf of the patient. This model acknowledges that the ill patient may not be capable of totally free and informed consent or autonomy, by virtue of anxiety, fear, or lack of knowledge. It is around this issue that psychiatrists have become most involved. They are often asked to assess patient competence to consent, especially when there is a question of impairment of judgment or decision-making capacity. Thus, psychiatrists may be said to act in a paternalistic fashion when asked to render opinions that potentially limit patient autonomy.

The nature of the covenantal relationship and the principle of beneficence call into question many current medical practices that involve the physician in activities that may not do "good" for the patient. These practices include the role of the physician in the rationing of health care, as a gatekeeper or guardian of society's resources (Nadelson 1986; Pellegrino and Thomasma 1988). Although the rationing of health care is attractive from an economic point of view, serious ethical questions are raised if the physician cannot be trusted by the patient to act in the patient's interests. If the physician becomes a double or triple agent, acting for a government, an insurance company, and an employer and presumably for the patient as well, the covenantal relationship is compromised.

CONFLICT BETWEEN ROLES: PHYSICIAN, INDIVIDUAL PATIENT, AND SOCIETY

The physician in today's society finds it increasingly difficult to differentiate his or her role and responsibilities as the agent of the patient from those as an agent of society. The conflict between these roles occurs in many aspects of practice. It is particularly evident in laws requiring that confidentiality be breached by reporting child abuse, threats of harm to another individual, or certain illnesses, such as sexually transmitted diseases, to appropriate authorities. Protecting the confidentiality of physician-patient relationships runs counter to social concern about the public good in these situations, and confidentiality may not be upheld as an overriding ethical principle (Freudenheim 1991).

The compromising of confidentiality has many potential repercussions, including the possibility that patients will no longer trust their physicians with certain types of information or seek appropriate or necessary care. These issues have been raised most often around the requirement to report HIV-positive individuals in order to trace contacts and advise them about risks, or in reporting patients who have made threats of violence or who have committed child abuse or other crimes of violence.

Another aspect of these conflicting roles that involves important ethical considerations includes pressure on physicians to make decisions based on nonclinical indications. For example, a physician may be pressured for economic reasons, such as increasing the reimbursement to a hospital, to recommend a certain treatment or to admit or discharge a patient when, in the physician's clinical judgment, this is not the best approach. Physicians may also be asked to take responsibility for treatments they have not personally recommended or administered because other personnel who may not be legally qualified have been the direct caretaker of the patient. This request places the physician in an ethical (and legal) dilemma and potentially harms the patient, often without the patient's knowledge or consent (Nadelson 1986). In the United States, these practices affect women patients more than men, because women use health care facilities more often and are more likely to be poor and to be treated by a number of different kinds of health care providers (National Institutes of Health 1990).

PATERNALISM AND INFORMED CONSENT

Historically, the organization of health care delivery was hierarchically based, with the physician dominating the system. The expectation that the physician, who in the past was usually male, was informed, authoritative, and protective conformed with traditional social roles of women and men (Notman and Nadelson 1978). Although the numbers of women physicians have increased, their relative absence from policy-making positions essentially preserves this traditional paternalistic perspective.

In many instances, decisions about an individual patient's care, or policy about resource use and priorities, have been based on this perspective, so that the best interests of the patient may be determined by others, often with little input from the patient himself or herself (Nadelson and Notman 1978, 1990). In the United States, this is best exemplified in policies related to reproduction, including the availability of sterilization or induced abortion, and allocation of resources for new technologies such as in vitro fertilization. A recent decision in the United States to prohibit the use of mifepristone (RU-486), an abortifacient that appears to have other possible medical uses, is a specific example. Among the potential uses of this drug are treatment of some types of breast cancer, brain tumors, Cushing's syndrome, and endometriosis (Wickenden 1990). The decision was based on the values and beliefs of those with decision-making authority, not of those who would be most affected. The potential benefit of the other uses of this drug was not seriously weighed in making the decision. Another example is the recent judicial ruling that ordered a woman who was convicted of child abuse to have a birth control device implanted as a condition of her probation (Lewin 1991). These decisions have raised serious ethical and legal debate, which has not yet been resolved.

Recent discussion about medical and surgical care, including organ transplants and coronary artery bypass surgery, suggests that bias exists regarding criteria for the choice of suitable patients. Women and members of minority groups are less frequently offered these options in the United States (Abraham 1991; National Institutes of Health 1990). The sizable nonclinical variations that have been noted in rates of cesarean delivery also suggest that bias and lack of objective criteria may be larger problems in health care delivery than was previously thought. Recent data suggest that these nonclinical variations largely had to do with hospital ownership, teaching versus nonteaching hospitals, payment source, and volume of procedures performed. The documentation of gender bias in medical care and in research has led to the creation of an Office of Research on Women's Health by the U.S. government and to proposed legislation to address the "inadequacies in the treatment of women's health in three critical areas: research on women's health, access to services, and prevention activities . . . " (Markey 1990; National Institutes of Health 1990; Palca 1990).

The negative aspects of paternalism are also seen in research policy, exemplified by banning the use of fetal tissue for research. This was done because it was felt that more women would seek induced abortions if they felt there was a justification or that "good" use could be made of the products of conception. Not only is this supposition unsupported by data, but it reflects a patronizing and paternalistic view of women. The decision was made by government officials and was based more on political pressure than on ethical principles ("Doctors Plan to Review Fetal Tissue Research" 1991; Hilts 1991).

Failure to include those affected by decisions in the decision-making process is an aspect of paternalism. While there has been an increase in paternalism in the United States health care system (exemplified by the encroachment by government and insurance companies on policies involving medical care), there has been a decrease in paternalism in the individual physician-patient relationship. Expectations of patients that they be informed and participate in decisions regarding their own health care have affected this relationship, and the locus of decision making has shifted toward the patient and family, at least when it is not in the hands of the government or insurance companies. A recent article (Scheier 1991) stated that, in the past, physicians "were empowered to make health care decisions for the benefit of the patient because they understood that patient's condition better than any layperson. Now . . . the physician's role primarily is to explain the various options of treatment—the pros and cons. The physician is the adviser, not the decision-maker."

Paternalism, then, has shifted away from the physician into the hands of bureaucracies. This shift confuses the picture for patients who do not know to whom to turn or whom to blame, and intensifies discontent with the lack of responsiveness of the system. This situation is particularly important because of what we know about an individual's illness and his or her expectations of those who are caretakers and healers.

Illness engenders responses that may be at variance with an individual's usual behavior, especially since those who are ill become more dependent on others. The patient who perceives himself or herself as needing to be cared for by a strong, parental figure can become too compliant. At times of crisis and in gratitude for being helped, the patient may also surrender aspects of his or her autonomy (Notman and Nadelson 1978). Ethical questions can be raised when the patient is encouraged or required to be passive, and thus the patient may not make an informed decision (Kahana and Bibring 1964). These patient responses may further encourage the physician or the bureaucracy to maintain greater authority than may be in the best interest of the patient. This exercise of authority can prevent communication and the development of mutual respect between physician and patient, and can lead to disappointment, antagonism, and mistrust of the system and those providing care in it (Notman and Nadelson 1978).

One way of dealing with these reactions in patients has been to compel the physician or the health-providing agency to detail, in advance, the dangers and risks of a particular procedure or medication. Despite these efforts, however, barriers to communication arise from the nature of the relationship itself. An official recommendation, whether explicit or implicit, can overshadow a cautionary statement. The language may not be understood and the implications not heard, or they may be so frightening to the patient that in order to agree, he or she must ignore potential problems or complications. Thus, the authority of a physician or institution may prevent a patient from objectively assessing dangers, benefits, or alternatives, even if they are clearly stated. On the other hand, a patient may also compromise his or her care by developing a negative response to a paternalistic posture, being mistrustful and unwilling to accept advice or recommendations, or overreacting to a statement about risks and side effects (Notman and Nadelson 1978). These responses raise questions about how informed consent is understood and obtained from patients.

Since informed consent implies understanding and assent, a patient's inability to comprehend the language used by the physician, the insurer, or other health-providing agencies, whether due to educational level, mental illness, or other factors, can be seen as violating the principles of obtaining informed consent (Applebaum and Grisso 1988). Thus, those in authority influence the patient's perception of his or her options and alternatives and affect compliance and decision making (Nadelson and Notman 1978).

As in treatment, the agreement to participate in research may be influenced by a subject's perception of the experimenter as possessing superior knowledge and authority. Agreement may be given by a person who appears to be willing but who may not be able to make an objective decision (Nadelson and Notman 1978). Obviously, it is not possible to change the nature of the relationship entirely or perhaps even substantially, but every effort should be made to prevent distortion and promote mutual participation.

In the research area, an often-quoted example of ethically unacceptable research was a study on contraception in Mexican American women (Katz 1972). One group of women was given contraceptive pills and another was given placebos and a vaginal cream, known to be a less effective contraceptive. All of the women believed they were protected from pregnancy. The misuse of the trust of the subjects was deceitful; the subjects never gave informed consent, and the women were unknowingly exposed to the risk of unintended pregnancy. Just as it exists between a physician and a patient, the importance of a partnership built on mutual trust exists between a researcher and a subject (Nadelson and Notman 1978). The subject must understand the information given and make an informed choice to volunteer.

AUTONOMY AND REPRODUCTION

The special characteristics of women's reproductive roles lead to specific ethical considerations. Since decisions about childbearing, contraception, induced abortion, sterilization, and surgery involving reproductive organs have profound social consequences, the autonomy of a woman in deciding these questions is often challenged. From a historical perspective, debate about contraception and induced abortion has escalated when there are desires for population expansion (Nadelson and Notman 1978).

In most cultures, women have generally not been in a position to achieve their own goals if they are distinct from those of their family and society. Decisions about medical care or surgical procedures that have an impact on sexuality and childbearing are often made by others, including governments and families. For example, the question of whether sterilization or induced abortion is funded can determine whether a woman can make that choice. Decisions may reflect the personal, cultural, or religious values of the physician, the family, or society. A father may insist that his pregnant teenage daughter cannot have an abortion because he does not believe in it, or a gynecologist may assume that a woman past 40 would want a hysterectomy or sterilization because she would not want to expose herself to the risk of having a defective child. In these cases, the actions taken or assumptions made can compromise the woman's autonomy.

Recent cases involving consent for cesarean section extend the ethical dilemmas. Can a court grant permission to a hospital to perform an unwanted cesarean section on a woman who is competent to make a decision regarding her medical care? If so, the state is overriding her decision and inviting government-mandated participation by physicians in administering treatment. This not only deprives the woman of her liberty, but also changes the nature of physician participation and the basis of the covenant between physician and patient.

A recent, troubling ethical dilemma has involved genetic testing in pregnancy. When used to diagnose genetic disorders, it may lead to a decision to have an abortion. Many believe that abortion should not be performed for any reason, but even those who do not share this view are troubled by the potential use of abortion for social reasons, including family finances, unmarried status, or even sex selection. From an ethical perspective, any restriction can be said to limit a woman's autonomy and to place the interests of the mother in opposition to those of the fetus. When can they be considered equal persons? This question of determining when "personhood" can be said to exist is an important consideration in this ethical debate.

Since genetic testing by amniocentesis or chorionic villus sampling can also reveal the sex of the child, an induced abortion could take place if the baby were not of the desired sex. In those families and cultures where boys are more valued than girls, this could result in major changes in population demographics. The argument has also been made that, once these new technologies are available, control of their use is not possible. Thus, unethical or coercive practices could result, including forced abortion.

As society and medicine change, the physician must become accustomed to a range of new realities. These include the extensive use of reproductive technologies, the possibility of sexually transmitted diseases in a wide diversity of patients, and requests for artificial insemination for unmarried women and homosexual couples (Notman and Nadelson 1978; Stotland 1990). As I have suggested, the emergence of AIDS in mass segments of our society has also raised ethical considerations regarding testing, the right to privacy, and protection of others.

The use of in vitro fertilization, artificial insemination by donor, and surrogate motherhood has also stimulated ethical debate and legal action. The new technologies "raise the specter of reproduction totally controlled by females whose uteri, despite methods of laboratory fertilization, remain essential for growing fertilized ova to human status. Patriarchal dominance and male lineage are suddenly at risk. Affiliative rights and knowledge of parenthood, particularly of fatherhood as an aspect of identity, become unsure. Even the social mother can no longer state with certainty that this is her biological offspring" (Brody 1988, p. 202).

These technologies and their use raise questions about the role of biological versus social parents, the rights of children born from these procedures, and the nature of informed consent by all parties. A woman making a surrogate contract, for example, may have been coerced, or she may not be able to make an informed decision because she cannot predict her feelings after gestation. The advent of surrogacy has also brought into focus questions about whether women can be used as incubators and whether fetuses have become commodities, raising the specter of forced pregnancy presented by novelist Margaret Atwood (1986) in *The Handmaid's Tale*. Certainly, contractual surrogacy places pressure on poor women to "rent" their bodies.

An aspect of the use of emerging technology that is especially salient for psychiatrists is the expectation that they can predict the outcomes and psychological risks of surrogacy, despite the absence of data on psychological impact. Not only is information lacking on how those involved in surrogacy will fare, but there are no data on the outcome for children born into these families. There are also no guidelines or criteria for selection of surrogate mothers and families. Currently, arrangements are made by entrepreneurs with minimal ethical or legal constraints.

Debate about this subject has been polarized, and no clear principle or policies have been formulated. One recently articulated perspective that has attracted attention is that relationships, not genes, should determine parental rights and responsibilities (Rothman 1989). Rothman (1989) believes that gestational mothers, with 9 months of relationship before the birth of their babies, should have more rights than should fathers or adoptive parents. The priority she proposes would change as fathers or adoptive parents develop nurturing relationships with these babies.

Additional ethical questions involving the rights and status of children born through these new techniques remain unsettled. The right to know one's genetic, family, and medical background has been controversial in cases of adoption; certainly it is in cases of surrogacy or artificial insemination. There is a potential conflict between the interests of the "parents" in privacy and the right of the child to know.

Techniques that allow freezing of embryos, with the potential for their later use, raise additional ethical dilemmas when couples divorce or die, or when they seek to terminate the "life" of the embryo. A new kind of paternalism also arises when procedures and technologies are reserved for specific types of individuals or situations, for example, in vitro fertilization only when there is an organic impediment to conception or when the women are married heterosexuals (van Hall 1988).

Substance abuse during pregnancy has been another subject of recent ethical and legal controversy. In the past, the fetus was viewed as a potential threat to the mother's life and health, since pregnancy and childbirth were associated with substantial morbidity and mortality. In recent years, this view has shifted, so that mothers are now seen as potential threats to their offspring and as not necessarily acting in the offspring's best interests. This change in perspective has led to legal action and even prison sentences for pregnant women who are alcoholic or addicted to drugs. This pits the autonomy of the mother against the interests of the fetus. In addition, it has changed the nature of the obstetrician-patient relationship. In this situation, when the obstetrician is treating both the mother and fetus as "the patient," the mother's autonomy can be compromised. The fetus is accorded both rights and "personhood," as is the mother. They obviously cannot be entirely equal, bringing into question, as suggested above, when and whether the "personhood" of the fetus can be differentiated from that of the mother (Blank 1986; Bowes and Selgestad 1981; Cole 1990; Harrison 1990; Johnsen 1987; Landwirth 1987; Lenow 1983; McNulty 1987–1988; Murray 1987; Rhoden 1987).

Another controversy involving pregnant women concerns consent for in utero treatment of their fetuses and whether failure to consent constitutes fetal abuse. Here a distinction between the moral and legal responsibilities of the mother has been made. It is generally held that a pregnant woman cannot be coerced to accept treatment to benefit her fetus. The physician's ethical duty according to the American Medical Association (1990a) is to be noncoercive and to accept the informed decision of the patient.

SEXUAL INTERACTIONS BETWEEN PHYSICIANS AND PATIENTS

An issue of increasing concern in the United States today is sexual interactions between physicians and patients (American Medical Association 1990b). Because of the intimate nature of the physician-patient relationship, a wide range of emotions, including sexual feelings, may be evoked, and there is a potential for overt sexualism of the interaction (Gabbard 1989). The incidence of sexual contact between physicians and patients is difficult to document, but those studies that have been done, coupled with recurring ethics complaints and lawsuits, suggest that it is not an infrequent occurrence (Derosis et al. 1987; Gartrell et al. 1986; Holroyd and Brodsky 1977; Kardener 1974; McCartney 1966; Perry 1976; Rapp 1987; Romeo 1978; Shepard 1971).

Between 5% and 10% of psychiatrists and psychologists have reported sexual contact with patients. Although there have been recent reports suggesting that the incidence of sexual contact is decreasing, it is not clear whether this reflects an actual decrease or a change in reporting patterns. No specific data are available on sexual interactions between patients and nonpsychiatric physicians, but one study has suggested that the figures may be comparable (Kardener et al. 1976). For psychiatrists in the United States, it has been estimated that about 88% of reported incidents of sexual misconduct involve male psychiatrists and female patients; 7.6% involve male psychiatrists and male patients; and 3.5% involve female psychiatrists and female patients (Gartrell et al. 1989; Simon 1989).

Desires for secrecy and the patient's dependency on the physician to protect his or her confidentiality complicate the ability to learn of this problem or to intervene (Dahlberg 1970; Marmor 1976). Many women fear being publicly exposed, especially if they have participated in a long-term sexual liaison, or they may feel betrayed or demeaned and do not want public acknowledgment of their activities (Nadelson 1989).

There are few reports of sexual involvement of female physicians with male patients. Physicians may become sexually involved with their patients for a variety of reasons. Women may appear to be seductive to a male physician who, due to depression, loneliness, disappointment, or stress, may be particularly vulnerable to being needed or sexually desired. These problems may lead him to respond sexually to a patient who enhances his feelings of importance and effectiveness or who is physically appealing. Some physicians who become involved in this behavior are sociopathic or compromised by alcoholism or substance abuse. Although a patient may misinterpret "warmth" and physical contact, such as hugging, by a physician as sexual advances when it is not so intended, it remains the physician's responsibility to be clear about the boundaries of the relationship (Nadelson 1989).

Given the nature of the transference in the physician-patient relationship, the patient's ability to give informed consent has been questioned (Herman et al. 1987; Kardener 1974; Kluft 1989). The analogy to rape and incest has been made by many clinicians (Gabbard 1989). This analogy is especially related to the transference aspects of the therapeutic interaction (Barnhouse 1978). Some states have specific laws based on these special characteristics. Since 1985, having sex with patients has been made a felony in seven states, and others are moving in this direction (Goleman 1990).

Although some physicians have claimed that the sexual interaction is "therapeutic" despite evidence to the contrary, it has been explicitly stated to be unethical and exploitative by the American Psychiatric Association (1989) and the American Medical Association (1990b). The ability of the physician to be objective and to give necessary care is compromised by breaching the therapeutic boundary.

At some times, the nature of the therapeutic relationship is not clear, for example, the physician who has consulted briefly on a patient or has provided care that does not involve an intense interpersonal relationship. Likewise, questions have been raised about when a patient ceases to be a patient and how long one can assume that the transference would be operative.

A number of clinical studies have stated that sexual relationships between caregivers and patients are harmful to patients and may have acute as well as long-term consequences (Bohoutsos et al. 1983; Burgess 1981; Feldman-Summers and Jones 1984; Herman et al. 1987; Kluft 1989; Pope and Bohoutsos 1986). In addition to the shame, guilt, and mistrust they experience, these patients have been reported to have posttraumatic stress disorder, anxiety and depressive disorders, sexual symptoms, and sleep disorders and are at higher risk for substance abuse. There have also been reports of increased suicide risk and admissions to psychiatric hospitals.

CONCLUSIONS

This chapter has briefly touched on some contemporary and emerging ethical issues, including those that especially affect women. The complex dynamics of the physician's relationship with the patient demand constant vigilance in order to be clear about the physician's role as the patient's advocate, as opposed to the agent of society, and about the special nature of the boundary of professional and personal relationships. For society, the changing role of women and the emergence of new technologies, especially those involving reproduction, have raised questions with profound ethical implications. It is also clear that culturally determined values and ethical values may clash. It appears at the moment that there is no consistency to medical decision making or a process for resolution. Perhaps the way forward lies in continued discussion, education, and mutual understanding.

REFERENCES

Abraham L: Transplants available—for young, white, wealthy men. American Medical News, January 7, 1991

Altman LK: AIDS testing of doctors is crux of thorny debate. The New York Times, December 27, 1990

American Medical Association Board of Trustees: Legal interventions during pregnancy: court-ordered medical treatments and legal penalties for potentially harmful behaviors by pregnant women. JAMA 264:2663–2670, 1990a

American Medical Association: Sexual misconduct in the practice of medicine. Report of the Council on Ethical and Judicial Affairs of the American Medical Association, presented to and passed by the House of Delegates in Miami, FL, December 19, 1990b

American Psychiatric Association: The Principles of Medical Ethics With Annotations Especially Applicable to Psychiatry. Washington, DC, American Psychiatric Association, 1989

Applebaum P, Grisso T: Assessing patients' capacities to consent to treatment. N Engl J Med 3219:1635–1638, 1988

Atwood M: The Handmaid's Tale. Boston, MA, Houghton Mifflin, 1986

Barnhouse RT: Sex between patient and therapist. J Am Acad Psychoanal 6:533–540, 1978

Beauchamp TL: Paternalism, in Encyclopedia of Bioethics. Edited by Reich WT. New York, Free Press, 1978, pp 1194–1201

Blank RH: Emerging notions of women's rights and responsibilities during gestation. J Leg Med 7:441–469, 1986

Bohoutsos J, Holroyd J, Lerman H, et al: Sexual intimacy between psychotherapists and patients. Professional Psychology: Research and Practice 14:185–196, 1983

Bowes WA, Selgestad B: Fetal versus maternal rights: medical and legal perspectives. Obstet Gynecol 58:209–214, 1981

Brody EB: Culture, reproductive technology and women's rights: an intergovernmental perspective. Journal of Psychosomatic Obstetrics and Gynaecology 9:199–205, 1988

Burgess A: Physician sexual misconduct and patients' responses. Am J Psychiatry 138:1335–1342, 1981

Cole HM: Legal interventions during pregnancy. JAMA 264:2663–2670, 1990

Dahlberg CC: Sexual contact between patient and therapist. Contemporary Psychoanalysis 6:107–124, 1970

Derosis H, Hamilton J, Morrison E, et al: More on psychiatrist-patient sexual contact. Am J Psychiatry 144:688–689, 1987

Doctors plan to review fetal tissue research. The Boston Globe, January 8, 1991

Englehardt HT Jr: The Foundations of Bioethics. New York, Oxford University Press, 1986

Feldman-Summers S, Jones G: Psychological impacts on sexual contact between therapist or other health care practitioners and their clients. J Consult Clin Psychol 52:1054–1061, 1984

Freudenheim M: Business and health: guarding medical confidentiality. The New York Times, January 1, 1991, p 1:42

Gabbard GO: Sexual Exploitation in Professional Relationships. Washington, DC, American Psychiatric Press, 1989

Gartrell H, Herman J, Olarte S, et al: Psychiatrist-patient sexual contact: results of a national survey, I: prevalence. Am J Psychiatry 143:1126–1131, 1986

Gartrell N, Herman J, Olarte S, et al: Prevalence of psychiatrist-patient sexual contact, in Sexual Exploitation in Professional Relationships. Edited by Gabbard GO. Washington, DC, American Psychiatric Press, 1989, pp 3–13

Goleman D: New guidelines issued on patient-therapist sex. The New York Times, December 20, 1990, p B2

Harrison M: Drug addiction in pregnancy: the interface of science, emotion and social policy. Paper presented at the annual meeting of the American Psychiatric Association, New York, May 17, 1990

Herman JL, Gartrell N, Olarte S, et al: Psychiatrist-patient sexual contact: results of a national survey, psychiatrists' attitudes. Am J Psychiatry 144:164–169, 1987

Hilts PJ: Groups set up panel on use of fetal tissue. The New York Times, January 8, 1991

Holroyd JC, Brodsky AM: Psychologists' attitudes and practices regarding erotic and nonerotic physical contact with patients. Am Psychol 32:843–849, 1977

Johnsen D: A new threat to pregnant women's autonomy. Hastings Center Reports, August 1987, pp 33–40

Kahana RJ, Bibring GL: Personality types in medical management, in Psychiatry and Medical Practice in a General Hospital. Edited by Zinberg NE. New York, International Universities Press, 1964, pp 108–123

Kardener SH: Sex and physician-patient relationship. Am J Psychiatry 131:1134–1136, 1974

Kardener SH, Fuller M, Mensh LN: Characteristics of "erotic" practitioners. Am J Psychiatry 133:1324–1325, 1976

Katz J (ed): Experimentation With Human Beings: The Authority of the Investigator, Subject, Professions, and State in the Human Experimentation Process. New York, Russell Sage Foundation, 1972

Kluft RP: Treating the patient who has been exploited by a previous therapist. Psychiatr Clin North Am 12:483–500, 1989

Landwirth J: Fetal abuse and neglect: an emerging controversy. Pediatrics 79:508–514, 1987

Lenow JL: The fetus as a patient: emerging rights as a person? Am J Law Med 9:1–29, 1983

Lewin T: Implanted birth control device renews debate over forced contraception. The New York Times, January 10, 1991, p A20

Markey EJ: Congress of the United States, House of Representatives, letter to Massachusetts constituents, December 9, 1990

Marmor J: The seductive psychiatrist. Psychiatry Digest 31:10–16, 1976

McCartney J: Overt transference. J Sex Res 2:227–237, 1966

McNulty M: Pregnancy police: the health policy and legal implications of punishing pregnant women for harm to their fetuses. New York University Review of Law and Social Change 16:277–319, 1987–1988

Murray TH: Moral obligations to the not-yet born: the fetus as patient. Clin Perinatol 14:329–343, 1987

Nadelson C: Health care directions: who cares for patients? (presidential address). Am J Psychiatry 143:949–955, 1986

Nadelson CC: Afterword, in Sexual Exploitation in Professional Relationships. Edited by Gabbard GO. Washington, DC, American Psychiatric Press, 1989, pp 229–231

Nadelson C, Notman MT: Women as patients and experimental subjects, in Encyclopedia of Bioethics. Edited by Reich WT. New York, Free Press, 1978, pp 1713–1720

Nadelson C, Notman MT: The doctor/patient relationship: ethical issues, in The Free Woman: Women's Health in the 1990s. Edited by van Hall E, Everserd W. Carnforth, England, Parthenon Publishing Group, 1990, pp 894–905

National Institutes of Health: Report, September 10, 1990

Newman L, Brody EB: Editorial. Journal of Psychosomatic Obstetrics and Gynaecology 9:155–158, 1988

Notman MT, Nadelson CC: The woman patient: medical and psychological interfaces, in The Woman Patient. Edited by Notman MT, Nadelson CC. New York, Plenum, 1978, pp 1–7

Palca J: Women left out at NIH. Science 248:1601–1602, 1990

Pellegrino ED, Thomasma DC: For the Patient's Good: The Restoration of Beneficence in Health Care. New York, Oxford University Press, 1988

Perry JA: Physicians' erotic and nonerotic physical involvement with patients. Am J Psychiatry 133:838–840, 1976

Pope K, Bohoutsos J: Sexual Intimacy Between Therapists and Patients. New York, Praeger, 1986

Rapp MS: Sexual misconduct. Can Med Assoc J 137:193–194, 1987

Rhoden NK: Cesareans and samaritans. Law, Medicine and Health Care 15:118–125, 1987

Romeo S: Dr. Martin answers his accusers. Knave, June 1978, pp 14–38

Rothman BK: Recreating Motherhood: Ideology and Technology in a Patriarchal Society. New York, WW Norton, 1989

Scheier R: Who lives? who dies? who decides? American Medical News, January 7, 1991, pp 3–4

Shepard M: The love treatment: sexual intimacy between patients and psychotherapists. New York, Wyden, 1971

Simon R: Sexual exploitation of patients: how it begins before it happens. Psychiatric Annals 9:104–112, 1989

Stotland NL: Psychiatric Aspects of Reproductive Technology. Washington, DC, American Psychiatric Press, 1990

van Hall EV: Manipulation of human reproduction. Journal of Psychosomatic Obstetrics and Gynaecology 9:207–231, 1988

Wickenden D: Drug of choice: the side effects of RU 486. The New Republic, November 26, 1990, pp 24–27

Chapter 25

PSYCHIATRIC CONSULTATION TO OBSTETRICS AND GYNECOLOGY

Nada L. Stotland, M.D.

❖ ❖ ❖ ❖ ❖ ❖ ❖ ❖ ❖ ❖ ❖ ❖ ❖ ❖

T his volume is devoted to the consideration of the psychiatric aspects of obstetrics and gynecology and the complementary issues in psychiatry surrounding female reproduction. Each chapter concerns a portion of that clinical field. This chapter addresses a process to supplement the others' content. Given the countless clinical and research areas in which psychiatry and obstetrics-gynecology each have an important contribution to make to patient care and education and the discovery of new knowledge, what are the processes and structures through which the collaboration can actually take place? The sites range from the laboratory and classroom to the operating room and the seats of government. The methods include written materials, formal lectures, conjoint or consultative work in office or at bedside, joint committees, and the formation of multispecialty organizations that develop programs, activities, and publications of mutual interest.

HISTORY

The history of psychosomatic medicine and consultation psychiatry could be said to stem from issues in obstetrics and gynecology. The term *hysteria* derives from ancient Greece, where it was used as a diagnosis for patients whose physical symptoms that could not otherwise be explained were attributed to the wanderings of the uterus from its normal position of the pelvis to other locations in the body (Pomeroy 1975). Reproductive organs, functions, and events evoke powerful affects. Freud conceptualized development in terms of psychosexual stages and considered the formation of a successful heterosexual relationship, including procreation, to be a hallmark of normal maturity (Freud 1931).

One of the landmark psychosomatic collaborations of the 20th century was the research of Benedek, a psychiatrist and psychoanalyst, and Rubinstein, a gynecologist. They studied women during the course of psychoanalysis that had been undertaken for reasons unrelated to the menstrual cycle. While the patients kept track of their menstrual periods, the gynecologist monitored urinary levels of newly discovered female hormones. The psychoanalyst recorded evidence in the patients' dreams and associations of their moods and thought content (Benedek and Rubinstein 1942). They concluded that the hormonal changes that are characteristic of the ovulatory phase are associated with affects and thoughts of nurturance and interest in sexual intercourse. It would seem that cyclic changes of this kind would enhance the likelihood of conception and therefore the preservation of the species.

During the 1940s and 1950s, psychoanalysis was a dominant force in psychiatry in the United States. The awesome power of psychodynamic understanding to make sense of human feelings and behavior was impressive, and there were attempts to utilize it in arenas from international relations to preschool education. Since many or most psychoanalysts were also physicians, there was considerable interest in applying psychoanalytic knowledge and technique to medical diagnosis and treatment, and thereby also in enhancing the integration of medicine and psychiatry. Such an integration was otherwise somewhat threatened by psychoanalysts' distance from, and even rejection of, the rest of clinical medicine and its techniques (Alexander 1950; Dunbar 1954). Others used psychoanalytic technique for the intensive study of patients with various medical illnesses (Alexander 1950; Dunbar 1954). They described constellations of personality traits and unconscious motives and conflicts that underlie several major disease entities. Physical symptoms were conceptualized in terms of neurotic compromise. For example, the asthmatic patient's wheezing was a cry for the mother. The hypertensive patient's cardiovascular changes resulted from unexpressed, unconscious rage. Infertility resulted from unconscious rejection of motherhood. Therapeutic interventions based on these etiologic formulations were reported to have positive effects. In some major medical centers, psychiatrists and psychoanalysts were assigned to some or all of the medical units to work with medical colleagues and patients.

Over the years, for a variety of reasons, these arrangements eroded. Improvements in research methodology called into question many of the above conclusions. One basic problem was the fact that many groups of patients were studied after they had suffered from their illnesses for many years. There was no way to know whether the psychodynamics that had been revealed in their diagnostic interviews were the cause or the result of their years of pain and disability. Suppressed feelings of neediness and anger were to be expected under the circumstances. In any case, the connections between personality types and medical disorders did not hold up.

Over time, researchers discovered genetic, infectious, and other factors that played major etiologic roles in hitherto mysterious signs and symptoms. For example, the ability to examine the fallopian tubes through laparoscopy and microscopy revealed evidence in some women of damage that had resulted from prior pelvic infections and that could be surgically repaired. These discoveries led some clinicians and patients to feel that psychodynamic explanations were simply a "wastebasket," a fanciful etiologic last resort, for conditions not yet conquered by "real" science. What was worse, they stigmatized the sufferers as neurotic, immature, and responsible for their own symptoms.

Other factors that played a role in the decline of psychiatric and psychodynamic involvement in medical care include funding, personnel, the development of other mental health disciplines, and the burgeoning of biologic approaches to psychiatry (Fenton and Guggenheim 1981). Some of these approaches, such as the dexamethasone suppression test, were used by psychiatrists but were understood to supplant the need for the understanding of childhood experience, feelings, and motivations. Psychoactive medications were quickly adopted into the armamentarium of nonpsychiatric physicians, who write the vast majority of prescriptions for them.

At the same time, evidence of synergistic relationships between biological and psychosocial factors in the genesis and phenomenology of illness continued to appear. A prospective study of military recruits revealed that accurate predictions could be made about which recruits were susceptible to peptic ulcers under the stress of combat. It was found that mind and body do work together, but in ways more complex and numerous than first supposed. Life events can precipitate mood and neurohumoral changes that affect immune response. Eating disorders and reproductive dysfunctions are related. "Infertile" couples may not be having sexual intercourse or may be using a schedule or technique that precludes conception; there has been a failure to meet the biological essentials for conception, but that failure stems from ignorance, interpersonal strains, or external constraints. A problem like this one may seem to be beyond the bounds of both gynecology and psychiatry, but this very situation continues to baffle clinicians and patients and to lead to needless expenditures and medical interventions. The consulting psychiatrist can prevent this situation by alerting the infertility team to incorporate a few simple screening questions into the initial diagnostic process (Christie and Pawson 1987).

Consultation-liaison psychiatry remains a function that reinforces and capitalizes on psychiatry as a medical discipline (Lipowski 1986). To a significant extent, consultation-liaison is a subspecialty of psychiatry. There are several "psychosomatic" and "consultation-liaison" organizations that publish journals and hold meetings. There are even sub-subspecialty groups that address issues related to specific medical conditions: oncology, nephrology, acquired immunodeficiency syndrome (AIDS), and obstetrics and gynecology. (The latter are discussed below.) However, few, if any, medical care institutions aspire to assign a psychiatrist to each clinical specialty or inpatient unit. Most of the clinical problems discussed in this volume are addressed by psychiatrists in general practice, in another subspecialty (e.g., child and adolescent psychiatry, geriatrics, forensics), or in consultation-liaison psychiatry as a whole, rather than by psychiatrists who spend all their time consulting to obstetrician-gynecologists. This chapter provides an overview of clinical issues and consultation-liaison activities for the psychiatrist, including multidisciplinary collaboration and research, teaching, and participation in subspecialty organizations.

CLINICAL AND CULTURAL SUBSTRATE OF OBSTETRIC-GYNECOLOGIC PRACTICE

The provision of psychiatric consultation and liaison to another medical specialty must be informed by some familiarity with the content and style of that specialty's practice (Stotland and Garrick 1990). Although obstetrician-gynecologists share many clinical issues with all other physicians (including psychiatrists), they also face some challenges that are unique to their specialty. Most of the subspecialties of obstetrics and gynecology attract practitioners who enjoy active intervention and expect their interventions to result in relatively prompt and positive clinical outcomes. This stance serves them well for much of their clinical work but leads to frustration in many of the situations in which psychiatric consultation is sought: failure of the patient to comply with medical recommendations, evidence of behavior that is actively self-destructive or threatens the well-being of the fetus, questions about a woman's ability to assume responsibility for a newborn, depression and grief, physical complaints without diagnosable physical foundation, and intense transference reactions to the gynecologist (Stotland 1988).

Residents in obstetrics and gynecology face a particularly daunting challenge. In just 4 years of training, they must absorb and master a huge body of medical information. The subspecialties of the field, with which they must have a working acquaintance, include highly technical areas such as gynecologic oncology, reproductive endocrinology, and perinatology. There are numerous invasive and noninvasive diagnostic techniques, including ultrasonography, intrapartum fetal monitoring, chorionic villus sampling, and amniocentesis. Diagnostic and therapeutic approaches to infertility are extremely complex.

At the same time, the resident must master surgical technique, with demands ranging from the extreme time pressure of the surgical delivery of a fetus in extremis to the delicacy of microsurgical fallopian tube repair and the plastic reconstruction of sexual organs extirpated because of malignancy. Their field overlaps significantly not only with general surgery and oncology, but with pediatrics, urology, and infectious disease. The knowledge base and technical procedures are changing so fast that residents must alter their thinking almost as soon as they acquire it. At the same time, the public funding on which much of academic medicine relies is notably scanty in the area of obstetrics. Financial constraints may restrict the numbers of residents in programs and further increase the already heavy clinical burden and number of nights on call.

This load of clinical work involves the care of patients facing problems and interventions with tremendous emotional valence. Obstetrics and gynecology, especially in the hospital, where most psychiatric consultation and liaison work takes place, involves not only routine pelvic examination screening and normal deliveries, which are in themselves emotionally demanding on patient and staff, but also the care of patients who have been raped, who have given birth to extremely small or damaged infants, who seek termination of pregnancy via induced abortion, whose pregnancies are threatened by medical or psychiatric illness, who have sexually transmitted diseases that threaten their fertility or survival, who have malignancies, and who have difficulties with their sexual or reproductive functions. As this description implies, there is little or no time for obstetrician-gynecologists, especially for residents, to talk to these patients at length; to learn about the emotional dimensions of these clinical problems; to address skills for diagnosing, referring, and treating the psychiatric complications of these conditions; or even to acknowledge and accept the profound feelings that they engender in the treating physician (Adler 1972).

In addition, many of the most vexing ethical conflicts in clinical medicine face the obstetrician-gynecologist. Should a pregnant woman be forced to undergo an obstetric intervention in the interest of her fetus, or punished if her behavior results in fetal damage? Which patients, if any, should be admitted to artificial insemination, in vitro fertilization, or surrogate mother programs (Lantos 1990)? Are physicians obligated to provide induced abortions, and at what stages of gestation, and under what circumstances? What constitutes informed consent for sterilization?

Not uncommonly, obstetrician-gynecologists must repair medical damage caused by behavior that they find personally repugnant (e.g., cocaine abuse during pregnancy) or provide services of which they do not fully approve. When these ethical and emotional demands are placed on a sleep-deprived resident who is struggling to develop technical skills and who chose the specialty in the hopes of facilitating expeditious and happy outcomes, the result may be avoidance, depression, and rage. These emotions are often reflected in requests for psychiatric consultation and in the functioning of the health care team requesting them (Karasu et al. 1977).

Recent changes in the social context of medical practice have had a particularly problematic impact on obstetrician-gynecologists. The proliferation of malpractice litigation has hit obstetricians especially hard. In the state of Illinois, for example, nearly 100% of obstetricians will be sued by patients at some point during their careers. Charles and Kennedy (1985) have documented the interruption of practice, avoidance by colleagues, loss of self-esteem, changes in practice patterns, and suspicion of future patients caused by malpractice suits, even for the majority of doctors who will be found innocent of the charges brought against them. Physicians feel constrained to perform diagnostic and therapeutic interventions on preventive legal, rather than medical, grounds.

Obstetrics is also legally perilous because any allegedly damaged infant and its family make a wrenching spectacle in the courtroom, because the lifelong care of such an infant is so costly, and because the statute of limitations on bringing a lawsuit does not apply until the infant has reached the age of majority and has had the opportunity to realize the nature and cause of his or her disability. Advances in obstetric technique constitute a two-edged sword: the public expects the medical profession to be able to solve any problem and to produce a perfect outcome in every case, whereas the very patients who are at higher risk because of delayed childbearing are those who are most likely to seek legal recourse for any frustration.

The consumer movement of the last 10–15 years has also been highly focused on obstetrics and gynecology. Self-help groups, often highly critical of physicians' behaviors and traditional medical interventions, have proliferated. Finding physicians who were wanting in knowledge and attitude, mothers founded the La Leche League to promote breast-feeding (La Leche League 1987). Chapters were founded in countries all over the world, and the demographics of infant feeding changed. At about the same time, physical therapists, nurses, and nonmedical persons began to teach "prepared childbirth" classes. These classes educated expectant parents about the anatomy and physiology of pregnancy, labor, delivery, and the postpartum period (Bing 1973). They also, however, brought women and their significant others together to question and defy traditional medical authority. They encouraged patients to believe that they could and should comprehend medical questions and make informed choices about their own care. They encouraged them to substitute relaxation and distraction techniques, over which they had control, for dependence on analgesics and anesthetics, which were administered by professionals and could lead to iatrogenic complications. They also encouraged the preparation, participation, and support of significant others in the experience of labor and delivery, diminishing to a significant degree the central emotional role of the physician (Seiden 1978). Organizations and articles in the popular press question routine repeat cesarean delivery and the indications for the enormous number of hysterectomies performed in the United States as compared with other affluent countries. Books like *Our Bodies, Ourselves,* which was written by a women's collective, explain issues that had been the exclusive domain of obstetrician-gynecologists (Boston Women's Health Collective 1984).

All of these developments, like the increase in sensational malpractice litigation, aroused or gave voice to suspicion and hostility between patients and doctors (Arms 1975). Obstetrician-gynecologists have found it particularly painful and ironic that, after all their attempts to meet the demands of information and skills acquisition and provision of services in the interest of women's health, they should be viewed in the press and the consulting room as purveyors of needless and often damaging interventions and as dismissive of women and their autonomy over their reproductive organs and functions. At the same time, however, there is significant clinical and documentary foundation for women's complaints about their care (Friedman 1986; Hellerstein 1984; Scully and Bart 1973).

The American College of Obstetricians and Gynecologists established a public advisory committee and makes available to members a kit for surveying their practices to determine patient satisfaction. The beleaguered practitioner is generally very appreciative of the psychiatric consultant's empathy for this difficult situation. The consultant can also help patients to utilize the self-help, family support, and behavioral techniques that they may have acquired in preparing for labor when they are faced with complications or other illnesses. Muscular relaxation and distraction-imaging are useful in a wide variety of situations, as are access to information and the ability to assert oneself constructively in a frightening confrontation with authority.

CONSULTATION-LIAISON MECHANISMS

The realities of practice and developments in knowledge and technique in the specialty of obstetrics and gynecology can be assimilated by the liaison psychiatrist by attending grand rounds and other conferences in the obstetrics and gynecology department. The psychiatrist can also use the occasion of the conference to meet members of the department and to make comments on psychiatric aspects of the cases and issues discussed. Often "curbstone" consultations will be sought and referrals made for formal inpatient and outpatient consultations.

The psychiatrist may also elect to participate in inpatient-care rounds regularly or to be present at or available to one or more outpatient clinics. On rounds or in a clinic, the psychiatrist can get an excellent sense of the ethos of the service and the personalities and level of psychological sophistication of the students, house, and professional staff, as well as the typical psychosocial and psychiatric problems of the patients. The psychiatrist's participation underscores the integration of psychiatric with medical concerns and offers the opportunity for helpful comments and interventions without the necessity for formal psychiatric consultation. The psychiatrist can help the members of the service learn to recognize early signs of psychiatric disorders before they develop into difficult management problems or emergencies, as well as to decide when and how to call for formal consultation.

In most academic and large community hospitals, services include family planning, sometimes with a separate section for adolescents;

normal and high-risk prenatal care; infertility diagnosis and treatment; general gynecologic care; gynecologic cancer diagnosis and treatment; and services in other subspecialty areas. In a busy department, there will be far too many services and clinics for even the most energetic and dedicated psychiatrist. Interested residents, fellows, and even medical students taking senior electives in consultation psychiatry can add to the psychiatric presence, get valuable experience, and develop subspecialty practice and research interests. This sort of program, however, requires an investment of time by faculty or senior consultants that is approximately equivalent to the time that would be required for the direct provision of services. In addition, the liaison is disrupted by the inevitable rotation and graduation of trainees.

Formal teaching is an important component of the substance and technique of liaison work. Whereas busy obstetrician-gynecologists are not often seeking extra classroom hours, the staff members in charge of resident conferences and grand rounds are almost always eager to fill the endless procession of time slots. The audience, although wary of unrealistic demands on physicians' time and psychological sophistication, is generally interested in scientifically stimulating and clinically useful information about common psychiatric problems such as anxiety and affective disorders. It is best to come prepared both with new findings about neurotransmitters, imaging, or psychopharmacology and with specific and easily implemented suggestions for screening, diagnosis, referral, and treatment. Nonpsychiatric physicians are often uncertain about how to distinguish among the various categories of mental health professionals and when to refer to each.

For example, it is not enough to recommend that screening for major psychiatric illness be a part of prenatal care. Obstetricians appreciate, and are more likely to use, a short list of questions to add to their admission history ("Have you ever been referred or referred yourself to see a psychiatrist, psychologist, or social worker?" "Have you ever been admitted to a hospital for psychiatric treatment?"). Other suggestions include the wording of questions about sexual practices and exposure to sexually transmitted diseases; criteria for prescription of antidepressants and referral for psychiatric care; assessment for organic brain syndromes; and assessment of competence to consent for surgery, to care for oneself, and to care for an infant.

Obstetrician-gynecologists are also interested in the psychological aspects of issues in their areas of expertise: induced and spontaneous abortion; pregnancy, labor, and delivery; new reproductive technologies; and malignancies.

INTERDISCIPLINARY ORGANIZATIONS AND ACTIVITIES

Issues in psychosomatic obstetrics and gynecology are discussed in many forums today. Symposia can be found on the programs of any major psychiatric or obstetric meeting. There are also national and international organizations devoted entirely to the field. They include the American and International Societies for Psychosomatic Obstetrics and Gynecology, which publishes the *International Journal of Psychosomatic Obstetrics and Gynecology*. The American Society holds yearly meetings in early spring; the International Society, meetings approximately every 3 years. There are also groups devoted to specific topics such as postpartum psychiatric illness (the Marce Society). Participation in these organizations acquaints members with the range of work being done and the people who are doing it. Membership consists of professionals in both mental health and obstetrics and is interdisciplinary, including physicians, psychologists, nurses, social workers, and midwives.

The American College of Obstetricians and Gynecologists has recently founded the Jacobs Institute for Women's Health, which publishes the quarterly journal *Women's Health Issues*. Members of many professional and consumer groups have also come together to address the policy and legislative implications of a number of the interdisciplinary issues discussed below. For example, the American Medical Association, the American Psychiatric Association, and the American College of Obstetricians and Gynecologists were among the participants in an amicus curiae brief in the *Webster v. Reproductive Health Services* abortion case decided by the Supreme Court in 1989.

ISSUES FOR THE FUTURE

At the interface of psychiatry and obstetrics and gynecology lie a number of emerging and emergent social, policy, and ethical, as well as medical, problems. They include the impact of the abuse of alcohol and crack cocaine on the fetus, with its attendant issues of maternal versus fetal rights, autonomy, punishment, and care; the unknown and sometimes notoriously problematic implications of surrogate motherhood and embryo freezing and transfer; the legislative and judicial restrictions on induced abortion; AIDS as a heterosexually and prenatally transmitted disease; and many others. Now that nearly all of the relevant groups are headquartered in Washington, DC, it is easy for representatives to meet and work together.

Interdisciplinary research in some of these areas has been significantly diminished by governmental restrictions on funding and even on the nature of the research performed. For example, very little research has been done on contraception for the last 10 or more years, despite the continued high incidence of unintended pregnancy. Little work has been published about induced abortion, despite the public's hunger for information about its psychological concomitants. Research involving fetal tissue has been banned.

At the level of clinical practice, funding is again a major issue. No longer do hospital and academic departments have the luxury of hiring psychiatric liaison-consultants to teach and spend time in clinical service areas. Patients' health insurance policies often severely limit their access to psychiatric services. Mental health care is increasingly singled out for "management" by companies that limit the choice and availability of services. Both faculty and trainees in medical schools are under increasing constraints to generate sufficient clinical income to pay their salaries, often while trying to fulfill a mission to take care of the medically indigent and uninsured. At the same time, obstetric-gynecologic subspecialty care often involves complex procedures that are far more expensive than psychiatric consultation. Once a good liaison relationship has been formed, the psychiatrist may be able to convince the infertility, oncology, or other service that psychiatric screening and support are equally important for clinical care and that patients and their insurance companies can be expected to pay for them equally.

Psychiatric consultation to obstetrics and gynecology is rich in breadth and depth. The consulting psychiatrist can participate in scientific developments at the cutting edge of human genetics and reproduction, in human events from the conception to the end of life, and from the most tragic and wrenching to the most heroic and joyous experiences. An awareness of the social context and the clinical realities facing the obstetric-gynecologic practitioner will help the consultant develop a consultative style and content that the consultee will appreciate and utilize in the interests of patients. Participation in interdisciplinary organizations and activities offers the interested psychiatrist the opportunity to meet and work with colleagues in other fields, to advance knowledge and care, and to act in concert in the public arena.

REFERENCES

Adler G: Helplessness in the helpers. Br J Med Psychol 45:315–326, 1972

Alexander F: Psychosomatic Medicine. New York, WW Norton, 1950

Arms S: Immaculate Deception: A New Look at Women and Childbirth in America. Boston, MA, Houghton Mifflin, 1975

Benedek T, Rubinstein B: The sexual cycle in women, in Psychosomatic Medicine Monographs, Vol 3. Washington, DC, National Research Council, 1942

Bing E: Six Practical Lessons for an Easier Childbirth. New York, Bantam, 1973

Boston Women's Health Collective: The New Our Bodies, Ourselves. New York, Simon & Schuster, 1984

Charles SC, Kennedy E: Defendant: A Psychiatrist on Trial for Medical Malpractice. New York, Free Press, 1985

Christie GL, Pawson ME: The psychological and social management of the infertile couple, in The Infertile Couple. Edited by Pepperel RS, Hudson B, Wood C. New York, Churchill Livingstone, 1987, pp 35–50

Dunbar HF: Emotions and Bodily Changes: A Survey of Literature on Psychosomatic Interrelationships. New York, Columbia University Press, 1954

Fenton BJ, Guggenheim FG: Consultation-liaison and funding: why can't Alice find Wonderland. Gen Hosp Psychiatry 7:255–260, 1981

Freud S: Female sexuality (1931), in The Standard Edition of the Complete Psychological Works of Sigmund Freud, Vol 21. Translated and edited by Strachey J. London, Hogarth Press, 1961, pp 223–243

Friedman EA: The obstetrician's dilemma: how much fetal monitoring and cesarean section is enough? N Engl J Med 315:641–643, 1986

Hellerstein D: The training of a gynecologist: how the "old boys" talk about women's bodies. Ms., November 1984, pp 136–137

Karasu TB, Plutchnik R, Conte H, et al: What do physicians want from a psychiatric consultation service. Compr Psychiatry 18:73–81, 1977

La Leche League International: The Womanly Art of Breastfeeding. Franklin Park, IL, Interstate Publishers, 1987

Lantos JD: Second-generation ethical issues in the new reproductive technologies: divided loyalties, indications, and the research agenda, in Psychiatric Aspects of Reproductive Technology. Edited by Stotland NL. Washington, DC, American Psychiatric Press, 1990, pp 87–96

Lipowski ZJ: Consultation-liaison psychiatry: the first half century. Gen Hosp Psychiatry 8:305–315, 1986

Pomeroy S: Goddesses, Whores, Wives and Slaves: Women in Classical Antiquity. New York, Schacken, 1975

Scully D, Bart P: A funny thing happened on the way to the orifice: women in gynecology textbooks, in Changing Women in a Changing Society. Edited by Huber J. Chicago, IL, University of Chicago Press, 1973, pp 283–288

Seiden A: The sense of mastery in the childbirth experience, in The Woman Patient, Vol 1. Edited by Notman M, Nadelson C. New York, Plenum, 1978, pp 87–105

Stotland N: Social Change and Women's Reproductive Health Care. New York, Praeger, 1988

Stotland NL, Garrick TR: Manual of Psychiatric Consultation. Washington, DC, American Psychiatric Press, 1990

Webster v Reproductive Health Services, 109 S.Ct. 3040 (1989)

Chapter 26

MINORITY WOMEN: ECOLOGICAL SETTING AND INTERCULTURAL DIALOGUE

Mindy Thompson Fullilove, M.D.

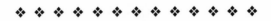

In the complex social organization of the human, the dominance of the societal factors becomes most patent. The physiological processes of fertilization and incubation, although the same in all societies, take place in social settings that vary historically, leading to damage, death, or survival of the fetus. In any one period of history, the supportive or destructive conditions in which fertilization and incubation take place vary with the class or social group to which the adults belong. Nurturance is accomplished by widely diversified procedures, depending on the society and the group within the society to which the child and parents belong. *It is no longer easy to generalize about the three processes as they occur in a particular species.* The physiology of reproduction in people is comparable in all settings. Different societal settings increase or decrease the probability of the survival of the offspring, as well as behavioral patterns involved in reproduction. It is possible that with the increased mastery by humans over environmental factors by means of improved technology, the very physiology of the processes of fertilization, incubation and nurturance may change.

Ethel Tobach, 1971[*]

---

[*]Reprinted from Tobach E: "Some Evolutionary Aspects of Human Gender." *American Journal of Orthopsychiatry* 41:710–715, 1971. Copyright 1971 by the *American Journal of Orthopsychiatry*. Used with permission.

The preparation of this chapter was supported in part by Centers Grant P-50-MH423520 from the National Institute of Mental Health and the National Institute on Drug Abuse.

MINORITY STATUS, CULTURE, AND WOMEN

Dr. Tobach, in the analysis cited above, reminds us that the physiology of reproduction is the same in all settings. As the settings vary, however, so too will the health and welfare of mother and infant be altered. As we turn to an examination of the sexual and reproductive health of minority women, we must consider the ways in which social setting shapes health. It is the thesis of this chapter that "minority status" has socioeconomic as well as cultural implications that act at separate points to determine the health of minority people. Although socioeconomic status has the largest impact on rates of disease and disability, it is culture that is most critical in the one-on-one interaction that occurs during the delivery of health care. Those with "minority status" are members of stigmatized races, religious and ethnic groups, or tribal groups. Although "race" is one of the factors associated with stigmatization, it is a social, rather than a genetic, construct that has meaning with regard to health (Cooper and David 1986).

Waves of migrants have come or have been brought to the United States over the past four centuries. Some of the incoming groups have been welcomed into the work force and into the power structure. Others have struggled for the very survival of their group. The stakes have been high: control over the wealth and bounty offered by a huge, well-endowed continent. Among the weapons of the battle have been those "isms," such as racism and religious intolerance, that have allowed people to deny the humanity of their competitors. In 1903, W. E. B. DuBois, the foremost black historian and commentator, stated that "the problem of the color line is the problem of the 20th century—the relation of the darker to the lighter men in Asia and Africa, in America, and the islands of the sea" (DuBois 1967, p. 23).

Almost 100 years later, despite battles for equality that have attracted international concern and attention, we still live in a world in which race, ethnicity, religion, and sex determine one's chance to live a healthy and productive life. In fact, the barriers of stigma create an ecology for minority people that is distinctly different from that of majority people. The minority woman, in her capacity for procreative and recreative sexuality, does not differ from her majority counterpart. Given that she lives under more adverse conditions, however, her ability to realize her wishes and dreams is more limited. Given her risk for ill health, the chances are great that she will have contact with the health care system, defined as it is by a culture and by rules that may be quite alien to her own.

At that moment, when the health care provider and the patient meet, the provider faces the challenge of establishing a dialogue that can assist in the diagnosis and treatment of illness. This dialogue is at the heart of health care. Through this communication, accurate information must be conveyed about the patient's symptoms, behaviors, and attempts at self-care. Eventually, it must enable the provider to convince the patient to follow a prescription for care. Finally, the dialogue is most truly a healing interaction when both provider and patient have felt affirmed and respected.

As we speak across cultural differences, we face barriers created by problems of meaning that are uniquely cultural. It is not, for example, inherently necessary that a handshake be soft or firm, except as prescribed by the traditions of individual cultures. Dr. S. Ahmad Hussain described an encounter at the Afghan Mission Hospital with a young man of the Puthan tribe from the mountainous area of Pakistan. Patient and doctor did not share a common philosophy of illness. When the young man appeared to be dying, the family decided to take him home. In their warrior tribe, a man must die either in battle or at home. This was adamantly opposed by the doctor, who thought that the absence of hospital-based care meant certain death for the young man. Yet, as the family explained and the doctor listened, respect—if not agreement—developed. Against all odds, the young man survived. On hearing that the doctor would be leaving for America, the young man went fishing early in the morning and then took a day-long bus ride in order to say good-bye and give the doctor a parting gift of six plump fish (Hussain 1990).

Dr. Hussain learned to look past the assumptions of his medical culture. However, when the barriers of culture intersect with the barriers of oppression—and even of genocide—then we face additional barriers of anger, fear, dissembling, and contempt. The characteristics of the intersection of culture with oppression are shaped by the history of the meeting. The story of Japanese people in the United States includes their internment in concentration camps during

World War II, when Americans did not trust the loyalty of Japanese to their new country. Chinese men came to America to work on the railroads and were forbidden to bring their wives. The old, single men remain part of the story of Chinatown in San Francisco and elsewhere. The almost complete annihilation of Native Americans by war and disease beginning immediately upon contact with white civilization ranks with the Holocaust as a horrific story of genocide. Vietnamese and Haitian boat people are just beginning to write the stories of their entry into the United States. No two groups will succeed or fail to exactly the same degree. Yet the relative achievement of each group will leave its mark on the health of its group's members, both male and female. This achievement will also shape the barriers to communication that will exist between the groups. This chapter examines markers of the health status of minority women, the sexual practices of minority women, a description of some ecological settings inhabited by minorities, and thoughts for improving health care.

HEALTH STATUS

Sexually Transmitted Diseases

Minorities suffer disproportionately from sexually transmitted diseases (STDs). There are striking differences in the rates of disease for each of the STDs noted here (Table 26–1); in particular, there is a marked difference between whites and blacks in the distribution of syphilis. Acquired immunodeficiency syndrome (AIDS), though not solely transmitted through sexual intercourse, is an STD of importance. AIDS case reports, which have routinely reported data by sex, document that, although there are fewer cases of AIDS among women, the vast majority of those cases have been diagnosed among minority women.

Although minorities face an excess risk for STDs, this risk is not uniformly distributed among minority populations. Patterns of STD transmission have a distinct geography that is closely related to the residential and socialization patterns of social-sexual groups, that is, networks of people connected by common sex partners. Thus, gonorrhea (Potterat et al. 1985), chlamydia (Zimmerman et al. 1990), and

AIDS (R. Wallace and Wallace 1990) all have distinctive (and different) patterns of geographical distribution.

Birth Outcomes

Two birth outcomes that are often viewed as critical indicators of health care are the survival of the mother and the survival of the infant. Women and their children from some minority groups fare worse than whites on both of these measures. In a recent study of maternal mortality, Atrash (Atrash et al. 1990) reported the rates of maternal mortality in the United States during the years 1979–1986. During that period, there was a marked downward trend in maternal mortality that was perhaps even more marked for minority women (Figure 26–1). Although minority women had a relative risk of maternal death 3.4 times higher than whites for 1974–1978, the relative risk had declined to 3 times that for whites for the years 1979–1986.

Infant mortality varies significantly by ethnicity. Becarra et al. (1991) examined infant mortality across ethnic groups. This study is notable because the authors attempted to divide Hispanics into subgroups defined by national origin—Mexico, Puerto Rico, Cuba, and other countries (Table 26–2). These data show that, although Hispanics—like blacks—have a higher risk for infant mortality than do

Table 26–1. United States population and reported cases of primary and secondary syphilis and gonorrhea

Characteristic	Year	White	Black	Hispanic	Other
		\% Distribution			
U.S. population[a]	1980	79.7	11.5	6.4	2.3
Syphilis[a]	1988	11.6	75.8	12.1	0.5
Gonorrhea[a]	1988	16.1	78.2	4.9	0.8
AIDS[b]	1990				
Men		63	26	14	0.0
Women		27	50	27	0.0

[a]Moran et al. 1989; [b]CDC AIDS Surveillance Report, June 1990.

whites, this risk is not uniform among different Hispanic subgroups. Puerto Rican infants, both those born in the United States and those born in Puerto Rico, face the highest risks. Cubans, by comparison, have rates of infant mortality that are significantly lower than those reported for white Americans or for the United States as a whole.

The heterogeneity of birth outcomes among Hispanics reflects access to prenatal and hospital delivery services, as well as the mothers' overall standard of living. The authors noted that only 57% of Puerto Rican women received prenatal care in the first trimester of pregnancy, compared to 82% of non-Hispanic whites. They found that out-of-hospital births were twice as likely among infants of Mexican American descent as in any other racial or ethnic group. They also noted that these statistics reflect the rapidly changing patterns of mi-

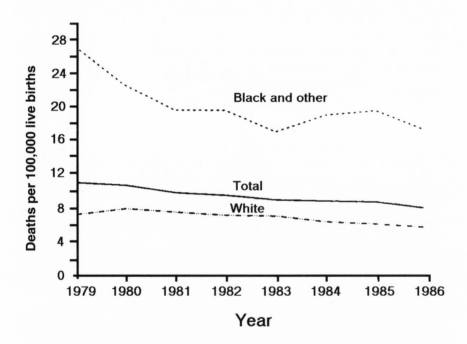

Figure 26–1.   Maternal mortality ratios by race and year, United States, 1979–1986.   *Source.* Reprinted from Atrash H, Koonin LM, Lawson HW, et al.: "Maternal Mortality in the United States, 1979–1986." *Obstetrics and Gynecology* 76:1055–1060, 1990. Reprinted with permission from the American College of Obstetricians and Gynecologists.

gration from Central and South America and the Caribbean, a subject discussed later in this chapter.

SEXUAL PRACTICES

Sex Roles

Across cultures, women are inferior to men in the control of wealth, the exercise of political power, access to education, and control of their own sexuality. A massive body of cultural rules attempt to limit women's sexual activity. A cross-cultural examination of gender rules reveals that they are more remarkable for their similarities than they are for their differences. Young girls often have as much freedom as young boys until the preadolescent period, when their schooling in their social role begins. Young adult women are expected to bear and

Table 26–2. Mortality risks among single-delivery infants by maternal race and ethnicity, United States, 1983 and 1984

Race/ethnicity	No. per 1,000[a]		
	Neonatal	Postneonatal	Infant
Non-Hispanics			
Whites	5.2	3.1	8.3
Blacks	10.9*	6.3*	17.2*
Other	6.1*	4.0*	10.1*
Hispanics	5.6*	3.1	8.7*
Mexicans	5.2	3.1	8.3
Puerto Ricans[b]	7.9*	3.7*	11.6
Cubans	5.0	2.0*	7.0*
Other	5.5	3.0	8.4
Puerto Rico	11.9*	3.0	14.9*
Total	6.4	3.6	9.8

[a]Neonatal and infant mortality risks calculated per 1,000 live births; postneonatal mortality risk calculated per 1,000 neonatal survivors.
[b]Excludes infants born in Puerto Rico (Puerto Rican islanders are reported as "Puerto Rico").
*Significantly different from risks for non-Hispanic whites ($P < .05$).
Source. Adapted from Becarra JE, Hogue JR, Atrash HK, et al.: "Infant Mortality Among Hispanics." *Journal of the American Medical Association* 265:217–221, 1991. Copyright 1991 American Medical Association. Used with permission.

nurture children, to limit their sexual activity to a single man, to provide for the nurturance of the family, to maintain kinship ties, to accept direction from men, and to follow rules for women's
comportment.

The linchpin in this model of women's servitude to the family is
the reproductive function of women. Although the cultural rules
would keep women "barefoot and pregnant in the kitchen," women
and their advocates have sought to assert women's control over their
own fertility. Older women, especially those who are past the reproductive years, may escape from the rules that oppress younger women.
It is not clear what processes enable some women to maintain their
integrity in their earlier years, but those who do assume positions of
leadership and authority that are uncontested by men. In fact, de la
Vega (1990), in describing women's roles in Latin cultures, emphasizes that the Latin woman has real power in the home, as the person
who provides the nurturance. As a growing number of Latin families
are headed by a single female parent, the woman's power increases,
though sometimes in conflict with the older ideas about women's sub-
servience to patriarchal rule.

Sexual Initiation

Sexual initiation is clearly a culturally defined behavior. Among
women, black women have traditionally been the most likely to initiate intercourse at an early age and often before marriage. Hispanic
women have been much more conservative in this regard. The figures
in Table 26–3, taken from the National Longitudinal Study of Youth,
are typical of those in national surveys examining these questions.
Black men are most likely to have been sexually active by age 19, followed by Hispanic men, black women and white men, and white
women. Hispanic women are least likely to have been sexually active
by this age, but even in this "least experienced" group, 50% of the
respondents had engaged in sexual intercourse.

Sexual Orientation

Sexual activity between members of the same sex occurs in all cultures, but, as much recent AIDS research has shown, the frame of ref-

Table 26–3. Estimated percentage of males and females born between 1963 and 1964 who had not engaged in sexual intercourse before their 19th birthday

Race/ethnicity	No. (%) of males	No. (%) of females
White	1,145 (23)	1,082 (34)
Black	207 (5)	203 (19)
Hispanic	381 (17)	95 (50)

Source. Adapted from the National Longitudinal Survey of Youth, 1963 and 1964 birth cohorts (Miller et al. 1990).

erence for understanding the behavior shifts dramatically across cultures. Native Americans, for example, define not only "men" and "women," but also a third gender that is neither male nor female. This creates the possibility that two "men" (as defined by Western definitions of gender) could have sex without it being perceived as "same-sex" sexual activity by the Native American definition. In some Hispanic cultures, a "man" is defined by certain gender-related behaviors. The act of penetration is a "manly" act, whether one penetrates a man or a woman. Therefore, a man who penetrates another man is having sex with a "feminine" person, not with another man.

What has been shown to be difficult for both men and women in minority cultures—perhaps even more than in white cultures—is the process of openly acknowledging a homosexual identity. Cochran and Mays (1988) have shown that homosexual and bisexual black women will not disclose their sexual orientations to health care providers, an omission that could be important to their health care. For members of some Asian cultures, the issues of shame surrounding homosexuality are reported to be intense. Even AIDS patients who are faced with the need for health care have been reported to avoid situations in which their sexual orientation might be revealed to family or friends.

Contraception and Sterilization

Numerous studies have queried young Americans about their attitudes toward birth control (Fullilove et al. 1990; Miller et al. 1990). What is remarkable about the data produced by these researchers is that adolescents routinely endorse reasons of all sorts for not using contraceptives: they are too young to get pregnant, it's the wrong time of the month, the contraceptives don't feel right, their parents wouldn't approve, they are afraid of contraceptives. The adolescents who were interviewed generally seemed willing to rationalize not using contraceptives, rather than becoming committed to their use. Prophylactics such as condoms and rubber dams are even less well understood and accepted than other contraceptives. Multiple studies from cities around the country document that only a fraction of adolescents are using condoms and even aggressive training is relatively ineffective in transforming young people into prophylactic users.

Despite the general presence of anti-contraceptive attitudes, minority teenage girls are at an even greater disadvantage. Compared with their white counterparts, they are

❖ Less well educated about reproductive physiology and birth control
❖ Likely to have a longer period of delay between the first sexual intercourse and the first use of contraception
❖ More likely to report a contraceptive failure

Later in life, contraception for minority couples becomes more established and effective. Even in Catholic communities—for example, in Mexico, under government family planning initiatives—the fertility rates have declined substantially in recent years. Some women who have completed their families select sterilization for birth control. The selection of the method is often related to the community-wide experience with sterilization. Rates of sterilization have been very high among Puerto Rican women. A study of Puerto Rican women living in New York City demonstrated that the choice of sterilization was influenced by many social and cultural factors, including the lack of temporary birth control methods, the large number of women who had been sterilized, the relatively long period during which women would be fertile but would not wish to have more children, and high levels of misinformation about the nature of the sterilization procedure (Lopez 1987). That study found that women who chose sterilization often had one or many family members—mothers, sisters, or aunts—who had done the same. By contrast, many black women view sterilization more suspiciously, as reports of coerced sterilization are not uncommon. In the most typical reports, poor women are threatened with loss of health care or other entitlements if they do not consent to sterilization. Thus, in some black communities, sterilization is viewed with hostility and fear.

Induced abortion, as a method of family planning, is widely used by minority women. What has been of interest in understanding their attitudes toward abortion is that, although women will choose to have an abortion, they do not identify with or support the goals of the abortion-rights movement. This apparent contradiction is perhaps explained by their view that, although they acknowledge a woman's right to choose, they do not endorse the loss of the new baby.

As a generalization, many studies of sexual attitudes and practices have suggested that many minority women are sexually conservative (Fullilove et al. 1990; Padilla and O'Grady 1987). It is not simple promiscuity that puts them at risk for illness; rather, it is the life settings in which they must live and work. In the next section, three minority experiences that have important implications for health and disease are described.

ECOLOGICAL SETTINGS

The three ecological settings described here are not intended to provide an exhaustive description of the settings in which minority people live and work. Rather, they are meant to enable the reader to compare and contrast the life of people living in each of these settings and the health care problems that occur within them.

Inner-City Disintegration and the Growth of the Underclass

The growth of the underclass has been described as a form of "American apartheid" (Massey 1990) that has been created by an interaction between rising rates of poverty and high levels of residential segregation. Where these social forces have intersected—for example, among blacks and Puerto Ricans in large urban areas of the Northeast and Midwest—they have acted to create an urban underclass that is persistently poor, spatially isolated, and disproportionately made up of minorities. Furthermore, the structures and social networks that enabled the poor to survive poverty have been weakened, if not decimated, by the same forces that have created the underclass itself.

As Sampson (1990), D. Wallace (1990), and others have pointed out, the growth of the underclass is the result not simply of economic decline, but rather of economic collapse in conjunction with the collapse of other complex social policies on housing, fire protection service, and transportation networks. As an example, Sampson (1990) cites the decision in Chicago to concentrate poor blacks in massive federal housing projects. He notes that ". . . with the concentration of poor blacks in housing projects, social transformation of the ghetto became profound. . . . Undeniably, family disruption in the black community is concentrated in public housing. In 1980, of the 17,178 families with children living in Chicago public housing projects, only 11% were married couple families. Teen-age pregnancy and out-of-wedlock births are similarly high" (p. 529).

Whereas Sampson's work has focused on the association between housing policies and crime rates, R. Wallace and Wallace (1990) have provided a similar analysis on the association between housing policies and health. Characteristic of the areas that house the urban underclass is a process of "contagious housing destruction," in which a significant proportion of the residential housing is destroyed through neglect, abandonment, and inadequate municipal services. The Taylor Homes in Chicago or the Latrobe Homes in New Orleans have a "snaggle-toothed" appearance that is characteristic of this contagious process.

In the South Bronx, contagious housing destruction was responsible for massive displacement of the poor. D. Wallace and Wallace (1990) describe this as follows:

> People had to move in such large numbers in so short a time that local communities were destroyed and local essential services imbalanced with respect to utilization. . . . These changes have two meanings: the breaking up of communities by forced migration and

the crowding of the poor into the remaining housing. . . . The old social networks which had coped with the effects of poverty and over-crowding had been destroyed in the migrations. Churches, social clubs, and political organizations died. The effects of overcrowding and increased poverty from rising rents had (and have) few mitigating influences. (p. 268)

In sum, the structure of families, of social networks, and of neighborhoods—that is, all aspects of the social networks of the poor—have been undermined.

A great deal of scholarship from many disciplines makes it clear that social networks are important for the maintenance of health. The social networks of the poor have several specific functions that ensure survival. First, the network acts as a "resource bank" in which members share whatever they have. These banks are critically important because they provide a mechanism to "tide one over" in times of scarcity. Second, the network collectively acts to raise the children. The parents are thus freed to solve the economic problems of the family without having to worry about inadequate supervision for the young ones. Third, the network acts to provide "reality testing" counterbalancing the stress, trauma, and negative messages that the poor receive. The social reality testing mitigates the potential narcissistic wound of a racist attack by reframing it. For example, black people will commonly say to each other, "White people will be white people," which acts to discount a racist act or message.

Given increasing poverty, increasing residential segregation, and destruction of social networks, it is not surprising that there have been massive increases in disease. In the case of the South Bronx, AIDS, tuberculosis, drug abuse, suicide, homicide, and many other illnesses and manifestations of illness can be mapped to the specific collapsing areas in which the urban underclass is struggling to make a life (D. Wallace and Wallace 1990).

Health Care at the Mexican-American Border

David C. Warner, a researcher at the Lyndon B. Johnson School of Public Affairs, University of Texas, Austin, has described the border between the United States and Mexico as comprising transborder metropolitan areas that have grown from sparsely populated desert into a region with 10 million inhabitants (Warner 1991). The transborder cities include Tucson, Arizona, and Nogales, Mexico, with a population of 1 million; San Diego, California, and Tijuana, Mexico, with a current population of 3.5 million; Rio Grande Valley and El Paso, Texas, and Juárez, Mexico, with a population of over 1 million; and Laredo, Texas, and Nuevo Laredo, Mexico, with 400,000 people. The region has a unique character because of its increasing interdependence: many of the region's problems cannot be solved by local municipalities without assistance from both federal governments, or from bi-national cooperation.

The disparities between the United States and Mexico create conditions that have enormous impact on the area. Of the many Mexicans who cross the border to find work in the United States, most are poor and many are illegal entrants. The receiving communities are taxed to supply health care, especially since there are few provisions for funding the health needs of illegal immigrants. As noted above, many Mexican American mothers deliver their babies out of the hospital. Warner (1991) points out the serious consequences of the major gaps in the services available to the poor: "In 1980, of the births occurring in Texas border counties, 6,215 of the 28,645 births to persons giving a Texas residence were out of the hospital, while 2,550 of the 4,216 listing a Mexico residence were out of the hospital" (p. 245).

Communicable diseases, including STDs, are a significant threat to the health of the population in the border area. STDs have long been a problem due to the cross-border use of "red light" districts and the increased difficulty of contact tracing. Of 1,502 cases of AIDS reported in Mexico through mid-1988, roughly 20% were thought to come from the six Mexican border states.

Finally, the border communities show all the problems attendant to rapid growth, uncontrolled development of industry, poverty, and instability. At the most extreme, the border residents live in *colonias,* or unincorporated settlements on both sides of the border. As Warner (1991) notes, "These communities often lack septic tanks, sewers, or running water, and outdoor privies commonly abut water wells, making most of the water unfit for consumption" (p. 242).

Cuban and Haitian Boat People

Lydia DeSantis, a researcher at the University of Miami, Florida, has written extensively on the problems of women arriving from Cuba and Haiti in 1980 (DeSantis 1989):

> The mass arrival in 1980 of 125,000 Cubans during the Mariel Sealift or "Freedom Flotilla" and the 36,000 Haitians who entered during the same year overwhelmed the health care, social, political and economic systems of Southeast Florida. Community agencies were already straining to meet the needs of other low-income groups in the area. The influx of Cuban "Marielitos" and Haitian "Boat People" caused health care professionals to become increasingly frustrated by the sheer numbers requiring curative and preventive health care. The frustration also resulted from lack of knowledge about the new immigrants, who differed from previous groups of Cubans and Haitians in their health care orientations, educational backgrounds, socioeconomic status, and social support systems. (p. 70)

The two groups entered the United States at the same time but differed on almost every other measure of education and economic prospects. The Cuban refugees comprised several subgroups, including families, gay men, and people with criminal histories or mental illness. Though poorer than earlier refugees from that country, all came from a society with universal literacy and an aggressive health care system based on Western biomedical medicine. The Cubans had received appropriate preventive health care—including vaccinations—while in Cuba and had learned to value a system of health care similar to that in the United States. Finally, Cuban refugees, for the most part, felt secure that they would be able to stay in the United States.

De Santis (1989) observed that the Cuban immigrant parents shared decision making and tended to bring the extended family into decisions about the child's health care. She hypothesized that efforts of the Cuban government toward sexual equality in the domestic realm had led to this male-female sharing of household functions. The Cuban mothers felt empowered to act on their children's behalf. If a child became ill, the mothers said, "It's the parents' fault. They did not love him enough" (p. 80).

The Haitian boat people, in contrast, came from one of the poorest countries in the world. They were often illiterate, rural people with a long tradition of folk medicine and little access to Western biomedical care. The Haitians, as a group, had a less secure status in the United States and feared they might be deported back to Haiti, where they faced death, torture, or other kinds of abuse. This group, though willing to use the United States health care system, did not share its philosophy.

Haitian mothers, who were historically responsible for child care in Haiti, continued to carry alone most of the responsibility in this domain. Few older women were available to assist these women in carrying out their responsibilities. DeSantis found that, in contrast to their Cuban counterparts, the Haitian women felt relatively powerless to affect their child's health. Though they did not believe that illness was preventable, they quickly sought treatment for the child once signs and symptoms were present.

IMPLICATIONS FOR PRACTICE AND PREVENTION

The preceding brief descriptions of three settings of minority life—the inner city, the Mexican-American border, and southeast Florida—are meant to suggest the variety of social and economic settings in which minority people find themselves, as well as to hint at the nature of the historical process that brought them there. Writers speaking on minority issues almost invariably emphasize the variation that characterizes minority populations and that must be the first assumption made in addressing another human being (Table 26–4). The task, given the diversity of human cultures and human experiences, is not to assume that any survey of "minority" behavior can prepare the practitioner for the task of cross-cultural communication. Rather than approach the situation with assumptions about behavior or attitudes, the practitioner must have a strategy for data collection.

First, the practitioner must be aware that 1) the patient has cultural expectations about roles and greetings and 2) the minority patient will be sensitive to signs of disrespect. Since one cannot know the assumptions of all the cultures one will contact, it is useful to behave

---

Table 26–4. We are not one people

Ernesto de la Vega

"It is difficult to speak of sexuality issues among Latinos in the United States as if they were just one homogeneous group of individuals. The U.S. Latino population—estimated to be more than 20 million people—includes individuals who speak many different languages and come from different regions, races, classes, and cultures of the Americas." (de la Vega 1990, p. 1)

Ronald M. Rowell

"The number and sheer depth of stereotypes about Indians create stress and anxiety for many Native Americans. At the root of such stereotypes is the mistaken view that we are 'one' people. Like Europeans, Native Americans are not one people, although our experiences with the outside world have helped to create a pan-Indian identity. One's tribe (nation)—Choctaw, Peoria, Tlingit, Malecite, Arikara, Okanagan, Snohomish, Caddo—is where one's primary ethnic identity lies. Each tribe has developed its own language, customs, and beliefs; each has had a different history; and each has exercised its own strategy for dealing with the relentless invasion of new peoples and with the catastrophic changes that have taken place in their traditional lifestyles." (Rowell 1990, p. 9)

Deborah A. Lee and Kevin Fong

"One must be sensitive to the lumping of Asians and Pacific Islanders together as one homogenous group. In addressing the health care/AIDS information and education needs of Asians and Pacific Islanders in the United States, it is necessary to recognize the cultural diversity of this population. There are at least 43 different Asian and Pacific Islander groups, from more than 40 countries and territories, who speak more than 100 different languages and dialects (some unwritten). Each group has a distinct culture and heritage." (Lee and Fong 1990, p. 16)

Robert Fullilove[a]

"People with black skin share a common motherland in Africa but, as a result of the diaspora, have lived on many continents and under many governments. Haiti, the West Indies, the United States, as well as all the countries of Africa, have been home to black people. Emerging from each homeland are people with cultures, beliefs and history that are as different as they are alike."

---

[a]From Robert Fullilove, American Public Health Association Annual Convention, New York, October 1990.

toward the patient as one would behave toward an honored member of one's own culture. It will never hurt the practitioner's image for the translator to clarify an act by saying, "That is how they show great respect in their culture." In contrast, it will be particularly injurious to the developing relationship for the patient to discover that she has been slighted or treated discourteously. Muriel Pettione, M.D., a senior attending physician at Harlem Hospital Center, a major hospital serving the black community in New York City, often points out how offensive it is for young residents to show signs of disrespect such as, for example, calling an older woman patient by her first name. Indeed, this kind of impropriety will destroy trust and injure communication.

Second, practitioners, who perforce must act without a manual of cultures, should use the services of "key informants"—as anthropologists call those members of the community who help them to understand a certain culture. Social workers, nurses, typists, taxi drivers—in fact, anyone with a command of the two cultures—can help the practitioner to understand the words and actions of the patient. With the help of the guide, the practitioner can assemble a working understanding of the life setting of the patient. Is the patient well-to-do or poor? Educated? Fluent in many languages and cultures? Residing in adequate housing and in a safe neighborhood? Involved in stable social and sexual relationships? Because such questions are a routine part of the biomedical examination as it is taught to health care practitioners, it is not important to elaborate in more detail on what to ask. Rather, it should be underscored that such questions provide information and prevent unwarranted—and perhaps stigmatizing—assumptions.

Finally, practitioners must be aware that they act within the context of cultural conflict. We have not, in the United States, succeeded in being a melting pot. Rather, some people have been incorporated into the dominant culture, whereas others have been blocked out. Therefore, individuals from different cultures do not necessarily meet as equals. The health care provider must take the responsibility for establishing a dialogue of equality. When that occurs, the provider-patient relationship will have a capacity for respect, understanding, and healing.

It is, in any event, rare that we have empathy for each other. Laurence Purdy, a pathologist in California, describes living through a serious earthquake (Purdy 1990). Just before the earthquake occurred, he had struggled to diagnose a specimen that eventually was identified as metastatic ovarian cancer. After the earthquake, he found that he wanted to go to meet the patient, which was unusual for him. For Purdy, the earthquake, which had shaken his belief in the world as secure, allowed him to empathize with the young woman with terminal cancer. He writes:

> Like all of us, (Sarah) had plans for the summer, for next year, for many years to come. Now she would have to plan for something else. She reminded me of the child I saw during the earthquake, screaming at God to ease up on it. A couple of nurses hugged him and tried to console him, but he was too shaken for human comfort, too aware that no human was mightier than what had just shaken the earth. He was alone in his fear, as I was, as Sarah is, each of us complacent about the security of our routine lives, taking everything—our health, our safety on terra firma—for granted, never knowing when the earth might all of a sudden shake the life from us or when the faults beneath our own surface may begin a unique, solitary, and frightening slippage. (p. 2883)

It seems that these transcendent human experiences have a unique importance, as they allow us to see across all the barriers of difference and to understand the sameness in human existence. As health care providers, we will encounter many of these powerful human events. With attention and concern, we can make many effective and empathic encounters.

References

Atrash H, Koonin LM, Lawson HW, et al: Maternal mortality in the United States, 1979–1986. Obstet Gynecol 76:1055–1060, 1990

Becarra JE, Hogue JR, Atrash HK, et al: Infant mortality among Hispanics. JAMA 265:217–221, 1991

Centers for Disease Control: AIDS Surveillance Report, June 1990

Cochran SD, Mays VM: Disclosure of sexual preference to physicians by black lesbian and bisexual women. West J Med 149:616–619, 1988

Cooper R, David R: The biological concept of race and its application to public health and epidemiology. J Health Polit Policy Law 11:97–116, 1986

de la Vega E: Considerations for reaching the Latino population with sexuality and HIV/AIDS information and education. SIECUS Report 18:1–8, 1990

DeSantis L: Health care orientations of Cuban and Haitian immigrant mothers: implications for health care professionals. Med Anthropol 12:69–89, 1989

DuBois WEB: The Souls of Black Folk. Greenwich, CT, Fawcett, 1967

Fullilove MT, Weinstein M, Fullilove RE III, et al: Race/gender issues in the sexual transmission of AIDS, in AIDS Clinical Review 1990. Edited by Volberding P, Jacobson MA. New York, Marcel Dekker, 1990, pp 25–64

Hussain SA: A parting gift. JAMA 263:1254, 1990

Lee DA, Fong K: HIV/AIDS and the Asian and Pacific Islander community. SIECUS Report 18:16–22, 1990

Lopez I: Sterilization among Puerto Rican women, in Cities of the United States: Studies in Urban Anthropology. Edited by Mullings L. New York, Columbia University Press, 1987, pp 269–291

Massey DS: American apartheid: segregation and the making of the underclass. American Journal of Sociology 96:329–357, 1990

Miller HG, Turner CF, Moses LE: AIDS: The Second Decade. Washington, DC, National Academy Press, 1990

Moran JS, Aral SO, Jenkins WC, et al: The impact of sexually transmitted diseases on minority populations. Public Health Rep 104:560–565, 1989

Padilla ER, O'Grady KE: Sexuality among Mexican Americans: a case of sexual stereotyping. J Pers Soc Psychol 52:5–10, 1987

Potterat JJ, Rothenberg RB, Woodhouse DE, et al: Gonorrhea as a social disease. Sex Transm Dis 12:25–32, 1985

Purdy LJ: Aftershock. JAMA 263:2883, 1990

Rowell RM: Native Americans, stereotypes and HIV/AIDS: our continuing struggle for survival. SIECUS Report 18:9–15, 1990

Sampson RJ: The impact of housing policies on community social disorganization and crime. Bull N Y Acad Med 66:526–533, 1990

Tobach E: Some evolutionary aspects of human gender. Am J Orthopsychiatry 41:710–715, 1971

Wallace D: Roots of increased health care inequality in New York. Soc Sci Med 31:1219–1227, 1990

Wallace D, Wallace R: The burning down of New York City. Anthropos, 1990, pp 256–272

Wallace R, Wallace D: Origins of public health collapse in New York City: the dynamics of planned shrinkage, contagious urban decay and social disintegration. Bull N Y Acad Med 66:391–434, 1990

Warner DC: Health issues at the US-Mexican border. JAMA 265:242–247, 1991

Zimmerman HL, Potterat JJ, Dukes RL, et al: Epidemiologic differences between chlamydia and gonorrhea. Am J Public Health 80:1338–1342, 1990

INDEX

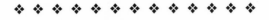

*Page numbers printed in **boldface** type refer to tables or figures.*

Psychological Aspects of Women's Health Care

Estriol, 116
Estrogen-androgen preparations, 364–365
Estrogen receptors, 429
Estrogens. See also Estradiol; Estriol; Estrone
  bone density and, 236
  cardiovascular disease and, 236
  interaction with psychotropic drugs, 184–186
  mood and, 233–234
  neurobiological effects of, 230
  ovarian secretion of, menopause and, 229
  peripheral effects of, 231
  in postpartum period, 116
  in pregnancy, 56
  in pseudocyesis, 62
  in puberty, 100
  replacement therapy. See Hormone replacement therapy (HRT)
  tryptophan metabolism and, 59
Estrone, 229
Ethics, medical, 499–500
  changing codes of, 486–488
  decision making and, 485–486
  informed consent and, 489–493
  paternalism and, 489–493
  role conflict and, 488–489
17α-Ethinyltestosterone derivatives, 199
Ethnic women. See Minority women
Etopside (VP-16), **298**
Extrapyramidal symptoms, in neonate, 80

❖ F ❖

Factitious disorders, in pregnancy, 61
FAE (fetal alcohol effects), 398
Failure to thrive, 420
Fallopian tube obstruction, 199

Family crisis intervention model, 50–51
FAS (fetal alcohol syndrome), **41**, 396
Fathers
  expectant
    birth of son and, 376
    fathers of, 378
    feelings of, 376–377
    guilt and fear during delivery, 378–379
    in high-risk pregnancy, 30
    marital relationship and, 378
    pressure on, 377–378
  intrapsychic consequences of perinatal loss, 148–149
  involvement with child, marital relationship, and, 379–380
  in postpartum period, 379
Fear, sexually transmitted diseases and, 271
Fear-tension-pain syndrome, 20
Female identity
  gynecologic surgery and, 267
  high-risk pregnancy and, 25
  pregnancy and, 15, 18, 102
Female life expectancy, 228
Female sexual disorders, 367–368
  differential diagnosis of, 354–357
  nomenclature for, 352–353
  prevalence of, 353–354
  psychiatric collaboration for, 351–352
  psychiatric drugs and, 366–367
  psychotherapeutic treatment of, 357–360
Fertility
  cessation at menopause, 332
  eating disorders and, 415–417
  knowledge of, 15
Fertilization, 519
Fetal alcohol effects (FAE), 398
Fetal alcohol syndrome (FAS), **41, 396**

Orgasm, sexual *(continued)*
  female inhibited, 356–357
Orthostatic hypotension, 72
Osteoporosis, 236
Ovarian cancer, hysterectomy and,
  279
Ovarian hyperstimulation
  syndrome, 198
Ovaries, estrogen production of,
  menopause and, 229–230
Ovulation, recovery from eating
  disorders and, 416
Ovulation-inducing agents, 197–198
Oxytocin, 116

❖ **P** ❖

Pain
  in breast cancer, 440–441
  in cancer, 296, 299–301
  chronic gynecologic forms of. *See
    also* Pelvic pain, chronic
  management of, 259–263
  psychological aspects of,
    254–259
  types of, 249–252
  of labor, prevention techniques
    for, 20
Panic disorder
  menstrual cycle and, 173
  in pregnancy, 59
Pap smear, abnormalities of, 269
Paracetamol, 183
Parental notification laws for
  minors, abortion and, 107–108
Parents, overinvolved dedication of,
  for malformed infant, 49
Parlodel (bromocriptine), 198
Passivity, female, 340
Paternalism, 486–487, 489–493,
  495–496
Pathological grief, in perinatal loss,
  153–157

Patient, choice of physician and, 6
Patient autonomy, 486
PCP. *See* Pneumocystis carinii
  pneumonia
Pelvic examination, 3
Pelvic exenteration, 305, 365
Pelvic inflammatory disease, 268
Pelvic malignancies, 3
Pelvic pain, chronic, 263
  definition of, 255–256
  diagnosis and treatment of,
    253–254
  in dyspareunia, 250–251
  in general pelvic pain, 251–252
  psychopathology of, 254–255
Pelvic relaxation, gynecologic
  surgery for, 277–278
Penis envy, 16, 336–337
Pentamidine, 318
Pergonal (human menopausal
  gonadotropins), 198
Perinatal death, psychological
  reactions to, 48
Perinatal Grief Scale, 140
Perinatal loss
  bereavement stages and, 144
  caregivers, roles of, 150–153
  definition of, 140
  epidemiology of, 140–141
  etiology of, 142–143
  grief in, 139–140
    complicated, risk factors for,
      153–154
    special aspects of, 145
  interpersonal consequences of,
    149–150
  intrapsychic consequences of
    for father, 148–149
    for mother, 145–148
  pathological grief in, 153–155,
    156–157
  psychiatric intervention for,
    155–157

for genetic reasons, 46–47
selective, 47–48
for sex selection, 48
third trimester of, 19
bleeding in, 23. *See also*
Abruptio placentae
psychotropic drug effects in, 75
unplanned
hyperemesis gravidarum and, 63
psychosocial circumstances of,
221
Pregnancy-related disorders
hyperemesis gravidarum, 62–64
pseudocyesis, 61–62
Premature self-delivery, in
schizophrenia and psychotic
disorders, 58
Prematurity, perinatal loss and, 141
Premenopausal period, 235
Premenstrual syndrome (PMS)
cultural aspects of, 169–170
definition of, 174–175
historical aspects of, 171–172
hormones in, 177–178
impact on male, 384–395
negative images of, 165
research on
findings in, 175, 177–178
legal issues in, 180
methodologic issues in, **178,**
178–180
political issues in, 180
symptoms, prevalence of, 175, 177
treatment of, gynecologic
methods for, 186–187
Premenstrual tension (PMT), 171
Prenatal care
adolescent pregnancy and,
108–110
obstacles to, 109
refusal of, in schizophrenia and
related psychotic disorders,
57–58

Prenatal child abuse, 401
Prenatal clinics, liaison psychiatrist
for, 109–110
Prenatal genetic testing
diagnostic, 42–44
indications for, 40, **41**
pregnancy loss after, 45–46
results, waiting time for, 40, **42**
timing of testing for, 40, **42**
Preoperative preparation, for
gynecologic surgery, 273–274
Prepregnancy period, risk of
hereditary disorders and, 38–39
Preterm delivery, perinatal loss and,
142
Primary dysmenorrhea, 172
Procarbazine, psychiatric side
effects of, 297, **298**
Profile of Mood States, 430
Progesterone
catecholamines and, 56
monoamine oxidase activity and,
59
in postpartum period, 116
for premenstrual syndrome, 187
vitamin B6 deficiency and, 59
Progesterone antagonist (RU-486),
169
Progesterone receptors, 429
Prolactin
in postpartum period, 116
in pseudocyesis, 62
Propranolol, 183, 297
Prospective ratings, **178,** 178–179
Protein, total, in pregnancy, 72
Provera (medroxyprogesterone
acetate), 199
Pseudocyesis, 61–62
Psychiatric disorders
incidence of, after induced
abortion, 218–219
late luteal phase dysphoric
disorder and, 175